Progress in
Thoracic
Anesthesia

Edited by

Peter D. Slinger, M.D., F.R.C.P.C.

University of Toronto
The University Health Network
Toronto, Ontario, Canada

With 22 contributors

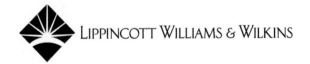 LIPPINCOTT WILLIAMS & WILKINS

Progress in Thoracic Anesthesia

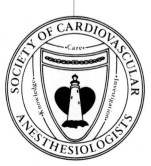

A Society of
Cardiovascular Anesthesiologists
Monograph

Accurate indications, adverse reactions, and dosage schedules for drugs are provided in this book, but it is possible that they may change. The reader is urged to review the package information data of the manufacturers of the medications mentioned.

Printed in the United States of America
(**ISBN** 0781758092)

03 04 05 06 07
1 2 3 4 5 6 7 8

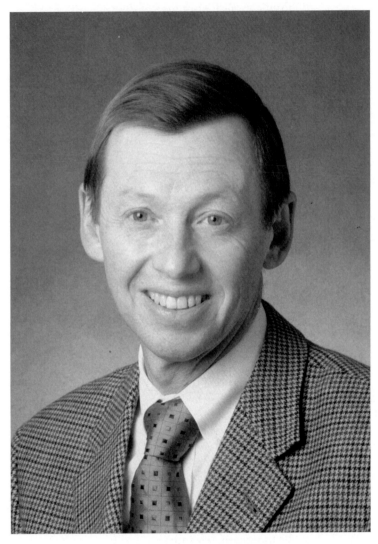

Peter D. Slinger, M.D., F.R.C.P.C.

Preface

Monograph: "A learned treatise on a small area of learning" (1)

For the past several years, the Society of Cardiovascular Anesthesiologists (SCA) has commissioned the production and distribution of an annual monograph on a topic the Publications Committee of the SCA believes will be useful to the membership for continuing medical education (CME). This monograph includes and extends the information that is presented in the "Monograph Panel" at the annual meeting of the SCA.

This year, I had the honor of being asked by the Publications Committee to organize a monograph on "Progress in Thoracic Anesthesia." Four of the authors of this current monograph (Drs. Klafta, Grichnik, Sullivan, and Keshavjee) presented during the Panel Session at the SCA meeting in Miami in April 2003. It was an excellent session, and I thank them for their participation. They are joined by 10 other authors in this text version of the monograph. In addition, we will post a World Wide Web (WWW)-based, audiovisual supplement to this monograph linked to the SCA website. This will be a prototype for a more complex WWW–based audiovisual CME by the SCA in the future.

I have been very pleasantly surprised by the willingness of the collaborators to be part of this project. I would particularly like to point out the contributions of several authors from outside North America. Their interest has impressed on me the influence that the SCA has internationally, as a focus for all anesthesiologists involved in cardiac, thoracic, and vascular surgery.

In this monograph, we have tried to give the readers an impression of the current length and breadth of anesthesia for thoracic surgery as well as some idea of what to expect in the future. The spectrum of patients who present for thoracic surgery is continually evolving. I date the appearance of modern anesthesia for thoracic surgery to 1900, with the introduction of the "Negative Pressure Apparatus" of Sauerbruch (2). In the 50 years before that, since the introduction of ether, the early pioneers of anesthesia could not deal with the "pneumothorax problem"—that is, they could not keep patients alive breathing air/ether spontaneously from a mask during surgery in the open hemithorax.

The first half of the last century saw great strides in thoracic anesthesia: tracheal intubation, positive-pressure ventilation, bronchial blockers, and double-lumen tubes. The past 20 years, during which I have been involved with thoracic cases, have witnessed the introduction of routine pulse oximetry, end-tidal capnography, fiberoptic lung isolation, and thoracic epidural analgesia. Each of these advances has increased the safety of surgery in the open thorax and allowed us to accept even higher-risk patients for potentially curative procedures.

For the anesthesia pioneers, the primary indication for lung surgery and anesthesia was to deal with infectious processes in the pre-antibiotic era. During the later half of the last century, lung cancer, which is now the leading cause of cancer deaths in both sexes, came to dominate the thoracic operating room lists. The past decade has seen the beginnings of surgical therapies for end-stage lung disease. Yet, we can still be presented with a case of bronchopleural fistula or bronchiectasis, which was the standard daily fare for Sauerbruch and still is for Dr. Jacob (see Chapter 12). The spectrum of our practice has become amazingly wide when you contrast those cases with the work of Drs. McRae and Keshavjee in the lab trying to "buff-up" donor lungs for transplantation by transfecting them with immunosuppressive genes (see Chapter 5).

I would like to thank the SCA for giving me the opportunity to edit this monograph. I would also like to thank the chapter authors for their excellent contributions. I hope that we have managed to produce a "learned treatise." A surgeon I know has described the practice of anesthesia as "90% boredom and 10% panic." In thoracic anesthesia, we have rarely had such a wide and favorable split, but we are striving to catch up to the rest of the specialty.

Peter Slinger MD, FRCPC
Professor of Anesthesia
University of Toronto

References

1. Webster's Seventh New Collegiate Dictionary. Toronto: Thomas Allen & Son, 1969.
2. Mushin WM, Rendell-Baker L. The Origins of Thoracic Anesthesia. Wood Library–Museum of Anesthesiology, 1991; 48–50.

Contributors

John M. Alvarez, F.R.A.C.S.
Cardiothoracic Surgeon
Department of Cardiothoracic
  Surgery
Sir Charles Gairdner Hospital
Perth, Western Australia

David Amar, M.D.
Professor of Anesthesiology
Department of Anesthesiology
Memorial Sloan-Kettering Cancer
  Center
New York, New York

Jay B. Brodsky, M.D.
Professor
Department of Anesthesiology
Stanford University School of
  Medicine
Stanford, California

Katherine P. Grichnik, M.D.
Associate Clinical Professor of
  Anesthesiology
Department of Anesthesiology
Duke University Medical Center
Durham, North Carolina

Paul M. Heerdt, M.D., Ph.D.,
  F.A.H.A.
Associate Professor of
  Anesthesiology and Pharmacology
Director, Thoracic Anesthesia Service
  and Cardiothoracic/
  Cerebrovascular Research
  Laboratory
Weill Medical College of Cornell
  University
Associate Member, Memorial Sloan-
  Kettering Cancer Center

Rebecca Jacob, M.D., D.A.
Professor
Department of Anesthesia
Christian Medical College
Vellore, India

Rajiv Jhaveri, M.D.
Staff Anesthesiologist
Department of Anesthesiology
Washington Hospital Center
Washington, D.C.

Roger Johns, M.D.
Professor
Department of Anesthesiology and
  Critical Care Medicine
Johns Hopkins University
Baltimore, Maryland

Michael R. Johnston, M.D.,
   F.R.C.S.C.
Associate Professor of Surgery
University of Toronto
The University Health Network
Toronto, Ontario, Canada

Stephen T. Kee, M.D.
Associate Professor
Department of Anesthesiology
Stanford University School of
   Medicine
Stanford, California

Shaf Keshavjee, M.D., M.Sc.,
   F.R.C.S.C., F.A.C.S.
Director, Toronto Lung Transplant
   Program
Director, Thoracic Surgery Research
Professor and Chair, Division of
   Thoracic Surgery
University of Toronto
Toronto, Ontario, Canada

Jerome M. Klafta, M.D.
Associate Professor
Associate Chair for Education
Department of Anesthesia & Critical
   Care
University of Chicago
Chicago, Illinois

Younsuck Koh, M.D., Ph.D.
Professor of Medicine
Division of Pulmonary and Critical
   Care Medicine
Asan Medical Center
Seoul, Korea
New York, New York

Burkhard Lachmann, M.D.,
   Ph.D.
Professor of Anesthesiology
Department of Anesthesiology
Erasmus University
Rotterdam, The Netherlands

Jaideep Malhotra, M.D.
Instructor
Department of Anesthesiology
Weill Medical College of Cornell
   University
New York, New York

Karen McRae, M.D.C.M.,
   F.R.C.P.C.
Thoracic and Lung Transplant
   Anesthesia
University Health Network
Assistant Professor, Department of
   Anesthesia
University of Toronto
Toronto, Ontario, Canada

Peter J. Papadakos, M.D.,
   F.C.C.M.
Professor of Anesthesiology and
   Surgery
Director, Critical Care Medicine
University of Rochester School of
   Medicine and Dentistry
Rochester, New York

Stephen H. Pennefather,
   M.R.C.P., F.R.C.A.
Consultant in Cardiothoracic
   Anesthesia
Department of Anesthesia
Cardiothoracic Center
Liverpool, United Kingdom

Glenn N. Russell, F.R.C.A.
Consultant in Cardiothoracic
    Anesthesia
Department of Anesthesia
Cardiothoracic Center
Liverpool, United Kingdom

Peter D. Slinger, M.D.,
    F.R.C.P.C.
Professor of Anesthesia
University of Toronto
The University Health Network
Toronto, Ontario, Canada

Erin A. Sullivan, M.D.
Anesthesia for New Thoracic
    Endoscopic Procedures
Department of Anesthesiology
University of Pittsburgh Medical
    Center
Pittsburgh, Pennsylvania

Edda M. Tschernko, M.D.
Associate Professor
Department of Cardiothoracic and
    Vascular Anesthesia & Critical
    Care Medicine
Vienna General Hospital
University of Vienna
Vienna, Austria

Contents

Peter D. Slinger, MD, FRCPC
Michael R. Johnston, MD, FRCSC

1 | Preoperative Assessment for Lung Cancer Surgery

Preoperative anesthetic assessment before chest surgery is a continually evolving science and art. Recent advances in anesthetic management, surgical techniques, and perioperative care have expanded the envelope of patients now considered to be "operable" (Fig. 1.1) (1). This article is an update on preanesthetic assessment for pulmonary resection surgery in patients with cancer. The principles described will apply to all other types of nonmalignant pulmonary resections and to other chest surgery. The major difference is that in patients with malignancy, the risk:benefit ratio of canceling or delaying surgery pending other investigation/therapy is always complicated by the risk of further spread of the cancer during any extended interval before resection. This is never completely "elective" surgery.

Although 87% of patients with lung cancer will die of their disease, the 13% cure rate represents approximately 26,000 survivors per year in North America. Surgical resection is responsible for essentially all of these cures. A patient with a "resectable" lung cancer has a disease that is still local or local-regional in scope and that can be encompassed in a plausible surgical procedure. An "operable" patient is someone who can tolerate the proposed resection with acceptable risk (2). Several general points should be appreciated in the assessment of pulmonary resection patients:

1. Anesthesiologists are not gate keepers. It is rarely the anesthesiologist's function to assess these patients to decide who is or is not an operative

Progress in Thoracic Anesthesia, edited by Peter Slinger,
Lippincott Williams & Wilkins, Baltimore © 2004.

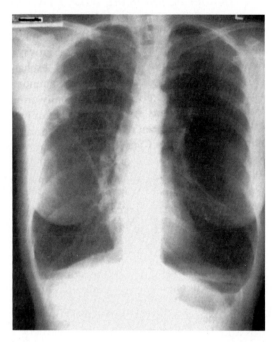

FIGURE 1.1 Preoperative chest radiograph of a 55-year-old woman with severe bullous emphysema and a carcinoma of the right upper lobe. Preoperative forced expiratory volume in 1 second was 25% of that predicted. Although this woman's pulmonary function does not meet traditional minimal criteria for a lung operation, she is now considered to be a potential candidate for bilateral combined cancer resection and emphysema surgery. [From Slinger and Johnston (1); with permission.]

candidate. In the majority of situations, the anesthesiologist will be seeing the patient at the end of a referral chain (from chest or family physician to surgeon). At each stage, a discussion of the risks and benefits of operation should have occurred. The anesthesiologist's responsibility is to use the preoperative assessment to identify those patients at elevated risk and then to use that risk assessment to stratify perioperative management and to focus resources on the high-risk patients to improve their outcome. This is the primary function of the preanesthetic assessment.

2. Although a large amount of research has been done on long-term survival (6 months to 5 years) after pulmonary resection surgery, a comparatively small volume of research is available on the short-term (<6 weeks) outcome of these patients. However, this area of research is currently very active, and several studies can be used to guide anes-

thetic management in the immediate perioperative period, when it has an influence on outcome.

3. Until very recently, preanesthetic management was part of a continuum, in which a patient was admitted preoperatively for testing and the management plan evolved as the test results were returned. Currently, the reality of practice patterns in anesthesia has changed. Today, a patient is commonly assessed initially in an outpatient clinic and often not by the member of the anesthesia staff who will actually administer the anesthesia. The actual contact with the responsible anesthesiologist may be only 10 to 15 minutes before induction. It is necessary to organize and to standardize the approach to preoperative evaluation for these patients into two temporally disjoint phases: the initial (clinic) assessment and the final (day-of-admission) assessment. Elements vital to each assessment will be described in this review.

4. An increasing number of thoracic surgeons are now being trained to perform "lung-sparing" resections, such as sleeve lobectomies or segmentectomies. The postoperative preservation of respiratory function has been shown to be proportional to the amount of functioning lung parenchyma that is preserved (3). To assess patients with limited pulmonary function, the anesthesiologist must understand these newer surgical options in addition to conventional lobectomy or pneumonectomy.

Prethoracotomy assessment naturally involves all the factors of a complete anesthetic assessment: past history, allergies, medications, upper airway, and so on. This article will focus on the additional information beyond a standard anesthetic assessment that the anesthesiologist needs to care for a patient having pulmonary resection.

PERIOPERATIVE COMPLICATIONS

To assess patients for thoracic anesthesia, it is necessary to understand the risks specific to this type of surgery. The major causes of perioperative morbidity and mortality in the thoracic surgical population are respiratory complications.

Major respiratory complications, such as atelectasis, pneumonia, and respiratory failure, occur in 15% to 20% of patients and account for most of the expected 3% to 4% mortality rate (4). The thoracic surgical population differs from other adult surgical populations in this respect; for other types of surgery, cardiac and vascular complications are the leading cause of early perioperative morbidity and mortality. Cardiac complications, such as arrhythmia, ischemia, and so on, occur in 10% to 15% of the thoracic population (5).

ASSESSMENT OF RESPIRATORY FUNCTION

The best assessment of respiratory function comes from a detailed history of the patient's quality of life. A completely asymptotic ASA class 1 or 2 patient with no limitation of activity and full exercise capacity probably does not need screening cardiorespiratory testing before pulmonary resection. Unfortunately, however, because of the biology of lung cancer, these individuals are a small minority of the patient population.

Because the anesthesiologist who will manage the case often has to assimilate a great deal of information about the patient in a short period of time, it is very useful to have objective, standardized measures of pulmonary function that can guide anesthetic management. It is also very useful to have this information in a format that can be easily transmitted between members of the health care team. Much effort has been spent to find a single test of respiratory function with sufficient sensitivity and specificity to predict outcome for all patients having pulmonary resection. It is now clear that no single test will ever accomplish this. Many factors determine overall respiratory performance (6, 7). It is useful to think of the respiratory function in three related but somewhat independent areas: respiratory mechanics, gas exchange, and cardiorespiratory interaction.

Respiratory Mechanics

Many tests of respiratory mechanics and volumes show correlation with postthoracotomy outcome: forced expiratory volume in 1 second (FEV_1), forced vital capacity, maximal voluntary ventilation, residual volume/total lung capacity ratio, and so on. It is useful to express these as a percentage of predicted volumes corrected for age, sex, and height (eg, FEV_1 %). Of these, the most valid single test for postthoracotomy respiratory complications is the predicted postoperative (ppo) FEV_1 %, which is calculated as

$$ppoFEV_1 \% = \text{preoperative } FEV_1 \% \times (1 - \% \text{ functional lung tissue removed}/100).$$

One method of estimating the percent of functional lung tissue is based on a calculation of the number of functioning subsegments of the lung that are removed (Fig. 1.2). Nakahara et al. (4) found that patients with a $ppoFEV_1$ of greater than 40% had no or minor postresection respiratory complications. Major respiratory complications were only seen in the subgroup with a $ppoFEV_1$ of less than 40% (although not all patients in this subgroup developed respiratory complications), and 10 of

Lung Subsegments

Total Subsegments = 42

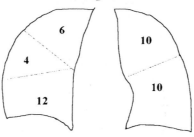

Example: Right lower lobectomy
Postoperative FEV1 decrease = 12/42 (29%)

FIGURE 1.2   The number of subsegments of each lobe are used to calculate the predicted postoperative pulmonary function. FEV_1 = forced expiratory volume in 1 second. [From Slinger and Johnston (1); with permission.]

10 patients with a ppoFEV$_1$ of less than 30% required postoperative mechanical ventilatory support. These key threshold ppoFEV$_1$ values (30% and 40%) are extremely useful to remember when managing these cases. The schema of Figure 1.2 may be overly complicated, and it can be useful just to simply consider the right upper and middle lobes combined as being approximately equivalent to each of the other three lobes, with the right lung being 10% larger than the left. These data of Nakahara et al. are from work during the 1980s, and recent advances, particularly the use of epidural analgesia, has decreased the incidence of complications in the high-risk group (8). However, ppoFEV$_1$ values of 40% and 30% remain useful as reference points for the anesthesiologist. The ppoFEV$_1$ is the most significant independent predictor of complications among a variety of historical, physical, and laboratory tests for these patients (5).

Lung Parenchymal Function

As important to the process of respiration as the mechanical delivery of air to the distal airways is the subsequent ability of the lung to exchange oxygen and carbon dioxide between the pulmonary vascular bed and the alveoli. Traditionally, arterial blood gas data, such as an arterial partial pressure of oxygen (PaO_2) of less than 60 mm Hg or an arterial partial pressure of carbon dioxide ($PaCO_2$) of greater than 45 mm Hg have been used as cutoff values for pulmonary resection. Cancer resections have now been successfully done (5), and even combined with volume reduction, in patients who do not meet these criteria (9), although the criteria remain useful as warning indicators of increased risk. The most useful test of the gas exchange capacity of the lung is the diffusing capacity for carbon monoxide (DLCO). Although the DLCO was initially thought just to reflect diffusion, it actually correlates with the total functioning surface area of alveolar-capillary interface. This simple, noninvasive test, which is included with spirometry and plethysmography by most pulmonary function laboratories, is a useful predictor of postthoracotomy complications. The corrected DLCO can be used to calculate a postresection value using the same calculation as for the FEV_1. A ppoDLCO of less than 40% predicted correlates with both increased respiratory and cardiac complications and is, to a large degree, independent of the FEV_1 (10).

Cardiopulmonary Interaction

The final and, perhaps, most important assessment of respiratory function is an assessment of the cardiopulmonary interaction. All patients should have some assessment of their cardiopulmonary reserves. The traditional, and still extremely useful, test in ambulatory patients is stair climbing (11). Stair climbing is done at the patient's own pace but without stopping, and it is usually documented as a certain number of flights. No exact definition exists for a "flight," but 20 steps at 6 inches per step is a frequent value. The ability to climb three or more flights is closely associated with decreased mortality and is somewhat associated with morbidity. The ability to climb less than two flights indicates very high risk.

Formal laboratory exercise testing has become more standardized and, thus, more valid, and it is currently the "gold standard" for assessment of cardiopulmonary function. Among the many cardiac and respiratory factors that are tested, the maximal oxygen consumption (VO_2max) is the most useful predictor of postthoracotomy outcome. Walsh et al. (12) have shown that in a high-risk group of patients (mean preoperative $FEV_1 = 41\%$ predicted), no perioperative mortality occurred if the preoperative VO_2max was greater than 15 mL/kg/min. This is a useful reference number for the anesthesiologist. Only 1 of 10 patients with a VO_2max of greater than 20 mL/kg/min had a respiratory complication. Exercise testing can be modified in patients who are not capable of stair climbing by using bicycle or arm exercises. Complete laboratory exercise testing is labor-intensive and expensive. Recently, several alternatives to exercise testing have been demonstrated to have potential as replacement tests for prethoracotomy assessment.

The 6-minute walk test (6MWT) shows an excellent correlation with VO_2max and requires little or no laboratory equipment (13). A 6MWT distance of less than 2,000 feet correlates to a VO_2max of less than 15 mL/kg/min and also correlates with a fall in oxygen saturation as measured by pulse oximetry (SpO_2) during exercise. Patients with a decrease of SpO_2 greater than 4% during exercise (stair climbing two or three flights or the equivalent) (14, 15) are at increased risk of morbidity and mortality. The 6MWT and exercise oximetry may replace VO_2max for assessment of cardiorespiratory function in the future. Both tests are still evolving, however, and for the present, exercise testing will remain the gold standard. Postresection exercise tolerance can be estimated based on the amount of functioning lung tissue that is removed. An estimated ppoVO_2max of less than 10 mL/kg/min may be one of the few remaining absolute contraindications to pulmonary resection. In a small series reported by Bollinger et al. (16), mortality was 100% (3/3 patients) in those with a ppoVO_2max of less than 10 mL/kg/min.

After pulmonary resection, a degree of right ventricular dysfunction occurs that seems to be in proportion to the amount of functioning pulmonary vascular bed that is removed (17). The exact cause and duration of this dysfunction remain unknown. Clinical evidence of this hemodynamic problem is minimal when the patient is at rest but dramatic when the patient exercises, leading to elevation of pulmonary vascular pressures, limitation of cardiac output, and absence of the normal decrease in pulmonary vascular resistance usually seen with exertion (18).

Ventilation Perfusion Scintigraphy

Prediction of postresection pulmonary function can be further refined by assessment of the preoperative contribution of the lung or lobe to be resected using ventilation/perfusion (V/Q) lung scanning (19). If the lung region to be resected is nonfunctioning or minimally functioning, the prediction of postoperative function can be modified accordingly. This is particularly useful in patients having pneumonectomy and should be considered for any patient with a ppoFEV$_1$ of less than 40%.

Split-Lung Function Studies

A variety of methods have been described to try and simulate the postoperative respiratory situation by unilateral exclusion of a lung or lobe with an endobronchial tube/blocker and/or by pulmonary artery balloon occlusion of a lung or lobe artery (20). These and other varieties of split-lung function testing have also been combined with exercise to try and assess the tolerance of the cardiorespiratory system to a proposed resection. Although these tests are currently used to guide therapy in certain individual centers, they have not shown sufficient predictive validity for universal adoption in potential patients for lung resection. One possible explanation for some predictive failures in these patients may be that the lack of a pulmonary hypertensive response to unilateral occlusion may represent a sign of a failing right ventricle that is misinterpreted as a good sign of pulmonary vascular reserve. Lewis et al. (21) have shown that in a group of patients with chronic obstructive pulmonary disease (COPD; ppoFEV$_1$ < 40%) having pneumonectomy, no significant changes were observed in the pulmonary vascular pressures intraoperatively when the pulmonary artery was clamped, but the right ventricular ejection fraction and cardiac output decreased. Echocardiography may offer more useful information than vascular pressure monitoring in these patients (22). It is conceivable that the future combination of unilateral occlusion studies with echocardiography may be a useful addition to this type of preresection investigation.

Flow-Volume Loops

Flow volume loops can help to identify the presence of a variable intrathoracic airway obstruction by providing evidence of a positional change in an abnormal plateau of the expiratory limb of the loop (23). This can result from compression of a main conducting airway by a tumor mass. Such a problem may warrant induction airway management with awake intubation or maintenance of spontaneous ventilation (24). However, in an adult patient who is capable of giving a complete history and who does not describe supine exacerbation of cough or dyspnea, flow-volume loops are not required as a routine preoperative test.

Combination Testing

No single test of respiratory function has shown adequate validity to be used as a sole preoperative assessment (5). Before surgery, an estimate of respiratory function in all three areas (mechanics, parenchymal function, and cardiopulmonary interaction) should be made for each patient. These three aspects of pulmonary function form the "Three-Legged Stool," which is the foundation of prethoracotomy respiratory assessment (Fig. 1.3). These data can then be used to plan both intra- and postoperative management (Fig. 1.4) and also to alter these plans when intraoperative surgical factors necessitate that a resection be made more extensive than originally thought. If a patient has a ppoFEV$_1$ of greater than 40%, it should be possible for that patient to be extubated in the operating room at the conclusion of surgery assuming that the patient is

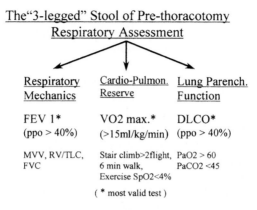

FIGURE 1.3 The "three-legged" stool of prethoracotomy respiratory assessment. An asterisk indicates the most valid test. DLCO = diffusing capacity of lung for carbon monoxide; FEV_1 = forced expiratory volume in 1 second; FVC = forced vital capacity; MVV = maximum voluntary ventilation; $PaCO_2$ = arterial partial pressure of carbon dioxide; PaO_2 = arterial partial pressure of oxygen; ppo = predicted postoperative; RV/TLC = residual volume/total lung capacity ratio; SpO_2 = oxygen saturation as measured by pulse oximetry; VO_2max = maximum oxygen consumption.

alert, warm, and comfortable ("AWaC"). Patients with a $ppoFEV_1$ of less than 40% will usually comprise approximately one-fourth of an average thoracic surgical population. If the $ppoFEV_1$ is greater than 30% and exercise tolerance as well as lung parenchymal function exceed the increased risk thresholds, then extubation in the operating room should

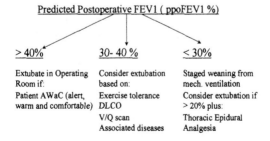

FIGURE 1.4 Anesthetic management guided by preoperative assessment and the amount of functioning lung tissue removed during surgery. DLCO = diffusing capacity of lung for carbon monoxide; FEV_1 = forced expiratory volume in 1 second; $ppoFEV_1$ = predicted postoperative forced expiratory volume in 1 second; V/Q = ventilation/perfusion.

be possible depending on the status of associated diseases (see below). Those patients in this subgroup who do not meet the minimal criteria for cardiopulmonary and parenchymal function should be considered for staged weaning from mechanical ventilation postoperatively so that the effect of the increased oxygen consumption of spontaneous ventilation can be assessed. Patients with a ppoFEV$_1$ of 20% to 30% and favorable predicted cardiorespiratory and parenchymal function can be considered for early extubation if thoracic epidural analgesia is used (see below). Otherwise, these patients should have a postoperatively staged weaning from mechanical ventilation. In the borderline group (ppoFEV$_1$ = 30–40%), the presence of several associated factors and diseases that should be documented during the preoperative assessment will enter into the considerations for postoperative management.

INTERCURRENT MEDICAL CONDITIONS

Age

There does not appear to be any maximum age that serves as a cutoff for pulmonary resection. If a patient is 80 years of age and has a stage I lung cancer, his or her chances of survival to age 85 are better with the tumor resected than without. The operative mortality in a group of patients 80 to 92 years of age was 3%, a very respectable figure, in a series reported by Osaki et al. (25). However, the rate of respiratory complications (40%) was double that expected in a younger population, and the rate of cardiac complications (40%), particularly arrhythmias, was nearly triple what should be seen in younger patients. Although the mortality rate from lobectomy in elderly patients is acceptable, the mortality rate from pneumonectomy (22% in patients > 70 years) (26), particularly right pneumonectomy, is excessive. Presumably, the reason for this is the increased strain on the right heart caused by resection of the proportionally larger vascular bed of the right lung.

Cardiac Disease

Cardiac complications are the second most common cause of perioperative morbidity and mortality in the thoracic surgical population.

Ischemia

Because the majority of patients having pulmonary resection have a history of smoking, they already have one risk factor for coronary artery disease (27). However, elective pulmonary resection surgery is generally regarded as an "intermediate risk" procedure in terms of perioperative cardiac ischemia (less than accepted "high-risk" procedures, eg, major emergency or vascular surgery) (28). The overall documented incidence of postthoracotomy ischemia is 5% and peaks on day 2 or 3 postoperatively (29). This is approximately the risk that would be expected from a similar patient population having major abdominal, orthopedic, or other procedures. Beyond the standard history, physical, and electrocardiogram, routine screening for cardiac disease does not appear to be cost-effective for all prethoracotomy patients (30). Noninvasive testing is indicated in patients with major (eg, unstable ischemia, recent infarction, severe valvular disease, significant arrhythmia) or intermediate (eg, stable angina, remote infarction, previous congestive failure, diabetes) clinical predictors of myocardial risk and also in elderly patients (28, 31). Therapeutic options to be considered in patients with significant coronary artery disease are optimization of medical therapy, coronary angioplasty, or coronary artery bypass, either before or at the time of lung resection (32). Timing of lung resection surgery after a myocardial infarction is always a difficult decision. Based on the data of Rao et al. (33) and generally confirmed by recent clinical practice, limiting the delay to between 4 and 6 weeks in a medically stable, fully investigated, and optimized patient seems to be acceptable after myocardial infarction.

Arrhythmia

Dysrhythmias, particularly atrial fibrillation, are a well-recognized complication of all pulmonary resection surgery (34). Factors known to correlate with an increased incidence of arrhythmia are the amount of lung tissue resected, age, intraoperative blood loss, and intrapericardial dissection (35, 36). Prophylactic therapy with digoxin has not been shown to prevent these arrhythmias. However, diltiazem has recently shown some promise (37).

Renal Dysfunction

Renal dysfunction after pulmonary resection surgery is associated with a very high incidence of mortality. Golledge and Goldstraw (38) reported a perioperative mortality rate of 19% (6/31) in patients who developed any significant elevation of serum creatinine in the postthoracotomy period, compared to 0% (0/99) in those who did not show any renal dysfunction. The factors, which were highly associated ($p < 0.001$) with an elevated risk of renal impairment, are listed in Table 1.1. Other factors that were statistically significant but less strongly associated with renal impairment included preoperative hypertension, chemotherapy,

TABLE 1.1   Factors Associated With an Increased Risk of
Postthoracotomy Renal Impairment

Previous history of renal impairment.
Diuretic therapy.
Pneumonectomy.
Postoperative infection.
Blood loss requiring transfusion.

ischemic heart disease, and postoperative oliguria (<33 mL/h). Non-steroidal anti-inflammatory agents (NSAIDs) were not associated with renal impairment in this series. Clearly, however, they are a concern in patient with an increased risk of renal dysfunction who is having thoracotomy. The high mortality rate in patients having pneumonectomy, either from renal failure or postoperative pulmonary edema, emphasizes the importance of fluid management in these patients (39) and the need for close and intensive perioperative monitoring, particularly in those patients who are on diuretics or who have a history of renal dysfunction.

Chronic Obstructive Pulmonary Disease

The most common concurrent illness in the thoracic surgical population is COPD, which incorporates three disorders: emphysema, peripheral airways disease, and chronic bronchitis. Any individual patient may have one or all of these conditions, but the dominant clinical feature is impairment of expiratory airflow (40). The severity of COPD has traditionally been assessed on the basis of the FEV_1 % of predicted values. The American Thoracic Society currently categorizes as follows:

1. Stage I: >50% predicted (this category previously included both "mild" and "moderate" COPD).
2. Stage II: 35–50% predicted.
3. Stage III: <35% predicted.

Stage I patients should not have significant dyspnea, hypoxemia, or hypercarbia, and other causes should be considered if these are present. Recent advances in the understanding of the COPD that are relevant to anesthetic management include respiratory drive, nocturnal hypoxemia, right ventricular dysfunction, and combined cancer and emphysema surgery.

Respiratory drive

Major changes have occurred in our understanding of the control of breathing in patients with COPD. Many stage II or III patients with COPD have an elevated $PaCO_2$ at rest. It is not possible to differentiate these "CO_2 retainers" from nonretainers on the basis of history, physical examination, or spirometric pulmonary function testing. This CO_2 retention seems to be related more to an inability to maintain the increased work of respiration required to keep the $PaCO_2$ normal in patients with mechanically inefficient pulmonary function and not primarily caused by an alteration of respiratory control mechanisms. It was previously thought that patients with chronic hypoxemia/hypercapnia relied on a hypoxic stimulus for ventilatory drive and became insensitive to $PaCO_2$. This explained the clinical observation that patients with COPD who were in incipient respiratory failure could be put into a hypercapnic coma by administration of a high concentration of oxygen (FIO_2). Actually, only a minor fraction of the increase in $PaCO_2$ in such patients results from a diminished respiratory drive, because minute ventilation is basically unchanged (41). The $PaCO_2$ rises because a high FIO_2 causes a relative decrease in alveolar ventilation and an increase in alveolar dead space by the redistribution of perfusion away from lung areas with relatively normal V/Q matching to areas of very low V/Q ratio, because regional hypoxic pulmonary vasoconstriction is decreased and caused by the Haldane effect (42). However, supplemental oxygen must be administered to these patients postoperatively to prevent the hypoxemia associated with the unavoidable fall in functional residual capacity (FRC). The attendant rise in Paco2 should be anticipated and monitored. To identify these patients preoperatively, all stage II or III patients with COPD need an arterial blood gas.

Nocturnal hypoxemia

Patients with COPD desaturate more frequently and severely than normal patients during sleep (43). This results from the rapid/shallow breathing pattern that occurs in all patients during REM sleep. In patients with COPD breathing air, this causes a significant increase in the respiratory dead space/tidal volume ratio and a fall in alveolar oxygen tension and PaO_2. This is not the sleep-apnea-hypoventilation syndrome (SAHS). There is no increased incidence of SAHS in patients with COPD. In 8 of 10 patients with COPD, the oxygen saturation fell to less than 50% at some time during normal sleep, and this was associated with an increase in pulmonary artery pressure (44). This tendency to desaturate, combined with the postoperative fall in FRC and opioid analgesia, places these patients at high risk for severe postoperative hypoxemia during sleep.

Right ventricular dysfunction

Right ventricular dysfunction occurs in as many as 50% of patients with COPD (45). The dysfunctional right ventricle, even when hypertrophied, is poorly tolerant of sudden increases in afterload (46), such as the change from spontaneous to controlled ventilation (47). Right ventricular function becomes critical in maintaining cardiac output as the pulmonary artery pressure rises. The right ventricular ejection fraction does not increase with exercise in patients with COPD as it does in normal patients. Chronic recurrent hypoxemia is the cause of the right ventricular dysfunction and the subsequent progression to cor pulmonale. Patients who have episodic hypoxemia in spite of normal lungs (eg, central alveolar hypoventilation, SAHS, etc.) (48) develop the same secondary cardiac problems as patients with COPD. Cor pulmonale occurs in 40% of adult patients with COPD and an FEV_1 of less than 1 L and in 70% of those with an FEV_1 of less than 0.6 L (45). It is now clear that mortality in patients with COPD is primarily related to chronic hypoxemia (49). The only therapy that has been shown to improve long-term survival and to decrease right-heart strain in COPD is oxygen. Patients with COPD who have resting PaO_2 of less than 55 mm Hg should receive supplemental home oxygen, as should those who desaturate to less than 44 mm Hg with usual exercise (40). The goal of supplemental oxygen is to maintain a PaO_2 of 60 to 65 mm Hg. Compared to patients with chronic bronchitis, emphysematous patients with COPD tend to have a decreased cardiac output and mixed venous oxygen tension while maintaining lower pulmonary artery pressures (46). Pneumonectomy candidates with a $ppoFEV_1$ of less than 40% should have transthoracic echocardiography to assess right-heart function. Elevation of right-heart pressure places these patients in a very high-risk group (22).

Combined cancer and emphysema surgery

The combination of volume reduction surgery or bullectomy in addition to lung cancer surgery has been reported in emphysematous patients who would previously not have met minimal criteria for pulmonary resection because of their concurrent lung disease (Fig. 1.1) (50, 51). Although the numbers of patients reported are small, the expected improvements in postoperative pulmonary function have been seen and outcomes encouraging. This offers an extension of the standard indications for surgery in a small, well-selected group of patients.

PREOPERATIVE THERAPY OF COPD

Four treatable complications of COPD must be actively sought, and therapy should begin at the time of the initial prethoracotomy assessment. These complications are atelectasis, bronchospasm, chest infection, and pulmonary edema. Atelectasis impairs local lung lymphocyte and macrophage function, predisposing the patient to infection (52).

Pulmonary edema can be very difficult to diagnose on the basis of auscultation in the presence of COPD, and it may present very abnormal radiological distributions (eg, unilateral, upper lobes, etc.) (53). Bronchial hyperreactivity may be a symptom of congestive failure (54). All patients with COPD should receive maximal bronchodilator therapy as guided by their symptoms. Only 20% to 25% of patients with COPD will respond to corticosteroids. In a patient who is poorly controlled on sympathomimetic and anticholinergic bronchodilators, a trial of corticosteroids may be beneficial (55). It is not clear if corticosteroids are as beneficial in COPD as they are in asthma.

Physiotherapy

Patients with COPD have fewer postoperative pulmonary complications when a perioperative program of intensive chest physiotherapy is initiated preoperatively (56). It is uncertain if this benefit applies to other patients having pulmonary resection. Among the different modalities available (cough and deep breathing, incentive spirometry, positive end-expiratory pressure [PEEP], continuous positive airway pressure [CPAP], etc.), there is no clearly proven superior method (57). The important variable is the quantity of time that is spent with the patient and devoted to chest physiotherapy. Family members or non-physiotherapy hospital staff can easily be trained to perform effective preoperative chest physiotherapy, and this should be arranged during the initial preoperative assessment. Even in the patients with the most severe COPD, it is possible to improve exercise tolerance with a physiotherapy program (58). Little improvement is seen before 1 month. Among patients with COPD, those with excessive sputum benefit the most from chest physiotherapy (59).

A comprehensive program of pulmonary rehabilitation involving physiotherapy, exercise, nutrition, and education has been shown consistently to improve functional capacity for patients with severe COPD (60). These programs are usually several months in duration and are generally not an option in resections for malignancy, although for non-malignant resections in patients with severe COPD, rehabilitation should be considered. The benefits of short-duration rehabilitation programs before malignancy resection have not been fully assessed.

Smoking

Pulmonary complications are decreased in patients having thoracic surgery who are not smoking versus those who continue to smoke up until the time of surgery (61). However, patients having cardiac surgery showed no decrease in the incidence of respiratory complications unless smoking was discontinued for more than 8 weeks before surgery (62). Carboxyhemoglobin concentrations decrease if smoking is stopped for more than 12 hours (63). It is extremely important for patients to avoid smoking postoperatively. Smoking leads to a prolonged period of tissue hypoxemia. Wound tissue oxygen tension correlates with wound healing and resistance to infection (64)

Lung Cancer

At the time of initial assessment, patients with cancer should be assessed for the "4-M's" associated with malignancy: mass effects (65), metabolic abnormalities, metastases (66), and medications. The previous use of medications that can exacerbate oxygen-induced pulmonary toxicity, such as bleomycin, should be considered (67–69) (Table 1.2). Recently, we have seen several patients with lung cancer who received preoperative chemotherapy with *cis*-platinum and then developed an elevation of serum creatinine when they received NSAIDs postoperatively. For this reason, we now do not routinely administer NSAIDs to patients who have been treated recently with *cis*-platinum.

Postoperative Analgesia

The strategy for postoperative analgesia should be developed and discussed with the patient during the initial preoperative assessment. Many techniques have been shown to be superior to the use of on-demand parenteral (intramuscular or intravenous) opioids alone in terms of pain control (70). These include the addition of neuraxial blockade, intercostal/paravertebral blocks, interpleural local anesthetics, NSAIDs, and so on to narcotic-based analgesia. However, only epidural tech-

TABLE 1.2 Anesthetic Considerations in Patients with Lung Cancer (the "4 M's")

Mass effects: obstructive pneumonia, lung abscess, superior vena cava syndrome, tracheobronchial distortion, Pancoast's syndrome, recurrent laryngeal nerve or phrenic nerve paresis, chest wall or mediastinal extension
Metabolic effects: Lambert-Eaton syndrome, hypercalcemia, hyponatremia, Cushing's syndrome
Metastases: particularly to the brain, bone, liver, and adrenal
Medications: chemotherapy agents, pulmonary toxicity (bleomycin, mitomycin), cardiac toxicity (doxorubicin), renal toxicity (cisplatin).

niques have been shown consistently to have the capability to decrease postthoracotomy respiratory complications (71, 72). It is becoming more evident that thoracic epidural analgesia is superior to lumbar epidural analgesia. This seems to be caused by the synergy that local anesthetics have with opioids in producing neuraxial analgesia. Studies suggest that epidural local anesthetics increase segmental bioavailability of opioids in the cerebrospinal fluid (73) and that they increase the binding of opioids by spinal cord receptors (74). Although lumbar epidural opioids can produce similar levels of postthoracotomy pain control at rest, only the segmental effects of thoracic epidural local anesthetic and opioid combinations can reliably produce increased analgesia with movement and increased respiratory function after a chest incision (75, 76). In patients with coronary artery disease, thoracic epidural local anesthetics seem to reduce myocardial oxygen demand and supply in proportion (77), which is unlike the effects of lumbar epidural local anesthetics, which can cause a fall in myocardial perfusion and oxygen supply as diastolic pressure falls but heart rate and oxygen demand are unchanged. This has been shown to correlate with echocardiographic evidence of ischemia (78).

The risks and benefits of the various forms of postthoracotomy analgesia should be explained to the patient during the initial preanesthetic assessment. Potential contraindications to specific methods of analgesia, such as coagulation problems, sepsis, or neurologic disorders, should be determined. When a thoracic epidural cannot be placed because of problems with patient consent or other contraindications, our current second choice for analgesia is a paravertebral infusion of local anesthetic via a catheter placed intraoperatively in the open hemithorax by the surgeon. This is combined with intravenous patient-controlled opioid analgesia and NSAIDs (79).

If the patient is to receive prophylactic anticoagulants and epidural analgesia is used, appropriate timing of anticoagulant administration and neuraxial catheter placement need to be arranged. The American Society of Regional Anesthesia (ASRA) guidelines suggest an interval of 2 to 4 hours before or 1 hour after catheter placement for prophylactic heparin administration (80). Low-molecular-weight heparin precautions are less clear, but an interval of 12 to 24 hours before and 24 hours after catheter placement are recommended.

Premedication

Premedication should be discussed and ordered during the initial preoperative visit. The most important aspect of preoperative medication is to avoid inadvertent withdrawal of those drugs that are taken for concurrent medical conditions (eg, bronchodilators, antihypertensives, β-blockers, etc.). For some types of thoracic surgery, such as esophageal reflux surgery, oral antacid and H_2-blockers are routinely ordered pre-operatively. Although some theoretical concern exists in giving patients who may be prone to bronchospasm an H_2-blocker without an H_1-blocker, this has not been a clinical problem, and H_2-blockers are frequently used in patients with asthmatic symptoms triggered by chronic reflux. We do not routinely order preoperative sedation or analgesia for patients having pulmonary resection. Mild sedation, such as an intravenous short-acting benzodiazepine, is often given immediately before placement of invasive monitoring lines and catheters. In patients with copious secretions, an antisialogogue (eg, glycopyrrolate) is useful to facilitate fiberoptic bronchoscopy for positioning of a double-lumen tube or bronchial blocker. To avoid an intramuscular injection, this can be given orally or intravenously immediately after placement of the intravenous catheter. It is a common practice to use short-term intravenous antibacterial prophylaxis, such as a cephalosporin, in patients having thoracic surgery. If it is the local practice to administer these drugs before admission to the operating room, they will have to be ordered preoperatively. Consideration for those patients who are allergic to cephalosporin or penicillin will have to be made during the initial preoperative visit.

FINAL PREOPERATIVE ASSESSMENT

The final preoperative anesthetic assessment for most patients having thoracic surgery is carried out immediately before admission of the patient to the operating room. At this time, it is important to review the data from the initial prethoracotomy assessment (Table 1.3) and the results of tests ordered at that time. In addition, two other specific areas affecting thoracic anesthesia need to be assessed: the potential for diffi-

TABLE 1.3   Initial Preanesthetic Assessment for Thoracic Surgery

All patients: assess exercise tolerance, estimate ppoFEV₁ %, discuss postoperative analgesia, discontinue smoking
Patients with ppoFEV₁ < 40%: DLCO, V/Q scan, VO₂max
Patients with cancer: consider the "4 M's" (mass effects, metabolic effects, metastases, and medications)
Patients with COPD: arterial blood gas, physiotherapy, bronchodilators
Increased renal risk: measure creatinine and BUN

BUN = blood urea nitrogen; COPD = chronic obstructive pulmonary disease; DLCO = diffusing capacity of lung for carbon monoxide; ppoFEV₁ = predicted postoperative forced expiratory volume in 1 second; VO₂max = maximum oxygen consumption; V/Q = ventilation/perfusion.

TABLE 1.4   Final Preanesthetic Assessment for
Thoracic Surgery

Review initial assessment and test results.
Assess difficulty of lung isolation. (Examine chest radiograph and computed
   tomographic scan.)
Assess risk of hypoxemia during one-lung ventilation

cult lung isolation and the risk of desaturation during one-lung ventilation (OLV) (Table 1.4).

Difficult Endobronchial Intubation

Anesthesiologists are familiar with clinical assessment of the upper airway for ease of endotracheal intubation. In a similar fashion, each patient having thoracic surgery must be assessed for the ease of endobronchial intubation. During the preoperative visit, there may be
historical factors or physical findings that lead to suspicion of difficult
endobronchial intubation (eg, previous radiotherapy, infection, and
previous pulmonary or airway surgery). In addition, there may be a
written bronchoscopy report with detailed description of anatomical
features. However, fiberoptic bronchoscopy is not totally reliable for estimating potential problems with endobronchial tube positioning (81).
The single most useful predictor of difficult endobronchial intubation is
the plain-film chest radiography (Fig. 1.5) (82).

The anesthesiologist should view the chest radiographs before induction of anesthesia, because neither the radiologist's nor the surgeon's report of the radiograph is made with the specific consideration
of lung isolation in mind. A large portion of patients having thoracic
surgery will also have had a chest computed tomographic (CT) scan
done preoperatively. Because anesthesiologists have learned to assess
radiographs for potential lung isolation difficulties, it is also worthwhile to learn to examine the CT scan. Distal airway problems not detectable on the plain-film chest radiograph can sometimes be visualized on the CT scan: A side-to-side compression of the distal trachea,
the so-called "saber-sheath" trachea, can cause obstruction of the tracheal lumen of a left-sided double-lumen tube during ventilation of
the dependent lung for a left thoracotomy (83). Similarly, extrinsic
compression or intraluminal obstruction of a mainstem bronchus,
which can interfere with endobronchial tube placement, may only be
evident on the CT scan. The major factors in successful lower airway
management are anticipation and preparation based on the preoperative assessment.

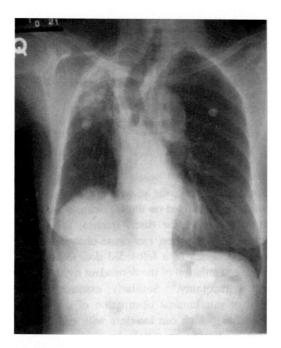

FIGURE 1.5   Preoperative chest radiograph of a 50-year-old woman with a history of previous tuberculosis, right upper lobectomy, and recent hemoptysis presenting for right thoracotomy possible completion pneumonectomy. The potential problems positioning a left-sided double-lumen tube in this patient are easily appreciated by viewing the radiograph but are not mentioned in the radiologist's report. [From Slinger and Johnston (1); with permission.]

Prediction of Desaturation During OLV

In the vast majority of cases, it is possible to determine which patients are most at risk of desaturation during OLV for thoracic surgery. The factors that correlate with desaturation during OLV are listed in Table 1.5. Identification of those patients most likely to desaturate allows the anesthesiologist and surgeon to make a more informed decision about the use of OLV intraoperatively. In patients at high risk of desaturation, prophylactic measures can be used during OLV to decrease this risk. The most useful prophylactic measure is the use of CPAP of 2 to 5 cm H_2O of oxygen to the nonventilated lung (84). Because this often tends to make the surgical exposure more difficult, particularly during video-assisted thoracoscopic surgery, it is worthwhile to identify those patients who will require CPAP early so that it can be discussed with the surgeon and instituted at the start of OLV.

TABLE 1.5   Factors That Correlate With an Increased Risk of Desaturation During One-lung Ventilation

High percentage of ventilation or perfusion to the operative lung on preoperative V/Q scan

Poor PaO_2 during two-lung ventilation, particularly in the lateral position intraoperatively

Right-sided surgery

Good preoperative spirometry (FEV_1 or FVC)

FEV1 = forced expiratory volume in 1 second; FVC = forced vital capacity; PaO_2 = arterial partial pressure of oxygen; V/Q = ventilation/perfusion.

The most important predictor of PaO_2 during OLV is the PaO_2 during two-lung ventilation. Although the preoperative PaO_2 correlates with the intraoperative OLV PaO_2, the strongest correlation is with the intraoperative PaO_2 during two-lung ventilation in the lateral position before OLV (85, 86). The proportion of perfusion or ventilation to the nonoperated lung on preoperative V/Q scans also correlates with the PaO_2 during OLV (87). If the operative lung has little perfusion preoperatively because of unilateral disease, the patient is unlikely to desaturate during OLV.

The side of the thoracotomy has an effect on PaO_2 during OLV. The left lung being 10% smaller than the right lung, there is less shunt when the left lung is collapsed. In a series of patients, the mean PaO_2 during left thoracotomy was approximately 70 mm Hg higher than during right thoracotomy (88).

Finally, the degree of obstructive lung disease correlates in an inverse fashion with PaO_2 during OLV. Other factors being equal, patients with more severe airflow limitation on preoperative spirometry will tend to have a better PaO_2 during OLV than patients with normal spirometry (89). The cause of this seemingly paradoxical finding seems to be related to the development of auto-PEEP during OLV in obstructed patients (90). Patients with normal healthy lungs having good elastic recoil and patients with increased elastic recoil, such as those with restrictive lung diseases, tend to benefit from applied PEEP during OLV, whereas those with COPD do not (91).

CONCLUSION

Recent advances in anesthesia and surgery have made it so that almost any patient with a resectable lung malignancy is now an operative candidate given a full understanding of the risks and after appropriate investigation. This necessitates a change in the paradigm used for preoperative assessment. Understanding and stratifying the perioperative risks allows the anesthesiologist to develop a systematic, focused approach to these patients, both at the time of the initial contact and immediately before induction, that can be used to guide anesthetic management.

References

1. Slinger PD, Johnston MR: Preoperative evaluation of the thoracic surgery patient. Semin Anesth Periop Med Pain 2002; 21:168–81.
2. Johnston MR. Curable lung cancer. Postgrad Med 1997; 101:155–65.
3. Brusasco V, Ratto GB, Crimi P, Sacco A, Motta G: Lung function after upper sleeve lobectomy for bronchogenic carcinoma. Scand J Thorac Cardiovasc Surg 1988; 22:73–8.
4. Nakahara K, Ohno K, Hashimoto J, et al.: Prediction of postoperative respiratory failure in patients undergoing lung resection for cancer. Ann Thorac Surg 1988; 46:549–52.
5. Reilly JJ: Evidence-based preoperative evaluation of candidates for thoracotomy. Chest 1999; 116:474S–476S.
6. Pierce RD, Copland JM, Sharpek, Barter CE: Preoperative risk evaluation for lung cancer resection: predicted postoperative product as a predictor of surgical mortality. Am J Resp Crit Care Med 1994; 150:947–55.
7. Epstein SK, Failing LJ, Daly BDT, Celli BR: Predicting complications after pulmonary resection. Chest 1993; 104:694–700.
8. Cerfolio RJ, Allen MS, Trastak VF, Deschamps C, Scanbon PD, Pairolero PC: Lung resection in patients with compromised pulmonary function. Ann Thorac Surg 1996; 62:348–51.
9. McKenna RJ, Fischel RJ, Brenner M, Gelb AF: Combined operations for lung volume reduction surgery and lung cancer. Chest 1996; 110:885–8.
10. Wang J, Olak J, Ferguson MK: Diffusing capacity predicts mortality but not long-term survival after resection for lung cancer. J Thorac Cardiovasc Surg 1999; 17:581–5.
11. Olsen GN, Bolton JWR, Weiman DS, Horning CA: Stair climbing as an exercise test to predict postoperative complications of lung resection. Chest 1991; 99:587–90.
12. Walsh GL, Morice RC, Putnam JB, et al.: Resection of lung cancer is justified in high risk patients selected by oxygen consumption. Ann Thorac Surg 1994; 58:704–10.
13. Cahalin L, Pappagianapoulos P, Prevost S, Wain J, Ginns L: The relationship of the 6-min walk test to maximal oxygen consumption in transplant candidates with end-stage lung disease. Chest 1995; 108:452–7.

14. Rao V, Todd TRJ, Kuus A, Beth KJ, Pearson FG: Exercise oximetry versus spirometry in the assessment of risk prior to lung resection. Ann Thorac Surg 1995; 60:603–9.
15. Ninan M, Sommers KE, Landranau RJ, et al.: Standardized exercise oximetry predicts postpneumonectomy outcome. Ann Thorac Surg 1997; 64:328–33.
16. Bollinger CT, Wyser C, Roser H, et al.: Lung scanning and exercise testing for the prediction of postoperative performance in lung resection candidates at increased risk for complications. Chest 1995; 108:341–8.
17. Reed CR, Dorman BH, Spinale FG: Mechanisms of right ventricular dysfunction after pulmonary resection. Ann Thorac Surg 1996; 62:225–32.
18. Van Miegham W, Demedts M: Cardiopulmonary function after lobectomy or pneumonectomy for pulmonary neoplasm. Respir Med 1989; 83:199–206.
19. Vesselle H: Functional imaging before pulmonary resection. Semin Thorac Cardiovasc Surg 2001; 13:126–135.
20. Tisi GM: Preoperative evaluation of pulmonary function. Am Rev Resp Dis 1979; 119:293–310.
21. Lewis JW Jr, Bastanfar M, Gabriel F, Mascha E: Right heart function and prediction of respiratory morbidity in patients undergoing pneumonectomy with moderately severe cardiopulmonary dysfunction. J Thorac Cardiovasc Surg 1994; 108:169–75.
22. Amar D, Burt M, Roistacher N, Reinsel RA, Ginsberg RJ, Wilson R: Value of perioperative echocardiography in patients undergoing major lung resection. Ann Thorac Surg 1996; 61:516–20.
23. Neuman GG, Wiengarten AE, Abramowitz RM, et al.: The anesthetic management of the patient with an anterior mediastinal mass. Anesthesiology 1984; 60:144–7.
24. Pullerits J, Holzman R: Anaesthesia for patients with mediastinal masses. Can J Anaesth 1989; 36:681–8.
25. Osaki T, Shirakusa T, Kodate M, et al.: Surgical treatment of lung cancer in the octogenarian. Ann Thorac Surg 1994; 57:188–93.
26. Mizushima Y, Noto H, Sugiyama S, et al.: Survival and prognosis after pneumonectomy in the elderly. Ann Thorac Surg 1997; 64:193–8.
27. Barry J, Mead K, Nadel EC, et al.: Effect of smoking on the activity of ischemic heart disease. JAMA 1989; 261:398–402.
28. Eagle KA, Berger PB, Calkins H: ACC/AHA guideline update for perioperative cardiovascular examination for noncardiac surgery—executive summary. Anesth Analg 2002; 94:1378–9.
29. Von Knorring J, Leptantalo M, Lindgren L: Cardiac arrhythmias and myocardial ischemia after thoracotomy for lung cancer. Ann Thorac Surg 1992; 53:642–7.

30. Ghent WS, Olsen GN, Hornung CA, et al.: Routinely performed multigated blood pool imaging (MUGA) as a predictor of postoperative complication of lung resection. Chest 1994; 105:1454–7.

31. Miller JI: Thallium imaging in preoperative evaluation of the pulmonary resection candidate. Ann Thorac Surg 1992; 54:249–52.

32. Rao V, Todd TRS, Weisel RD, et al.: Results of combined pulmonary resection and cardiac operation. Ann Thorac Surg 1996; 62:342–7.

33. Rao TKK, Jacob KH, El-Etr AA: Reinfarction following anesthesia in patients with myocardial infarction. Anesthesiology 1983; 59:499–505.

34. Ritchie AJ, Danton M, Gibbons JRP: Prophylactic digitalisation in pulmonary surgery. Thorax 1992; 47:41–3.

35. Didolkar MS, Moore RH, Taiku J: Evaluation of the risk in pulmonary resection for bronchogenic carcinoma. Am J Surg 1974; 127:700–705.

36. Van Nostrand D, Ejelsberg MO, Humphrey EW: Preresectional evaluation of risk from pneumonectomy. Surg Gynecol Obstet 1968; 127:306–12.

37. Amar D, Roistacher N, Burt ME, et al.: Effects of diltiazem versus digoxin on dysrhythmias and cardiac function after pneumonectomy. Ann Thorac Surg 1997; 63:1374–81.

38. Golledge J, Goldstraw P: Renal impairment after thoracotomy: incidence, risk factors and significance. Ann Thorac Surg 1994; 58:524–8.

39. Slinger PD. Postpneumonectomy pulmonary edema: is anesthesia to blame? Curr Opin Anaesthesiol 1999; 12:49–54.

40. American Thoracic Society: Standards for the diagnosis and care of patients with chronic obstructive pulmonary disease. Am J Resp Critic Care Med 1995; 152:S78–121.

41. Parot S, Saunier C, Gauthier H, Milic-Emile J, Sadoul P: Breathing pattern and hypercapnia in patients with obstructive pulmonary disease. Am Rev Resp Dis 1980; 121:985–91.

42. Hanson CW III, Marshall BE, Frasch HF, Marshall C: Causes of hypercarbia in patients with chronic obstructive pulmonary disease. Crit Care Med 1996; 24:23–8.

43. Douglas NJ, Flenley DC: Breathing during sleep in patients with obstructive lung disease. Am Rev Respir Dis 1990; 141:1055–70.

44. Douglas NJ, Calverley PMA, Leggett RJE, Brash HM, Flenley DC, Brezinova V: Transient hypoxaemia during sleep in chronic bronchitics and emphysema. Lancet 1979; i(8106):1–4.

45. Klinger JR, Hill NS: Right ventricular dysfunction in chronic obstructive pulmonary disease. Chest 1991; 99:715–23.

46. Schulman DS, Mathony RA: The right ventricle in pulmonary disease. Cardiol Clin 1992; 10:111–35.

47. Myles PE, Madder H, Morgan EB: Intraoperative cardiac arrest after unrecognized dynamic hyperinflation. Br J Anaesth 1995; 74:340–1.

48. MacNee W: Pathophysiology of cor pulmonale in chronic obstructive pulmonary disease. Am J Respir Crit Care Med 1994; 150:833–52.
49. Cote TR, Stroup DF, Dwyer DM, Huron JM, Peterson DE: Chronic obstructive pulmonary disease mortality. Chest 1993; 103:1194–7.
50. DeMeester SR, Patterson GA, Sundareson RS, Cooper JD: Lobectomy combined with volume reduction for patients with lung cancer and advanced emphysema. J Thorac Cardiovasc Surg 1998; 115:681–5.
51. McKenna RJ Jr, Fischel RJ, Brennar M, Gelb AF: Combined operations for lung volume reduction and lung cancer. Chest 1996; 110:885–8.
52. Nguyen DM, Mulder DS, Shennib H: Altered cellular immune function in atelectatic lung. Ann Thorac Surg 1991; 51:76–80.
53. Huglitz UF, Shapiro JH: Atypical pulmonary patterns of congestive failure in chronic lung disease. Radiology 1969; 93:995–1006.
54. Susaki F, Ishizaki T, Mifune J, Fugimura M, Nishioku S, Miyabo S: Bronchial hyperresponsiveness in patients with chronic congestive heart failure. Chest 1990; 97:534–8.
55. Nisar M, Eoris JE, Pearson MG, Calverly PMA: Acute bronchodilator trials in chronic obstructive pulmonary disease. Am Rev Respir Dis 1992; 146:555–9.
56. Warner DO: Preventing postoperative pulmonary complications. Anesthesiology 2000; 92:1467–71.
57. Stock MC, Downs JB, Gauer PK, Alster JM, Imreg PB: Prevention of postoperative pulmonary complications with CPAP, incentive spirometry and conservative therapy. Chest 1985; 87:151–7.
58. Niederman MS, Clemente P, Fein AM, et al.: Benefits of a multidisciplinary pulmonary rehabilitation program. Chest 1991; 99:798–804.
59. Selsby D, Jones JG: Some physiological and clinical aspects of chest physiotherapy. Br J Anaesth 1990; 64:621–31.
60. Kesten S: Pulmonary rehabilitation and surgery for end-stage lung disease. Clin Chest Med 1997; 18:174–81.
61. Dales RE, Dionne G, Leech JA, et al.: Preoperative prediction of pulmonary complications following thoracic surgery. Chest 1993; 104:155–9.
62. Warner MA, Diverti MB, Tinker JH: Preoperative cessation of smoking and pulmonary complications in coronary artery bypass surgery. Anesthesiology 1984; 60:383–90.
63. Akrawi W, Benumof JL: A pathophysiological basis for informed preoperative smoking cessation counselling. J Cardiothorac Vasc Anesth 1997; 11:629–40.
64. Jonsson K, Hunt TK, Mathes SJ: Oxygen as an isolated variable influences resistance to infection. Ann Surg 1988; 208:783–7.

65. Gilron I, Scott WAC, Slinger P, Wilson JAS: Contralateral lung soiling following laser resection of a bronchial tumor. J Cardiothorac Vasc Anesth 1994; 8:567–9.
66. Mueurs MF: Preoperative screening for metastases in lung cancer patients. Thorax 1994; 49:1–3.
67. Ingrassia TS III, Ryu JH, Trasek VF, Rosenow EC III: Oxygen-exacerbated bleomycin pulmonary toxicity. Mayo Clin Proc 1991; 66:173–8.
68. Thompson CC, Bailey MK, Conroy JM, Bromley HR: Postoperative pulmonary toxicity associated with mitomycin-C therapy. South Med J 1992; 85:1257–9.
69. Van Miegham W, Collen L, Malysse I, et al.: Amiodarone and the development of ARDS after lung surgery. Chest 1994; 105:1642–5.
70. Kavanagh BP, Katz J, Sandler AN: Pain control after thoracic surgery: a review of current techniques. Anesthesiology 1994; 81:737–59.
71. Licker M, de Perrot M, Hohn L, et al.: Perioperative mortality and major cardiopulmonary complications after lung surgery for non-small cell carcinoma. Eur J Cardiothorac Surg 1999; 15:314–9.
72. Ballantyne JC, Carr DB, de Ferranti S, et al.: The comparative effects of postoperative analgesic therapies on pulmonary outcome: cumulative meta-analysis of randomized, controlled trials Anesth Analg 1998; 86:598–612.
73. Hansdottir V, Woestenborghs R, Nordberg G: The pharmacokinestics of continous epidural sufentanil and bupivacaine infusion after thoracotomy. Anesth Analg 1996; 83:401–6.
74. Tejwani GA, Rattan AK, Mcdonald JS: Role of spinal opioid receptors in the antinociceptive interactions between intrathecal morphine and bupivacaine. Anesth Analg 1992; 74:726–34.
75. Hansdottir V, Bake B, Nordberg G: The analgesic efficiency and adverse effects of continous epidural sufentanil and bupivacaine infusion after thoracotomy. Anesth Analg 1996; 83:394–400.
76. Mourisse J, Hasenbos MAWM, Gielen MJM, Moll JE, Cromheedse GJE: Epidural bupivacaine, sufentanil or the combination for post thoracotomy pain. Acta Anaesthesiol Scand 1992; 36:70–4.
77. Saada M, Catoire P, Bonnet F, et al.: Effect of thoracic epidural anesthesia combined with general anesthesia on segmental wall motion assessed by transesophageal echocardiography. Anesth Analg 1992; 75:329–35.
78. Saada M, Duval A-M, Bonnet F, et al.: Abnormalities in myocardial wall motion during lumbar epidural anesthesia. Anesth Analg 1989; 71:26–33.
79. Karmakar MK: Thoracic paravertebral block. Anesthesiology 2001; 95:771–80.

80. Liu SS. ASRA Consensus Statements. Neuraxial analgesia and anticoagulation. Reg Anesth 1998; 23:S1–7.
81. Alliaume B, Coddens J. Deloof T: Reliability of auscultation in positioning of double-lumen endobronchial tubes. Can J Anaesth 1992; 39:687–91.
82. Saito S, Dohi S, Tajima K: Failure of double-lumen endobronchial tube placement: congenital tracheal stenosis in an adult. Anesthesiology 1987; 66:83–5.
83. Bayes J, Slater EM, Hadberg PS, Lawson D: Obstruction of a double-lumen tube by a saber-sheath trachea. Anesth Analg 1994; 79:186–9.
84. Slinger P, Triolet W, Wilson J: Improving arterial oxygenation during one-lung ventilation. Anesthesiology 1988; 68:291–5.
85. Slinger P, Suissa S, Triolet W: Predicting arterial oxygenation during one-lung anaesthesia. Can J Anaesth 1992; 39:1030–5.
86. Flacke JW, Thompson DS, Read RC: Influence of tidal volume and pulmonary artery occlusion on arterial oxygenation during endobronchial anesthesia. South Med J 1976; 69:619–26.
87. Hurford WE, Kokar AC, Strauss HW: The use of ventilation/perfusion lung scans to predict oxygenation during one-lung anesthesia. Anesthesiology 1987; 64:841–4.
88. Lewis JW, Serwin JP, Gabriel FS, Bastaufar M, Jacobsen G: The utility of a double-lumen tube for one-lung ventilation in a variety of noncardiac thoracic surgical procedures. J Cardiothorac Vasc Anesth 1992; 6:705–10.
89. Katz JA, Lavern RG, Fairley HB, et al.: Pulmonary oxygen exchange during endobronchial anesthesia, effect of tidal volume and PEEP. Anesthesiology 1982; 56:164–70.
90. Myles PS: Auto-PEEP may improve oxygenation during one-lung ventilation. Anesth Analg 1996; 83:1131–2.
91. Slinger PD, Kruger M, McRae K, Winton T: The relation of the static compliance curve and positive end-expiratory pressure to oxygenation during one-lung ventilation. Anesthesiology 2001; 95:1096–1102.

Jerome M. Klafta, MD

2 | Advances in Lung Isolation for Chest Surgery

Effective lung isolation (or, synonymously, lung separation) is central to the conduct of one-lung anesthesia for many intrathoracic surgical procedures. During the past several years, considerable progress has been made in our ability to provide safe and reliable lung isolation and one-lung anesthesia to our patients, especially those whose anatomy or comorbidities present significant challenges. I have organized and will discuss these developments as follows:

1. Device modifications and innovations.
2. Improved understanding and refinement of techniques.
3. Novel approaches to lung isolation.

DEVICE MODIFICATIONS AND INNOVATIONS

Double-Lumen Tubes

Common sizes of double-lumen tubes (DLTs) for adults include 35, 37, 39, and 41 French (F), but 26-, 28-, and 32-F sizes are now also available from some manufacturers. The 26-F size from Rusch is appropriate for children as young as 8 years, and tube selection guidelines for lung isolation in children have been published (1, 2). The particular dimensions and design characteristics of adult DLTs vary somewhat between manufacturers (Rusch, Duluth Ga; Portex, Keene, NH; Kendall, Mansfield,

Progress in Thoracic Anesthesia, edited by Peter Slinger,
Lippincott Williams & Wilkins, Baltimore © 2004.

Mass; Mallinckrodt, St. Louis, MO), but the left-sided Broncho-Cath from Mallinckrodt is the most popular DLT in the United States.

In 1994, the left-sided Broncho-Cath tube was redesigned: The bronchial curve was made tighter, an inverted cuff was placed closer to the tip of the bronchial lumen, and the bevel of the bronchial lumen tip was eliminated. The nonbeveled tip made inserting the tube through the glottic opening difficult, however, despite adequate laryngoscopic views (3, 4). In 2001, Mallinckrodt reintroduced a beveled edge on the tip of the tube, changed the inside of the Y-adapter for smoother passage of a fiberoptic bronchoscope (FOB), and shortened the connector to reduce dead space.

Univent Tubes

The Univent tube (Fuji Systems, Tokyo, Japan), an alternative device for providing one-lung ventilation (OLV) first introduced in 1982, also underwent design modifications in 2001. The manufacturer reports that the new TCB (Torque Control Blocker) Univent has a more flexible shaft that is easier to direct into the target bronchus and a blocker made from a softer, medical-grade silicone material that is more compliant than the material used in the previous model. Univent tubes for adults in sizes 6.0 to 9.0 (corresponding to the inner diameter of the ventilating lumen) require a cuff inflation volume of 6 to 8 cc. Pediatric Univent tubes in sizes 3.5 and 4.5 (cuffed and uncuffed) are now available. All Univent tubes are latex-free.

Arndt Endobronchial Blockers

The Arndt endobronchial blocker, or wire-guided endobronchial blocker (Cook Critical Care, Bloomington, Ind), is a fairly recent addition to the armamentarium of lung separation devices (5–7). This system minimizes some of the traditional difficulties associated with the use of Fogarty embolectomy catheters as independent bronchial blockers (BBs) and with Univent tubes. A patient's lungs can be conveniently ventilated while the blocker is fiberoptically positioned through the Arndt multiport airway adapter. The guidewire loop that protrudes through the blocker's tip is used to couple the blocker to the FOB, which can be directed fiberoptically to the desired location in the bronchial tree. The blocker's 1.4-mm lumen can be used to insufflate oxygen or suction gas from the blocked lung after the wire loop is removed. The balloon of the blocker may be less likely to dislodge than that of a Fogarty catheter because of its elliptical shape and high-volume, low-pressure cuff. The smallest single-lumen tube (SLT) for use with this blocker coaxially (inner diameter =7.5 mm) has a corresponding outer diameter that compares favorably with that of the typical DLTs and Univent tubes used for small adults. This blocker is also latex-free.

Since the introduction of this device in 1999, Cook Critical Care has changed the color of the blocker catheter from blue to yellow to contrast with the blue balloon and facilitate recognition with the FOB. A spherical balloon, in addition to the current elliptical balloon, is also available in the adult (9-F) size. A 5-F pediatric blocker has been available since 2001 and can be used inside SLTs as small as 4.5 mm. A midsize, 7-F catheter is now available and permits the utilization of a larger-diameter FOB or a smaller-diameter SLT for coaxial use. Most recently, "Murphy eye" side holes have been introduced into the distal end of the 9-F adult catheter to circumvent suctioning difficulty if the end hole abuts the bronchial mucosa (George Arndt, personal communication, 2002). Characteristics of available blockers are described in Table 2.1.

Airway Exchange Catheters

In the setting of a difficult airway, an airway exchange catheter (AEC) may be used to exchange an SLT for a DLT preoperatively or a DLT for an SLT postoperatively. Cook Critical Care manufactures AECs specifically designed for DLT exchanges. These differ from conventional AECs in that they are longer (100 cm) and have centimeter markings that extend to 50 cm. The 11- and 14-F sizes will fit inside small and large DLTs, respectively. An extrafirm variety (colored green) became available in 2002.

TABLE 2.1   Arndt Endobronchial Blockers

Size (F)	Smallest single-lumen tube inner diameter for coaxial use (mm)	Length (cm)	Cuff shape	Average cuff inflation volume (cc)
9	7.5	78 & 65	Elliptical	6.0–12.0
			Spherical	4.0–8.0
7	6.0	65	Spherical	2.0–6.0
5	4.5	65 & 50	Spherical	0.5–2.0

Data from Cook Critical Care.

IMPROVED UNDERSTANDING AND REFINEMENT OF TECHNIQUES

Right-Sided DLTs

The perceived or real difficulty in achieving adequate OLV with right-sided DLTs is confirmed by the fact that they are used much less frequently than left-sided DLTs: 94% of Broncho-Cath sales are left-sided (Sherri Cowan, personal communication 2002). Use of left-sided DLTs is generally encouraged because of the greater margin of safety in positioning them (8). In the hands of practitioners familiar with the use of right-sided DLTs and facile with fiberoptic bronchoscopy, however, successful and reliable OLV is possible (9). When right- and left-sided DLTs were compared for left-sided thoracic surgery in 40 patients, no right upper lobes collapsed, and the difference in the time to place the tubes was clinically insignificant (3.37 vs 2.08 minutes) (10). Although their routine use in thoracic surgery is controversial (11, 12), right-sided DLTs are indicated when a patient requires a DLT but has an anatomic abnormality of the left mainstem bronchus, such as an exophytic or stenotic lesion or a left tracheobronchial disruption. Regardless of the reasons for using a DLT, the right mainstem bronchial length must be at least 10 mm to accommodate the lateral aspect of the bronchial cuff (13). This length may be determined bronchoscopically or by chest radiography or computed tomography (CT). Attempting to position a right-sided DLT in a patient whose right mainstem bronchus is too short is almost certainly doomed to failure.

Placement and Positioning of DLTs

Precise positioning of a DLT is most reliably achieved with the benefit of an FOB. In comparisons of fiberoptic positioning of DLTs with conventional methods, more than one-third of left-sided DLTs were malpositioned after blind intubation and the inspection-and-auscultatory method (14). In a recent study of 200 patients, the incidence of malpositioning (0.5-cm deviation from the ideal position) was 46%, among those in whom DLT placement was judged correct by clinical assessment. Of those malpositioned, 32% were "critical" malpositions, defined as those in which the left endobronchial limb allowed no clear view of the left upper or lower lobe bronchus, those in which the right endobronchial limb allowed no clear view of the right upper lobe bronchus, or those in which intratracheal dislocation of more than half the endobronchial cuff occurred (15).

Visually unassisted or "blind" placement of left DLTs may result in initial intubation of the wrong bronchus in 7% to 30% of cases using the modified Broncho–Cath (15, 16). Reliable and reproducible methods of placing left-sided DLTs (and, with slight modification, right-sided DLTs) on the first attempt using an FOB have been described (17).

When 50 patients undergoing thoracic surgery with left-sided DLTs were positioned from supine to lateral, the tube tended to move outward by an average of approximately 1 cm (18). Inflation of the endobronchial cuff before lateral positioning did not decrease the incidence or the amount of overall change in distance. *Because of the tendency for carinal shift and DLT movement upward with lateral positioning, keeping the bronchial cuff at least 1 cm inside the left mainstem bronchus before turning the patient laterally is advantageous.* In another study of 61 patients, the incidence of proximal repositioning was reduced significantly (43% vs 16%) after patients were turned from supine to lateral when the left Broncho-Cath was initially inserted with the proximal edge of its bronchial cuff 5 mm beyond the tracheal carina (19).

Confirming Lung Separation

A number of reasons support use of use a "just seal" or minimum occlusive seal technique (13, 20, 21) to inflate the bronchial cuff of a DLT or BB. First, a cuff that is inflated beyond a minimum occlusive pressure may result in tracheobronchial ischemic complications or even rupture (20, 22). Second, an overinflated bronchial cuff or BB is more likely to dislodge or herniate over the tracheal carina and, thus, interfere with contralateral ventilation. Third is the ability to immediately and definitively verify lung separation. That "moment of truth" when the thoracoscopic port is inserted or the hemithorax is opened is thoroughly predictable. If lung collapse is slow or incomplete, documented lung separation assures the anesthesiologist that manipulation of the DLT or BB or their cuffs will not improve the situation. Attention can then be focused on other maneuvers that will improve the surgical exposure: manual compression, suction, time, or intrahemithoracic CO_2 insufflation (23). The positive-pressure or bubble test for achieving a bronchial cuff minimum occlusive seal and confirming lung separation is depicted in Figure 2.1 (13).

Neither an airtight bronchial seal nor cuff pressure of 25 cm H_2O guarantees protection against aspiration (24). Fluid may leak along the longitudinal folds in the cuff wall (25). Thus, even though an airtight seal is the desired end point in the vast majority of indications for lung separation (ie, enhanced surgical exposure), it may not be sufficient to prevent the spread of blood and secretions. An airtight seal does not guarantee a watertight seal. Water-soluble (KY jelly) lubricant on the cuff of an SLT and a cuff seal of 30 cm H_2O reduced aspiration of dye (26); aspiration occurred in 11% of the group with the lubricated cuff and in 83% of the group without the lubricated cuff.

Air Bubble Method for Detection of Cuff Seal/Leak

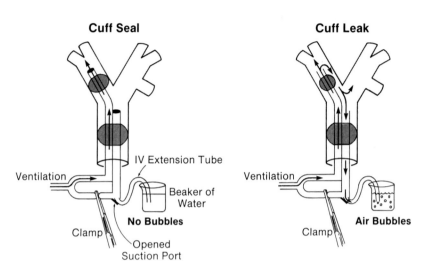

FIGURE 2.1 Air bubble method for detection of cuff seal/leak. [From Benumof (13); with permission.]

Comparisons of Lung Isolation Techniques

Several recent studies have compared the effectiveness of lung isolation techniques. Campos and Kernstine (27) prospectively compared the effectiveness of lung isolation with a left Broncho-Cath, TCB Univent tube, and the Arndt endobronchial blocker in 64 patients undergoing elective right- or left-sided thoracic surgery. No statistically significant differences were found among the three groups in frequency of tube malpositions, number of required bronchoscopies, or overall quality of lung isolation as assessed by the surgeon (blinded to technique). Once lung isolation was achieved, the Arndt blocker took slightly longer to place (3 minutes, 34 seconds) compared to the DLT (2 minutes, 8 seconds) or Univent (2 minutes, 38 seconds), inclusive of time to place the SLT, although 86- and 46-second differences are hardly of clinical significance. Complete lung collapse took longer with the Arndt blocker (26 minutes, 2 seconds) than with the DLT (17 minutes, 54 seconds) or Univent (19 minutes, 28 seconds) and more frequently required suction assistance.

Two European studies compared the left Broncho-Cath DLT with Rusch 6-F blockers not originally designed for this use. When 35 patients undergoing right- or left-sided, video-assisted thoracoscopic procedures were randomly allocated into groups, it took marginally longer to place a left BB (4 minutes, 13 seconds) than a right BB (2 minutes, 25 seconds) or a left DLT (2 minutes, 16 seconds) (28). Quality of the lung collapse was worse in the right BB group than in the other two groups. Left BBs were more difficult to place initially than right BBs, and one DLT could not be positioned correctly. Ender et al. (29) compared these two techniques in 159 patients who required left-lung collapse for minimally invasive direct coronary artery bypass procedures. The median times for intubation and correct placement, oxygenation during OLV, and effectiveness of lung collapse were the same between groups. In the BB group, 4% of the BBs could not be placed, and these patients were managed with a DLT.

Limiting Diameter of the Upper Airway

A cadaver study (30) found that in 76% of women and 68% of men, the effective diameter of the larynx at vocal cord level was greater than that of the cricoid, but in no case was it found to be less. Stated another way, in these same percentages of patients, the cricoid cartilage was of a *smaller* effective diameter than the larynx at the vocal cord level. This result suggests the conventional teaching that the glottic opening is the limiting diameter in normal adult airways may not be correct, and it may explain why resistance to passage of a DLT sometimes occurs *beyond* the glottis.

Size Selection of DLTs

Assuming that the main body of a DLT will fit through the glottic opening and the trachea, an appropriately sized DLT is the largest tube that will fit in the mainstem bronchus, with only a small air leak being detectable when the cuff is deflated (31). The presence of some air leakage ensures that the tube is not tightly impacted in the bronchus. Thus, the

TABLE 2.2   Outer Diameters (mm) of the Bronchial Component of Plastic Left-Sided Double-Lumen Tubes*

Manufacturer	Double-lumen tube size			
	35 F	37 F	39 F	41 F
Mallinckrodt	9.5	10.0	10.1	10.6
Rusch	9.4	10.1	10.8	11.5
Sheridan	9.3	9.9	9.9	10.7
Portex	9.7	10.2	11.2	12.0

From Hannallah et al. (31); with permission.
*Others have demonstrated that there is significant variability in these diameters for all DLT sizes (33).

goal is to select a DLT with a bronchial end having an outer diameter 1 to 2 mm smaller than the diameter of the intubated bronchus to allow for the size of the deflated cuff (32). Published diameters of the bronchial components of various DLTs appear in Table 2.2.

The tip diameters of different DLTs are known, but the diameter of the left mainstem bronchus in any given patient is more difficult to determine. Although many practitioners select 41- and 39-F DLTs for tall and short men, respectively, and 39- and 37- or 35-F DLTs for tall and short women, respectively, considerable interindividual variability is found in left mainstem diameters, and gender and height have relatively weak predictive value (31, 32). Because prediction is imprecise, measurement of the left mainstem diameter on chest radiographs is appealing; however, this is practical only 50% of the time (31). Other alternatives include measuring left mainstem diameter on chest CT (34, 35) or three-dimensional CT scan reconstruction (36). Brodsky et al. (37) measured the more readily obtainable tracheal diameter on chest radiographs at the level of the clavicles and used a previously described, mean left bronchial to tracheal width ratio of 0.68 to calculate the left mainstem diameter. Their predictions worked well, but those of others did not (38). More recently, a slightly larger left bronchial to tracheal width ratio of 0.75 for men and of 0.77 for women using three-dimensional chest CT scan reconstructions was reported (39).

Attempting to select an appropriately sized DLT is important, but perhaps equally important clinically is recognizing when a DLT is too large (ie, the bronchial lumen will not fit in the bronchus or forms an airtight seal with no air in the cuff) or too small (ie, >3 cc of air in the bronchial cuff are required to create a seal) and then adjusting the DLT size accordingly.

NOVEL APPROACHES TO LUNG ISOLATION

Novel approaches to lung isolation involve lung separation and the difficult airway, the patient with a tracheostomy, selective lobar blockade, and unconventional uses of BBs.

Lung Separation and the Difficult Airway

General Approach

A thorough working knowledge regarding the physical details of all the devices and techniques available for lung separation is necessary to safely and effectively manage this challenging subset of patients. Airway difficulties may arise from the upper airway (more common) or the lower airway. Upper airway anatomic or pathologic features that render conventional rigid laryngoscopy for placement of SLTs difficult are even more problematic for placement of DLTs and Univent tubes because of their size and shape (40). Awake fiberoptic intubation with a DLT or SLT may be the best option in cases of known or anticipated difficult intubation (17, 41), and fortunately, several options are available for achieving lung separation once an SLT has been successfully placed. The Arndt endobronchial blocker in particular represents a significant advancement in the treatment of these patients (5–7) and is especially useful when a nasal intubation is required (see earlier discussion) (42).

Lower airway difficulties are encountered with anatomical variation or distortion of the tracheal or bronchial anatomy. Distortion can occur with strictures, extraluminal compression, deviation, or intraluminal masses. These features will influence the selection of the bronchus to be targeted and the choice of a BB or DLT. Lower airway difficulties can be detected or predicted using diagnostic bronchoscopy before intubation or preoperative imaging studies. An algorithm for airway treatment options in these patients is presented in Figure 2.2 (43).

DLTs

The tracheal cuffs of DLTs are particularly vulnerable to being torn by a patient's teeth when a DLT is being placed with the aid of rigid laryngoscopy in those with prominent dentition, a small mouth opening, or

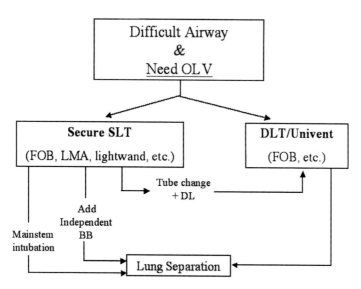

FIGURE 2.2 Approach to lung separation options in patients with a difficult airway. BB = bronchial blockers; DL = direct laryngoscopy; FOB = fiberoptic bronchoscope; LMA = laryngeal mask airway; OLV = one-lung ventilation; SLT = single-lumen tube. [From Klafta and Ovassapian (43); with permission.]

limited neck extension. Several proposed solutions to this problem include a retractable protective sheath (44), a lubricated Penrose drain (Davol Inc, Cranston, RI), (45), lubricated teeth guards (46), and manipulation of the tube during laryngoscopy (47).

Oral fiberoptic intubation with a DLT is well described in both awake and asleep patients (46, 48, 49). A patient's mouth opening and oropharyngeal size must be large enough to accommodate a DLT for orotracheal intubation. Placement requires good topical anesthesia, adequate conscious sedation, and assistance in maintaining soft-tissue support. Soaking a DLT in a warm water bath just before intubation and using sufficient lubrication will minimize its rigidity (49). Concurrent direct laryngoscopy may be required to elevate the supraglottic tissues to facilitate passage of a DLT through the glottic opening after the fiberoptic scope is in the trachea (17, 50).

Univent Tubes

Some anesthesiologists consider a Univent tube easier to place and position than a DLT (51), particularly in patients with upper airway abnormalities (52). Others, however, do not (4). The internal diameter of the ventilating lumen in a size 8.5 or 9.0 Univent tube will accommodate an adult 5.0-mm bronchoscope (51), which then precludes the need to change tubes after diagnostic bronchoscopy. Although it is also suitable for fiberoptic intubation, the Univent tube has several limitations. First, unlike the polyvinyl chloride construction of the SLT and DLT, the Univent tube is constructed of a polymeric silicone material that will not soften in a warm water bath. As such, its curved shape is fixed, which may be a disadvantage when sliding it over a bronchoscope. Second, the fixed concavity often makes the leading edge of the tube impinge on the vocal cords, thus impeding its passage into the trachea. A successful nasal intubation with a 7.0 Univent tube has been described, despite its size and rigidity (53).

SLTs

Using an SLT to intubate a mainstem bronchus is another option for achieving lung separation, and it is frequently the preferred technique in children who are too small for DLTs (54). The advantages of this approach include its simplicity and the rapidity with which lung separation can often be achieved, particularly when the right lung must be ventilated. Blind advancement of an SLT rarely results in a left mainstem intubation, but rotating an in situ SLT 180° while turning the patient's head to the right will improve the success rate of left mainstem intubation to approximately 92% (55). Fiberoptic guidance of an SLT into the appropriate mainstem bronchus is probably the easiest and most reliable technique. If significant amounts of blood or secretions preclude fiberoptic visualization, using fluoroscopy to visualize and direct the radiopaque bronchoscope is another option (56).

Disadvantages of SLTs for lung separation include frequent exclusion of right upper lobe ventilation when an SLT is in the right mainstem bronchus. Left upper lobe ventilation can also be excluded when the left mainstem bronchus is relatively short (57). Regardless of which lung is ventilated, neither independent suctioning nor application of continuous positive airway pressure to the nonventilated lung is possible. Finally, if the nasotracheal route is used, most SLTs will not be long enough to provide reliable mainstem intubation.

The Patient with a Tracheostomy

Although the presence of a tracheostomy greatly simplifies airway management for most anesthetics, it presents an interesting challenge when lung separation is required. As with orotracheal intubation, use of a DLT (17), Univent tube (58), or BB through the tracheostomy stoma is an option, despite the fact that these tubes are not specifically designed for this use. Depending on the details of a patient's anatomy, such as stomal diameter, distance between the skin and the anterior tracheal wall, and stoma-to-carinal distance, both DLTs and Univent tubes may be difficult to place and position precisely and atraumatically.

Another way to achieve lung separation in the patient with a tracheostomy is using a BB, either coaxially or alongside an SLT or tracheostomy tube through the stoma (59) or through the mouth (60). Blind or fiberoptically directed mainstem intubation with an SLT inserted through the stoma is another option, although this has the usual limitations associated with mainstem intubations.

Selective Lobar Blockade

Selective lobar blockade is a strategy for partial lung isolation in patients who cannot tolerate the exclusion of an entire lung's ventilation. Selective lobar ventilation following contralateral pneumonectomy was achieved using an Arndt blocker in one patient and a left DLT in the right mainstem bronchus in another (61). A Univent tube was used in three patients to selectively block the right upper, middle, and middle and lower lobes (62). Similar techniques have been described in children (63). In a separate, randomized study of 30 patients undergoing lobectomy, oxygenation was improved with selective lobe collapse compared with total lung collapse, with or without continuous positive airway pressure to the nonventilated lung (64).

Unconventional Uses of BBs

A BB was placed through the tracheal lumen of an ill-fitting, right-sided DLT to force the bronchial cuff into position (65) and through the bronchial lumen of a left-sided DLT that was too large to fit in the left mainstem bronchus (66, 67). In another patient, a Fogarty catheter was used to block an aberrant tracheal bronchus in combination with a Univent tube during a right thoracotomy (68). A double-endobronchial blocker technique has been described in nine patients (69); in this technique, two BBs were placed through an SLT for situations in which one BB could not be adequately positioned.

These examples of creative solutions to problems encountered with use of DLTs or conventional BB techniques highlight the fact that various methods of lung separation are, in fact, complementary in certain clinical situations.

SUMMARY

Effective lung isolation is the foundation for successful OLV. Appreciating the physical details of different lung isolation devices, developing expertise in fiberoptic bronchoscopy, and maintaining a broad repertoire of techniques will promote success in providing safe and effective lung separation even in the most challenging patients.

References

1. Hammer GB, Fitzmaurice BG, Brodsky JB: Methods for single-lung ventilation in pediatric patients. Anesth Analg 1999; 89:1426–9.
2. Hammer GB: Pediatric thoracic anesthesia. Anesth Analg 2001; 92:1449–64.
3. Brodsky JB, Macario A: Modified Bronchocath double-lumen tube. J Cardiothorac Vasc Anesth 1995; 9:784–5.
4. Campos JH, Reasoner DK, Moyers JR: Comparison of a modified double-lumen endotracheal tube with a single-lumen tube with enclosed bronchial blocker. Anesth Analg 1996; 83:1268–72.
5. Arndt GA, Kranner PW. Rusy DA, et ai.: Single-lung ventilation in a critically ill patient using a fiberoptically directed wire-guided endobronchial blocker. Anesthesiology 1999; 90:1484–6.

6. Arndt GA, Buchika S, Kranner PW, et al.: Wire-guided endobronchial blockade in a patient with a limited mouth opening. Can J Anaesth 1999; 46:87–9.

7. Arndt GA, DeLessio ST, Kranner PW, et al.: One-lung ventilation when intubation is difficult—presentation of a new endobronchial blocker. Acta Anaesthesiol Scand 1999; 43:356–8.

8. Benumof JL, Partridge BL, Salvatierra C, Keating J. Margin of safety in positioning modern double-lumen endotracheal tubes. Anesthesiology 1987; 67:729–38.

9. Campos JH, Massa F, Christoper F. Is there a better right-sided tube for one-lung ventilation? A comparison of the right-sided double-lumen tube with the single-lumen tube with enclosed bronchial blocker. Anesth Analg 1998; 86:696–700.

10. Campos JH, Massa FC, Kernstine KH. The incidence of right upper-lobe collapse when comparing a right-sided double-lumen tube versus a modified left double-lumen tube for left-sided thoracic surgery. Anesth Analg 2000; 90:535–40.

11. Campos JH, Gomez MN: Pro: right-sided double-lumen endotracheal tubes should be routinely used in thoracic surgery. J Cardiothorac Vasc Anesth 2002; 16:246–8.

12. Cohen E. Con: right-sided double-lumen endotracheal tubes should not be routinely used in thoracic surgery. J Cardiothorac Vasc Anesth 2002; 16:249–52.

13. Benumof JL: Anesthesia for Thoracic Surgery. 2nd ed. Philadelphia: WB Saunders, 1995; 330–89.

14. Pennefather SH, Russell GN: Placement of double lumen tubes—time to shed light on an old problem (editorial). Br J Anaesth 2000; 84:308–10.

15. Klein U, Karzai W, Bloos F, et al.: Role of fiberoptic bronchoscopy in conjunction with the use of double-lumen tubes for thoracic anesthesia: a prospective study. Anesthesiology 1998; 88:346–50.

16. Brodsky JB, Macario, A, Cannon WB, Mark JB: "Blind" placement of plastic left double-lumen tubes. Anaesth Intensive Care 1995; 23:583–6.

17. Ovassapian A: Fiberoptic Endoscopy and the Difficult Airway. 2nd ed. Philadelphia: Lippincott-Raven, 1996; 117–56.

18. Desiderio DP, Burt M, Kolker AC, et al.: The effects of endobronchial cuff inflation on double-lumen endobronchial tube movement after lateral decubitus positioning. J Cardiothorac Vasc Anesth 1997; 11:595–8.

19. Fortier G, Cote D, Bergeron C, Bussieres JS: New landmarks improve the positioning of the left Broncho-Cath double-lumen tube—comparison with the classic technique. Can J Anaesth 2001; 48:790–4.

20. Guyton DC, Besselievre TR, Devidas M, et al.: A comparison of two different bronchial cuff designs and four different bronchial cuff inflation methods. J Cardiothorac Vasc Anesth 1997; 11:599–603.

21. Hannallah MS, Benumof JL, McCarthy PO, Liang M: Comparison of three techniques to inflate the bronchial cuff of left polyvinylchloride double-lumen tubes. Anesth Analg 1993; 77:990–4.

22. Fitzmaurice BG, Brodsky JB: Airway rupture from double-lumen tubes. J Cardiothorac Vasc Anesth 1999; 13:322–9.

23. Brock H, Rieger R, Gabriel C, et al.: Hemodynamic changes during thoracoscopic surgery. The effects of one-lung ventilation compared with carbon dioxide insufflation. Anaesthesia 2000; 55:10–6.

24. Hannallah MS, Gharagozloo F, Gomes MN, Chase GA: A comparison of the reliability of two techniques of left double-lumen tube bronchial cuff inflation in producing water-tight seal of the left mainstem bronchus. Anesth Analg 1998; 87:1027–31.

25. Seegobin RD, van Hasselt GL: Aspiration beyond endotracheal cuffs. Can Anaesth Soc J 1986; 33:273–9.

26. Young PJ, Patil A, Haddock A, Blunt MC: The protective effect of cuff lubrication against pulmonary aspiration (abstract). Anesthesiology 2000; 93:A1365.

27. Campos JH, Kernstine KH: A comparison of a left-sided Broncho-Cath® with the torque control blocker Univent and the wire-guided blocker. Anesth Analg 2003; 96:283–9.

28. Bauer C, Winter C, Hentz JG, et al.: Bronchial blocker compared to double-lumen tube for one-lung ventilation during thoracoscopy. Acta Anaesthesiol Scand 2001; 45:250–4.

29. Ender J, Bury AM, Raumanns J, et al.: The use of a bronchial blocker compared with a double-lumen tube for single-lung ventilation during minimally invasive direct coronary artery bypass surgery. J Cardiothorac Vasc Anesth 2002; 16:452–5.

30. Seymour AH, Prakash N: A cadaver study to measure the adult glottis and subglottis: defining a problem associated with the use of double-lumen tubes. J Cardiothorac Vasc Anesth 2002; 16:196–8.

31. Hannallah MS, Benumof JL, Ruttimann UE: The relationship between left mainstem bronchial diameter and patient size. J Cardiothorac Vasc Anesth 1995; 9:119–21.

32. Slinger P. Choosing the appropriate double-lumen tube: a glimmer of science comes to a dark art (editorial). J Cardiothorac Vasc Anesth 1995; 9:117–8.

33 Russell WJ, Strong TS: Dimensions of double-lumen tracheobronchial tubes. Anaesth Intensive Care 2003; 31:50–3

34. Chow MYH, Liam BL, Thng CH, Chong BK: Predicting the size of a double-lumen endobronchial tube using computed tomographic

scan measurements of the left main bronchus diameter. Anesth Analg 1999; 88:302–5.

35. Hannallah M, Benumof JL, Silverman PM, Kelly LC, Lea D: Evaluation of an approach to choosing a left double-lumen tube size based on chest computed tomographic scan measurement of left mainstem bronchial diameter. J Cardiothorac Vasc Anesth 1997; 11:168–71.

36. Eberle B, Weiler N, Vogel N, Kauczor HU, Heinrichs W: Computed tomography-based tracheobronchial image reconstruction allows selection of the individually appropriate double-lumen tube size. J Cardiothorac Vasc Anesth 1999; 13:532–7.

37. Brodsky JB, Macario A, Mark JBD: Tracheal diameter predicts double-lumen tube size: a method for selecting left double-lumen tubes. Anesth Analg 1996; 82:861–4.

38. Chow MYH, Liam BL, Lew TWK, Chelliah RY, Ong BC: Predicting the size of a double-lumen endobronchial tube based on tracheal diameter. Anesth Analg 1998; 87:158–60.

39. Brodsky JB, Malott K, Angst M, Fitzmaurice BG, Kee SP, Logan L: The relationship between tracheal width and left bronchial width: implications for left-sided double-lumen tube selection. J Cardiothorac Vasc Anesth 2001; 15:216–7.

40. Wilson RS. Lung isolation: tube design and technical approaches. Chest Surg Clin N Am 1997; 7:735–51.

41. Patane PS, Sell BA, Mahla ME: Awake fiberoptic endobronchial intubation. J Cardiothorac Anesth 1990; 4:229–31.

42. Campos JH: Current techniques for perioperative lung isolation in adults. Anesthesiology 2002; 97:1295–301.

43. Klafta JM, Ovassapian A: Lung separation and the difficult airway. Probl Anesth 2001; 13:69–77.

44. Coppa GP, Brodsky JB: A simple method to protect the tracheal cuff of a double-lumen tube (letter). Anesth Analg 1998; 86:675.

45. Marymont J, Szokol J, Fry W: Method to prevent damage to the tracheal cuff of a double-lumen endotracheal tube during laryngoscopy (letter). J Cardiothorac Vasc Anesth 1999; 13:371.

46. Erb JM: A less difficult method to protect the tracheal cuff of a double-lumen tube (letter). Anesth Analg 1998; 87:1217.

47. Fortier G, St Onge S, Bussieres J: Two other simple methods to protect the tracheal cuff of a double-lumen tube (letter). Anesth Analg 1999; 89:1064.

48. Ovassapian A: Fiberoptic positioning of right-sided double-lumen endobronchial tubes. J Bronchol 1994; 1:1–8.

49. Ovassapian A, Klafta J: Double-lumen endobronchial tubes and the difficult intubation (abstract). Proceedings of the 12th World Congress of Anesthesiologists, Montreal, Canada, June 4–9, 2000; 1.4.06.

50. Benumof JL: Difficult tubes and difficult airways (editorial). J Cardiothorac Vasc Anesth 1998; 12:131–12.

51. Gayes JM: Pro: one-lung ventilation is best accomplished with the Univent endotracheal tube. J Cardiothorac Vasc Anesth 1993; 7:103–7.

52. Slinger P: Con: the Univent tube is not the best method of providing one-lung ventilation. J Cardiothorac Vasc Anesth 1993; 7:108–12.

53. Gozal Y, Lee W: Nasal intubation and one-lung ventilation (letter). Anesthesiology 1996; 84:477.

54. Hammer GB, Fitzmaurice BG, Brodsky JB: Methods for single-lung ventilation in pediatric patients. Anesth Analg 1999; 89:1426–9.

55. Kubota H, Kubota Y, Toyoda Y, et al.: Selective blind endobronchial intubation in children and adults. Anesthesiology. 1987; 67:587–9.

56. Klafta JM, Olson JP: Emergent lung separation for management of pulmonary artery rupture. Anesthesiology 1997; 87:1248–50.

57. Lammers CR, Hammer GB, Brodsky JB, et al.: Failure to separate and isolate the lungs with an endotracheal tube positioned in the bronchus. Anesth Analg 1997; 85:946–7.

58. Andros TG, Lennon PF: One-lung ventilation in a patient with a tracheostomy and severe tracheobronchial disease. Anesthesiology 1993; 79:1127–8.

59. Dhamee MS: One-lung ventilation in a patient with a fresh tracheostomy using the tracheostomy tube and a Univent endobronchial blocker. J Cardiothorac Vasc Anesth 1997; 11:124–5.

60. Veit AM, Allen RB: Single-lung ventilation in a patient with a freshly placed percutaneous tracheostomy. Anesth Analg 1996; 82:1292–3.

61. Ng J, Hartigan PM: Selective lobar bronchial blockade following contralateral pneumonectomy. Anesthesiology 2003; 98:268–70.

62. Hagihira S, Maki N, Kawaguchi M, Slinger P: Case 5–2002. Selective bronchial blockade in patients with previous contralateral lung surgery. J Cardiothorac Vasc Anesth 2002; 16:638–42.

63. Takahashi M, Yamada M, Honda I, et al.: Selective lobar-bronchial blocking for pediatric video-assisted thoracic surgery. Anesthesiology 2001; 94:170–1.

64. Campos JH: Effects of oxygenation during selective lobar versus total lung collapse with or without continuous positive airway pressure. Anesth Analg 1997; 85:583–6.

65. Nino M, Body SC, Hartigan PM: The use of a bronchial blocker to rescue and ill-fitting double-lumen endotracheal tube. Anesth Analg 2000; 91:1370–1.

66. Capdeville M, Hall D, Koch CG: Practical use of a bronchial blocker in combination with a double-lumen endotracheal tube. Anesth Analg 1998; 87:1239–41.
67. Soonthon-Brant V, Benumof JL: Unexpected small tracheo-bronchial tree size and separation of the lungs. J Cardiothorac Vasc Anesth 2002; 16:260–2.
68. Lee H, Ho Y, Cheng R, Shyr M: Successful one-lung ventilation in a patient with aberrant tracheal bronchus. Anesth Analg 2002; 95:492–3.
69. Amar D, Desiderio DP, Bains MS, Wilson RS: A novel method of one-lung isolation using a double endobronchial blocker technique. Anesthesiology 2001; 95:1528–30.

Katherine P. Grichnik, MD

Advances in the Management of
3 | One-Lung Ventilation

INTRODUCTION

Thoracic surgical volume is expanding, with an increased ability to care for patients having advanced surgical and respiratory disease. To optimally care for such patients, one should understand ventilation and perfusion changes with lateral positioning, the cause of intraoperative hypoxemia, and innovative strategies for one-lung ventilation (OLV).

VENTILATION AND PERFUSION IN THE LATERAL POSITION

Distribution of Ventilation

Comprehension of ventilation and perfusion abnormalities in the lateral position with two-lung ventilation (TLV) provides a basis for understanding superimposed OLV. In the classic diagrams of pressure-volume relationships for the distribution of ventilation, Benumof (1) eloquently depicted ventilation during surgery in the thorax (Fig. 3.1). With the change from an upright position to a lateral position, the nondependent lung behaves as the superior portion of the upright lung, and the dependent lung behaves as the inferior portion of the upright lung. With the induction of anesthesia, overall functional residual capacity (FRC) decreases(2–4), but with the lateral position, the nondependent lung moves

Progress in Thoracic Anesthesia, edited by Peter Slinger,
Lippincott Williams & Wilkins, Baltimore © 2004.

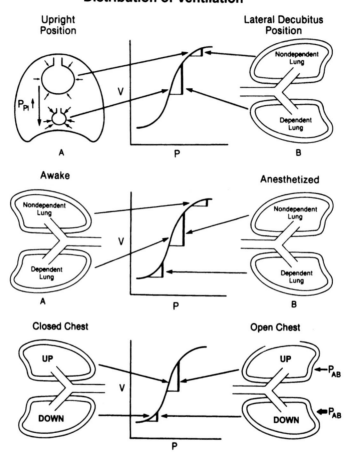

Awake, Closed Chest Distribution of Ventilation

FIGURE 3.1 Positional distribution of ventilation. The distribution of ventilation in various positions is related to a pressure (P)-volume (V) curve. A = upright position; B = lateral decubitus position; P_{AB} = pressure of abdomen; P_{PI} = pleural pressure. [From Benumof (1); with permission.]

to a more compliant portion of the pressure-volume curve and the dependent lung to a less compliant portion of the pressure-volume curve, resulting in gain of FRC for the nondependent lung and loss of FRC for the dependent lung (1, 5, 6). This leads to approximately 55% of the tidal volume (TV) being delivered to the nondependent lung in the lateral anesthetized position (7). With positive-pressure ventilation, gravitational influences on the distribution of ventilation are diminished. Furthermore, with anesthesia and muscle relaxation, a flaccid diaphragm allows abdominal contents to move cephalad, the mediastinum may push downward, and improper positioning may limit the lung movement—all three of which further decrease the proportion of the TV ventilation distributed to the dependent lung. Finally, with opening of the chest, further changes occur to increase nondependent lung compliance without significant change in dependent lung compliance. Thus, the FRC of the nondependent lung increases proportionally, with more of the TV directed to it.

Respiratory mechanical studies have traditionally been conducted in patients undergoing closed-chest procedures. However, Dechman et al. (8) illustrate the separate behavior of open- and closed-chest systems when the chest wall is removed as a significant mechanical force (Fig. 3.2) Patients undergoing supine closed-chest procedures were compared with patients undergoing supine median sternotomy (an "open-chest" procedure). The effect of the addition of positive end-expiratory pressure (PEEP) on lung elastance (the inverse of compliance; increased stiffness is indicated by increased elastance) was measured (9) In the closed chest, all levels of PEEP resulted in decreased elastance of the respiratory system, with little change in the elastance of the lung. In sharp contrast, any addition of PEEP to a patient having an open-chest procedure resulted in an increase in the elastance or stiffness of the lung. Preferential ventilation of the nondependent portions of the open lung with resultant overdistention may have led to movement of the lung to a less favorable position on the pressure-volume curve to increase stiffness. These mechanical principles must be kept in mind when considering TLV in the lateral position, because an entire lung is dependent and an entire lung is nondependent. The addition of PEEP to nondependent lung areas (supine or lateral) must be done with caution. In contrast, Klingstedt et al. (10) demonstrated an improvement in the distribution of ventilation to perfusion (V/Q) in the lateral position by adding PEEP only to the dependent lung.

Distribution of Perfusion

The traditional concepts of pulmonary blood flow have been well described by West (11) (Fig. 3.3). Gravity was proposed as the primary basis for the distribution of perfusion with more blood flow in the dependent areas of a lung compared to the superior areas of a lung. Similar to ventilation, with the lateral position the nondependent lung behaves as the superior portions of the upright lung and the dependent lung behaves as the inferior portions of the upright lung; it receives relatively more blood flow than the nondependent lung.

Two studies underscore the importance of gravitational effects with the distribution of blood flow and OLV. Wantabe et al. (12) demon-

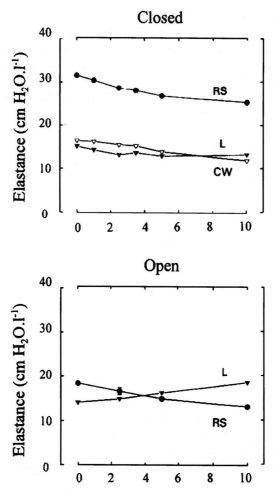

FIGURE 3.2   Effect of positive end-expiratory pressure on elastance. The change in elastance of a respiratory system under open- and closed-chest conditions is compared. Note that under the open-chest condition, the chest wall drops out as a variable. Lung elastance is the opposite of lung compliance and denotes an increase in lung stiffness. CW = chest wall; L = lung; RS = respiratory system. [From Dechman et al. (8); with permission.]

strated a fall in the arterial partial pressure for oxygen (PaO_2) with the onset of OLV during three different positions: supine, semilateral, and lateral (Fig. 3.4). Oxygenation was best preserved with the lateral position compared to the other positions in which the influence of gravity serves to divert blood flow to only the dependent, ventilated lung. Bardoczky et al. (13) also compared oxygenation with OLV in the lateral position versus the supine position at multiple levels of inspired oxygen.

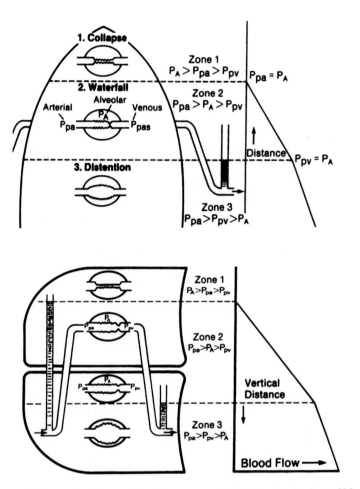

FIGURE 3.3   Zones of West. The classic zones of West depict the flow of blood in the lung as related to the alveolar pressure, the arterial pressure, and the venous pressure at various gravitational levels. Note the similarity of the zones in the upright and lateral positions such that in the lateral position, the nondependent lung behaves as the superior portions of the upright lung and the dependent lung behaves as the inferior portion of the upright lung. P_A = alveolar pressure; P_{pa} = pulmonary artery pressure; Ppas = pulmonary artery systolic pressure; P_{pv} = pulmonary vein pressure. [From West (11); with permission.]

The move from the supine to the lateral position improved oxygenation at all oxygen levels.

Nongravitational forces are also important, because the distribution of pulmonary perfusion is more diverse than can be explained by gravity alone. Hakim et al. (14) used single-photon emission computed tomography to study the distribution of blood flow in human lungs at

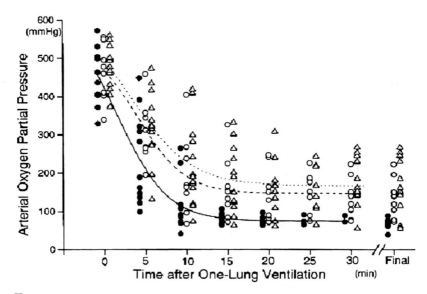

FIGURE 3.4 Arterial oxygen pressure as a function of position. Arterial oxygenation during one-lung ventilation is shown in the supine (Δ), semilateral (O), and lateral (•) positions. [From Wantabe et al. (12); with permission.]

a single lung level at a single level of gravity (Fig. 3.5). They found a central-to-peripheral distribution of blood flow along isogravitational planes. The gradients are postulated to result from the distance that blood must travel to reach a peripheral lung site, with dependence on the diameter and branching patterns of the pulmonary vasculature. Glenny (15) further explored pulmonary perfusion and conceptualized the geometry of the pulmonary vascular tree as having two components: a fixed structure, which is the primary determinant of regional perfusion; and a variable component, which is influenced by local factors. Glenny noted that:

1. Lung regions with high blood flow remained high-flow areas, and low-flow areas continued to have low blood flow, despite extreme changes in pulmonary artery pressure and cardiac output with exercise.
2. Heterogeneity in blood flow distribution was stable over long periods of time.
3. Gravity was only mildly influential in blood flow distribution when perfusion was investigated in upright versus inverted lungs.

Relevant to thoracic surgery, Mure et al. (16), using labeled microspheres in a canine model, found that blood flow changes little when moving from a supine to a lateral position. Other factors that may affect

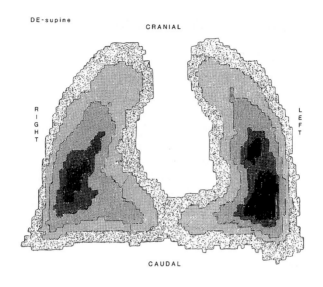

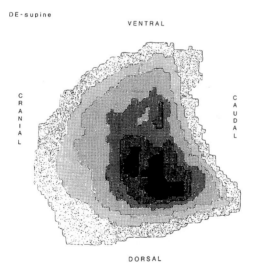

FIGURE 3.5 Isogravitational pulmonary blood flow. The assessment of pulmonary blood flow using single-photon emission computed tomography is shown. Note the central-to-peripheral distribution of blood flow along isogravitational planes. Darker areas represent higher blood flow, and lighter areas represent lower blood flow. [From Hakim et al. (14); with permission.]

pulmonary blood flow distribution in the lateral position include geometric differences in chest cavity dimensions, pre-existing pulmonary hypertension, and pre-existing abnormalities of lung volume (eg, emphysema).

INTRAOPERATIVE HYPOXEMIA

Onset of Hypoxemia

An absolute pulmonary shunt is created with the sudden cessation of ventilation of the nondependent lung in the face of continued perfusion to that lung. Concurrently, V/Q abnormalities resulting from lateral positioning, an open chest, gravitational and nongravitational forces, as well as a variety of patient and perioperative factors act to influence the onset, duration, and severity of hypoxemia.

Guenoun et al. (17) reconfirmed the time course for the onset of hypoxemia after the initiation of OLV (Fig. 3.6). Initially, the PaO_2 falls sharply, but it then declines less precipitously after 15 to 20 minutes of OLV, as seen in other studies (18).

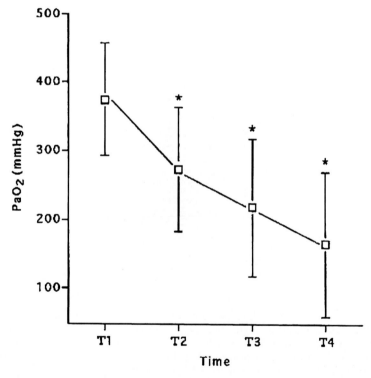

FIGURE 3.6 Fall in arterial partial pressure of oxygen (PaO_2) with one-lung ventilation (OLV) over time. T1 = 10 minutes of two-lung ventilation; T2 = 5 minutes of OLV in the lateral decubitus position; T3 = 15 minutes of OLV in the lateral decubitus position; T4 = 5 minutes after thoracotomy. [From Guenoun et al. (17); with permission.]

Prediction of Intraoperative Hypoxemia

It would be of great interest to be able to predict which patient would become hypoxic; this would allow us to attempt to prevent hypoxemia or to avoid OLV for a particular surgery. A collection of postulated factors is presented in Table 3.1 and are considered individually.

Some have found an inverse correlation between a good predicted postoperative forced expiratory volume in 1 second (FEV_1) and more hypoxemia intraoperatively (18) (Fig. 3.7). Explanations include:

1. A diseased lung may collapse more slowly, leading to a longer period of residual ventilation of the nondependent lung.
2. A diseased lung may already have been subject to reduced perfusion on the basis of intrinsic pathology and/or chronic hypoxic pulmonary vasoconstriction (HPV) such that OLV has little influence.
3. Once deflated, a diseased lung with emphysema may actually kink pulmonary vessels, thus limiting the perfusion to a nonventilated lung.
4. A diseased lung may develop intrinsic PEEP, which may augment dependent-lung FRC to limit the development of atelectasis and hypoxia.

This logic then applies to the observation that significant hypoxemia is sometimes seen in patients undergoing OLV for nonpulmonary surgery (presumably patients with otherwise-normal lung function).

Patients with a high percentage of perfusion to the operative lung suffer a high incidence of unacceptable PaO_2 as compared to patients with relatively less perfusion of the operative lung, who have a lower incidence of a low PaO_2 with OLV (19) (Fig. 3.8). When the percentage of blood flow to the operative lung on the preoperative scan to the operative lung was greater than 45%, the likelihood of hypoxemia was increased (20).

TABLE 3.1 Postulated Factors for the Risk of Hypoxemia During Thoracic Surgery

Preoperative percentage of predicted FEV_1 (Inverse correlation)
Thoracotomy for nonpulmonary surgery
Amount of perfusion to operative half of the thorax
Poor preoperative PaO_2
Cardiac output and pulmonary artery pressure
Hemoglobin
Elderly
Side of surgical procedure
Supine versus lateral position

FEV_1 = forced expiratory volume in 1 second; PaO_2 = arterial partial pressure of oxygen.

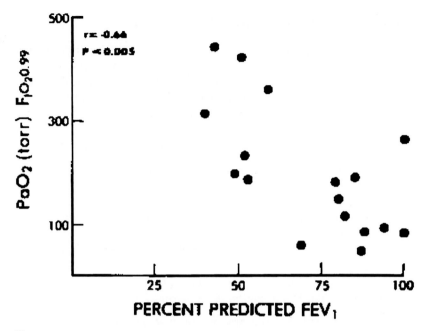

FIGURE 3.7 Arterial partial pressure of oxygen (PaO_2) during one-lung ventilation (OLV) as a function of predicted postoperative forced expiratory volume in 1 second (FEV_1). Note the relationship of a higher predicted postoperative FEV_1 with a lower intraoperative PaO_2 during OLV. FIO_2=fraction of inspired oxygen. [From Katz et al. (18); with permission.]

Slinger et al. (21) found that three factors were most important to predict desaturation after 10 minutes of OLV. These included the side of surgery, the PaO_2 on TLV, and the percentage of predicted FEV_1 (also an inverse correlation). The right lung receives 10% more blood flow than the left lung; thus, it may be more subject to hypoxemia under OLV conditions (21). The PaO_2 after induction of anesthesia under TLV is critical, because it reflects the reserve of the patient's respiratory system to maintain oxygenation in the face of general anesthesia, positive-pressure ventilation, and lateral position with a high fraction of inspired oxygen (FIO_2). Slinger et al. used these variables to construct an equation to predict hypoxemia after 10 minutes of OLV, and they successfully predicted arterial oxygen desaturation in 40% of patients determined to be at risk.

In another study, 92 patients were examined for 49 variables that could be related to intraoperative hypoxemia (17). Five significant factors were identified with a multivariate analysis:

1. Relative perfusion to the operative lung.
2. Age [PaO_2 usually decreases with age in awake humans, with increases in baseline V/Q mismatch (22, 23)].

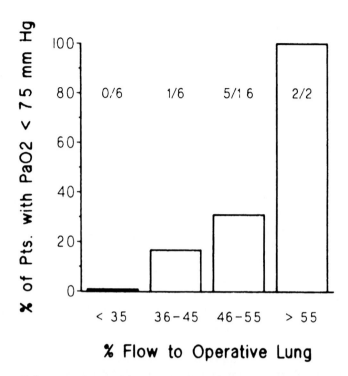

FIGURE 3.8 Proportion of patients with hypoxemia during one-lung ventilation grouped according to the relative preoperative perfusion to the operative lung. PaO_2 = arterial partial pressure for oxygen. [From Hurford et al. (19); with permission.]

3. Low to normal hematocrit (likely caused by improved rheological effects).
4. PaO_2 on TLV.
5. Lower mean arterial pressure when hypoxemic.

In the logistic regression analysis, only PaO_2 with TLV was determined to be an independent predictor. It was noted that most of the variables were not amendable to modification before or during surgery, with the exception of limiting mean arterial pressure to prevent increases in pulmonary artery pressure, which could inhibit HPV (24).

What Is Acceptable Hypoxemia?

With OLV, desaturation to 88% to 90% is common, and multiple authors have used this level as a threshold for intervention (21, 25, 26). However, no adequate studies have defined an acceptable level of arterial oxygen saturation during thoracic surgery. Treatment should be considered with mild desaturation to avoid significant declines in oxygenation while the intervention is being initiated. A minimum acceptable arterial oxygen saturation must be determined in the context of patient pathology and comorbid diseases.

Limiting Hypoxia: HPV

The principal mechanism for the limitation of hypoxemia is to decrease the pulmonary shunt, which is accomplished primarily through HPV, an acute or chronic reflex response of the pulmonary circulation to (segmental) alveolar hypoxia (27) This local phenomenon occurs within 1 minute, is maximal at 15 minutes, and is reversible; the magnitude of the response is proportional to the amount of lung that is rendered hypoxic (1, 28, 29). Hypoxic pulmonary vasoconstriction serves to divert pulmonary blood flow from low oxygen tension regions to better-aerated lung and is most pronounced in the precapillary arterioles. It is a unique response of the pulmonary vascular system, because it is the opposite of the vasodilatory effect of hypoxia on the systemic vasculature (30–32). It can limit what would theoretically be a 40% shunt to a 22% shunt (33).

A complex set of factors influence the HPV response. The response may be provoked by primary hypoxia or by atelectasis resulting in hypoxia. Small segments of hypoxic lung result in greater diversion of blood flow, whereas large segments of hypoxic lung result in greater increases in pulmonary artery pressures compared to blood flow diversion (34, 35). Small segments of hypoxic lung and ventilation with a low PaO_2 favor the PaO_2 as the main stimulus, whereas large segments of hypoxic lung and atelectasis favor the partial pressure of venous oxygen (PvO_2) as the main stimulus for HPV (36).

The mechanisms mediating HPV are less understood, but they appear to alter locally the balance of vasodilatory and vasoconstrictive compounds. Some proposed causes include mediators that inhibit prostaglandin synthesis, enhance leukotriene synthesis, or alter calcium-channel pathways and changes in nitric oxide (NO) production that enhance vasoconstriction (37–40). Potential humoral agents include endothelin, angiotensin II, NO, and adrenomedullin (41, 42). Archer and Michelakis (43) have proposed a biological system unit to explain HPV mechanisms (Fig. 3.9). Each unit consists of a sensor, a mediator, and one or more effectors, in this case to preserve the critical physiological variable of pulmonary PaO_2. In their definition, that the sensor must monitor a variable that is modified by mild hypoxia such that a biological adaptation could take place before energy depletion or tissue damage occurs. In their model, the sensor is in the pulmonary artery

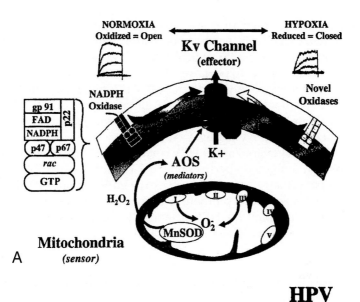

FIGURE 3.9 (A) Schematic for a biological sensor unit to preserve oxygenation in the pulmonary artery. The sensor resides in the pulmonary artery smooth muscle cells and uses the vascular redox system of the electron-transport chain of mitochondria. The mediators are activated oxygen species, such as hydrogen peroxide. The signal is transmitted by voltage-sensitive potassium channels, which control membrane potential as well as calcium entry and tone (the effector). (B) Flow chart of the biological response to hypoxia. AOS = activated oxygen species; FAD = flavin adenine dinucleotide; GTP = guanosine triphosphate; NADPH = reduced form of nicotinaminde-adenine dinucleotide phosphate. [From Archer and Michelakis (43); with permission.]

HPV

Hypoxia

↓

Decreased K⁺ channel current

↓

Depolarization

↓

Increased L-type Ca²⁺ Current

↓

Increased Ca²⁺ influx

↓

Increased Cytosolic Ca²⁺

↓

Biological Response
- Vasoconstriction
- Catecholamine Secretion
- Neural Activation

B

smooth muscle, the mediators are activated oxygen species, the signal is transmitted by voltage-sensitive potassium channels and the effector is the membrane potential to control calcium entry and tone. Vasoconstriction in response to hypoxia results. Supporting evidence for this theory is the known phenomenon that HPV is inhibited by antagonists of voltage dependent Ca^{2+} channels (44), although the magnitude of the effect may depend on the phase of HPV and the particular voltage-dependent calcium-entry pathway (45).

Physiological factors affect HPV. Increases in cardiac output lead to increases in pulmonary perfusion, which can inhibit HPV (46). Intermittent hypoxia may increase or decrease the HPV response (47, 48), but hyperoxia has no effect on pulmonary vascular resistance (49). Surgical manipulation may limit the HPV response, the magnitude of which is related to individual mediator release (50, 51).

Inhalational and Intravenous Anesthetic Affects on HPV

The anesthetic technique may affect the magnitude of the HPV response. In general, it is believed that intravenous anesthetic (IVA) agents have little effect of HPV but that inhalational anesthetics (IHA) directly inhibit HPV.

Effects on V/Q Matching Under TLV

Loeckinger et al. (52) examined the effects of IVA versus IHA during TLV without the influence of OLV (Fig. 3.10). Sevoflurane and isoflurane compared to midazolam increased blood flow to areas of low V/Q ratio, indicating that the IHA had vasodilated the basal poorly aerated lung, effectively shunting blood from the better-aerated areas. Pulmonary vascular resistance was not observed to change, making a specific HPV effect less likely. This finding challenges the explanation the IHA cause V/Q mismatch because of specific inhibition of HPV; a more global vasodilator response may contribute.

Experimental Effects of IHA and IVA

Isoflurane and enflurane are similar in having mild cardiovascular effects, causing bronchodilation, and inhibiting HPV experimentally (53–55). In a dog model, inhibition of HPV by isoflurane was independent of cardiac output and P_{VO_2} (56), and enflurane at one minimum alveolar concentration was found to inhibit HPV by 21.5% during OLV (57). Sevoflurane and desflurane are potent bronchodilators that can also inhibit HPV (58, 59). The HPV effect of sevoflurane is noted at

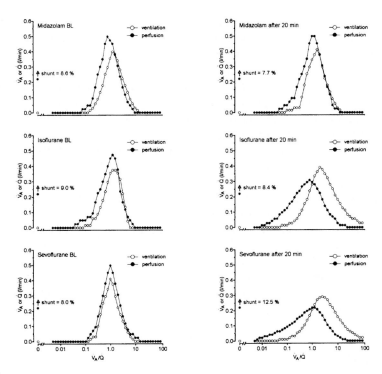

FIGURE 3.10   Inhalation agents compared to intravenous agents during two-lung ventilation. Midazolam was compared to sevoflurane and isoflurane during two-lung, open-chest conditions to examine the matching of ventilation to perfusion over time. Note that midazolam preserved ventilation to perfusion matching, whereas isoflurane and sevoflurane did not. $\dot{Q}$ = perfusion; V_A = alveolar ventilation. [From Loeckinger et al. (52); with permission.]

higher concentrations; thus, it may not be clinically relevant. Propofol has been reported to either not influence HPV (57) or actually to potentiate HPV (60, 61). Nitrous oxide can independently depress HPV (62, 63) and causes sympathetic nervous system activation (64, 65), which could secondarily inhibit HPV. Fentanyl and morphine are often used as a part of a balanced anesthetic technique and have little effect on HPV (66–68)

Contradictory Clinical Effects of IHA and IVA

Conflicting results have been obtained when comparing IHA techniques both to each other and to IVA techniques during OLV clinically (69–73). For example, Benumof et al. (69) demonstrated that PaO_2 was significantly less during IHA compared to IVA in patients undergoing thoracic surgery in a cross-over study. In support, Abe et al. (74) also found that propofol decreased shunt and improved oxygenation, in contrast to IHA. Propofol has been compared to IHA for thoracotomy and found to cause less impairment of postoperative lung function (75). Furthermore, the different IHA may have varying effects; one group found that desflurane preserved arterial oxygenation to a greater extent than isoflurane during anesthesia and OLV, suggesting a smaller effect on HPV compared to that of isoflurane (76).

Beck et al.(77), however, found that propofol and sevoflurane were not significantly different with respect to changes in shunt fraction in the lateral position under OLV (Fig. 3.11) Similarly, Yondov et al. (78) found no difference in intraoperative PaO_2 with a total IVA technique using propofol as compared to volatile anesthetics.

Interpretation of these studies is confounded by the effects of surgically induced lung trauma, the unpredictability of individual HPV responses, and other variable effects of IHA and IVA, such as depression of cardiac output with subsequent decreases in PvO_2 (79). The common conclusion appears to be that inhalational agents may inhibit HPV, but not to a clinically significant end point.

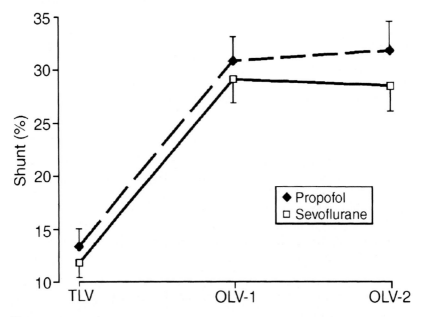

FIGURE 3.11 Sevoflurane versus propofol and shunt fraction during one-lung ventilation (OLV). No significant difference was found between sevoflurane and propofol during thoracic surgery with respect to shunt fraction. OLV-1 = supine OLV; OLV-2 = lateral OLV; TLV = two-lung ventilation. [From Beck et al. (77); with permission.]

Vasoactive Agents and HPV

The concept that vasodilators, such as sodium nitroprusside and nitroglycerin, blunt the HPV response (80–82) has been challenged (83, 84), because some authors have shown no change in shunt fraction or oxygenation with administration of sodium nitroprusside during thoracotomy (82). Prostaglandin $F_2\alpha$, inhibits HPV only when injected into the atelectatic lung pulmonary artery (85), has little effect when administered systemically (50). Dopamine and dobutamine may inhibit HPV indirectly by increasing cardiac output and PvO_2 (86, 87).

Novel Ideas for HPV Response

Novel approaches to augmentation and modification of an HPV response may be considered. It is known that sepsis and endotoxemia inhibit HPV (88), which could be caused by generation of reactive oxygen species (ROS) (89, 90). Scavengers of ROS are postulated to prevent or reverse the inhibition of HPV and to restore oxygenation. In an animal model, OLV of the right lung was introduced, resulting in increased left lung pulmonary vascular resistance, which is a surrogate for HPV (91) (Fig. 3.12). The left lung pulmonary vascular resistance was decreased by the administration of lipopolysaccharide to simulate endotoxemia, but ROS scavengers attenuated this impairment of HPV. The ROS scavengers were useful when given intraperitoneally or intratracheally. The intriguing questions to be explored are whether ROS are generated during OLV and whether ROS inhibitors could have a role in augmenting an HPV response intraoperatively.

Treatment of Hypoxia

Conventional treatment for hypoxemia should always be attempted initially: hand ventilation to assess dynamic compliance of the pulmonary system, optimization of ventilator settings, and confirmation of the correct endotracheal tube position. Insufflation of 1 to 2 L/min of oxygen through the open-lumen half of the double-lumen tube for the nonventilated lung (blow-by oxygen), continuous positive airway pressure (CPAP) to the nonventilated lung, and PEEP to the ventilated lung are standard therapies. Vascular clamping of the arterial supply to the tissue to be resected is most useful for large lung resections, especially pneumonectomy. Intermittent TLV may be necessary. Usually, CPAP is initiated before PEEP to avoid worsening of hypoxia from PEEP-induced compression of pulmonary blood vessels, which can promote diversion of blood flow to the nonventilated lung (1).

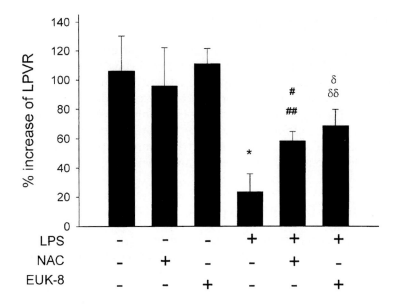

FIGURE 3.12 Preservation of the hypoxic pulmonary vasoconstriction (HPV) response with reactive oxygen species (ROS) scavengers. Endotoxemia was simulated with lipopolysaccharide (LPS) administration, which inhibited the increase in left pulmonary vein vascular resistance (LPVR) as a surrogate measure of an HPV response. The first column is the control column. The second and third columns demonstrate that *n*-acetylcystine (NAC; an ROS scavenger) and EUK-8 (a nonselective, manganese-containing ROS scavenger) had no independent effects on LPVR. The fourth column shows the effect of LPS, and the fifth and sixth columns show the effect of NAC or EUK-8 to restore LPVR or a HPV effect. Data are mean ± SD. ∗ = $P < 0.001$ versus saline-challenged mice; # = $P < 0.05$ versus endotoxin-challenged mice; ## = $P < 0.05$ versus saline-challenged mice treated with NAC; δ = $P < 0.01$ versus endotoxin-challenged mice; δδ = $P < 0.05$ versus saline-challenged mice treated with EUK-8. [From Baboolal et al. (91); with permission.]

Ishikawa et al. (92) reported an original method for improving oxygenation during OLV. They noted that a portion of patients responded to physical compression of the nonventilated lung during OLV after the onset of hypoxemia. This was not a uniform finding, however, and probably was caused by the redirection of blood flow toward the ventilated lung from kinking and compression of the nondependent lung vasculature.

Use of NO for Hypoxemia

Many groups have investigated the use of inhaled NO directed toward the dependent ventilated lung, with variable results (93, 94). Rocca et al. (95) found a benefit primarily in patients who had experienced profound hypoxemia during OLV. Inhaled NO improved oxygenation (PaO_2:FIO_2 ratio) and decreased pulmonary vascular resistance. However, other patient groups, such as those with a high documented shunt or pulmonary hypertension, did not benefit from NO. Sticher et al. (96) proposed that the dose of NO used in previous studies was inconsistent and excessive. In a porcine study, those authors found that OLV with hypoxia was most effectively improved by 4 ppm of NO as compared to higher doses (Fig. 3.13). The mechanism is unclear, however, and is probably related to large changes in V/Q matching, some of which may be aggravated by larger NO doses. Furthermore, NO is also proposed to be a mediator for inhibition of HPV in sepsis and endotoxemia when released within the nondependent, nonventilated lung (97). It remains to be proven that exogenous NO toward the dependent, ventilated lung is reproducibly effective in humans under OLV conditions in conjunction with the effects of anesthetic agents.

Others have proposed the use of inhaled prostacyclin as an alternative to NO, citing equal efficacy in patients having cardiac surgery, with acute respiratory distress syndrome (ARDS), and having a transplant (98). Hache et al. (99) and DeWet et al. (100) have found that inhaled prostacyclin decreases pulmonary artery pressures and variably improves PaO_2:FIO_2 ratios in patients having thoracotomies. Cost and ease of use may propel further study in thoracic surgery, because inhaled prostacyclin is reported to cost $150 day (compared to $3,000 per day for NO) with a simple delivery to the Y piece in the ventilatory circuit (100, 101).

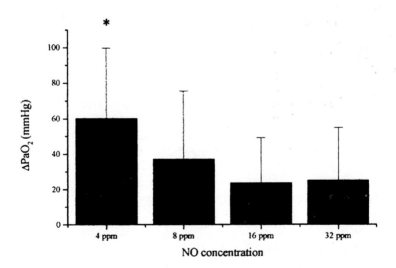

FIGURE 3.13 Improvement in oxygenation with nitric oxide (NO). Small doses of NO improve oxygenation to a greater degree than larger doses in a porcine model of one-lung ventilation. Nitric oxide was administered after hypoxia had occurred. ΔPaO_2 = improvement in arterial partial pressure for oxygen as the result of the NO administration. [From Sticher et al. (96); with permission.]

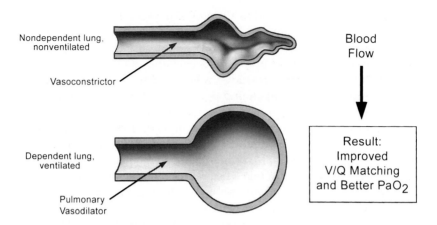

FIGURE 3.14   Model for optimization of hypoxic pulmonary vasoconstriction (HPV). Use of a pulmonary vasoconstrictor directed toward the nondependent lung and a pulmonary vasodilator directed toward the dependent lung is proposed to improve ventilation/perfusion (V/Q) matching during one-lung ventilation. [From Moutafis et al. (104); with permission.]

Almitrine is a systemic vasoconstrictor that has been used in patients with ARDS to potentiate HPV and improve oxygenation (102). A novel approach for hypoxia with OLV is to combine an inhaled vasodilator (NO) to the dependent, ventilated lung with an agent such as almitrine to promote vascular constriction in the nondependent, nonventilated lung to achieve better V/Q matching (103) (Fig. 3.14). In further studies, almitrine was used independently to ameliorate decreases in PaO_2 with OLV without significant hemodynamic changes (104). Almitrine may cause lactic acidosis, hepatic dysfunction (105), and peripheral neuropathies (106); thus, some have suggested phenylephrine as an alternative. The search for pharmacological solutions to hypoxemia is promoted by the increase in thoracoscopic procedures, during which traditional solutions to intraoperative hypoxemia, such as CPAP, may be less useful (107).

INTRAOPERATIVE VENTILATORY STRATEGIES FOR ONE-LUNG SURGERY

The Concept of Lung Protection

Traditionally, guidelines for the management of OLV have included use of a TV from 8 to 10 mL/kg to avoid dependent-lung atelectasis and maintenance of a minute ventilation to defend an arterial partial pressure for carbon dioxide ($PaCO_2$) of 40 mmHg. However, one can challenge these recommendations on the basis that relatively high TV to a single dependent lung and high respiratory rates may actually inflict harm. One potential deleterious event from a traditional ventilatory strategy is dynamic pulmonary hyperinflation. Most patients develop intrinsic PEEP with OLV (108, 109), and use of high TV may further exacerbate the inability of patients with diseased lungs to empty the dependent lung with each expiration. There may also be an increased risk of barotrauma with the use of a high driving pressure to achieve large TV. The ARDS literature suggests that acute lung injury is associated with "volutrauma" (ie, delivery of large TV during mechanical ventilation) (110–115).

The theory of lung protection from barotrauma and volutrauma is that allowing a lung to experience lower inspiratory and peak pressures while preventing cyclic alveolar collapse should ameliorate mechanical and inflammatory lung injury (116). Amato et al. (117) described lung protective strategies for use in medical patients with ARDS (Table 3.2). Those authors found improved survival, a higher rate of weaning from mechanical ventilation, and a lower rate of barotrauma. This technique was validated in a large, multicenter, randomized trial (118).

Anesthesiologists traditionally use PEEP in the dependent lung only after hypoxia has occurred as a therapeutic maneuver. It can be proposed that PEEP instituted at the beginning of OLV may prevent lung injury. In a sheep model of lung injury, use of PEEP at the initiation of OLV at two different levels was associated with a greater

TABLE 3.2 Lung Protective Strategy for Reduction of Barotrauma in Patients with Acute Lung Injury

Maneuver	Recommended value
Limit inspiratory driving pressure ($P_{PLAT} - PEEP_{TOTAL}$)	<20 cm H_2O
Limit peak airway pressure	<40 cm H_2O
Pressure-limited or pressure-support ventilation	Pressure-controlled inverse ratio ventilation if $FIO_2 > 0.5$
Relatively high PEEP (if $PEEP_{AUTO}$ occurs, then $PEEP_{TOTAL} = PEEP_{EXT} + PEEP_{AUTO}$)	$PEEP_{TOTAL}$ at 2 cm H_2O pressure $> P_{FLEX}$
Frequent lung recruitment measures	Hold continuous positive airway pressure at 30–40 cm H_2O pressure for 40 seconds
Respiratory rate	<30 breaths per minute

Data from Amato et al. (117).
FIO_2=fraction of inspired oxygen; P_{FLEX} = inflection point corresponding to the upward shift in the slope of the pressure-volume curve; P_{PLAT} = plateau pressure after inspiratory pause; $PEEP_{AUTO}$ = the difference between alveolar pressure at end expiration and airway pressure; $PEEP_{EXT}$ = PEEP applied externally to the respiratory circuit, $PEEP_{TOTAL} = PEEP_{EXT} + PEEP_{AUTO}$.

PaO$_2$:FIO$_2$ ratio and less shunt but also, more importantly, with less inflammation and histological injury (119).

To be comparable to OLV in humans, we must first assume a degree of lung injury with OLV during thoracic surgery, which would benefit from a lung protective strategy (120), and then that the addition of external PEEP would not be injurious to patients having OLV, who often develop intrinsic PEEP (108). Slinger and Hickey (121). demonstrated that external PEEP does not increase total PEEP or aggravate auto-PEEP if the expiratory time is appropriately long. Although this discussion is focused on lung injury, Slinger et al. (122) also showed that in some patients, addition of external PEEP will move the dependent-lung pressure-volume curve to a more favorable position with respect to preservation of FRC and can improve oxygenation in selected patients. The importance of measuring total PEEP whenever extrinsic PEEP was used is emphasized.

A rabbit model was used to investigate TLV, OLV protective ventilation, and OLV nonprotective ventilation (123). Protective ventilation resulted in less collapse and overdistention compared to greater lung water gain, more inflammation, and higher inspiratory pressures in the nonprotected group. A strategy of using PEEP from the start of surgery may necessitate the use of concurrent CPAP to oxygenate blood, possibly shunted from the dependent lung to the nondependent lung.

Permissive Hypercapnea

Use of a lung protective strategy may conflict with the goal of maintaining normocapnea, especially with the known increases in airway pressures and airflow resistance with lateral OLV. Permissive hypercapnea has been suggested in both medical disease and selected surgical procedures (124, 125). Sticher et al. (126) investigated patients undergoing OLV who were randomized to low-TV ventilation versus normal-TV ventilation; the PaCO$_2$ allowed to rise without intervention. The authors noted increases in cardiac index and pulmonary vascular resistance with decreases in systemic vascular resistance in the hypercapnea group, but no differences in oxygenation were noted.

Pressure-Controlled Ventilators

A pressure-controlled ventilator (PCV) may be advantageous to achieve a lung protection strategy during OLV. Limiting peak and plateau transalveolar airway pressures may limit mechanical lung trauma; combined with a decelerating flow pattern, the distribution of gas flow may improve (127). With this mode of ventilation, the TV varies but can be kept low by setting the maximum peak pressures allowed.

Turul et al. (128) compared use of a volume-controlled ventilator with PCV during OLV. They found that peak airway pressure, plateau pressure, and shunt increased during volume-controlled ventilation as compared to PCV. The PaO_2 was higher with PCV, and this correlated inversely with preoperative pulmonary function tests. Patients with the poorest preoperative pulmonary function derived the greatest benefit in oxygenation from PCV.

Flow-Volume Loops

Intraoperative flow-volume loops may also be used to assess individual patient responses to the multitude of therapies discussed. In-line flow-volume loops allow one to monitor for development of incomplete expiration caused by interrupted expiratory flow (129) (Fig. 3.15). Continual

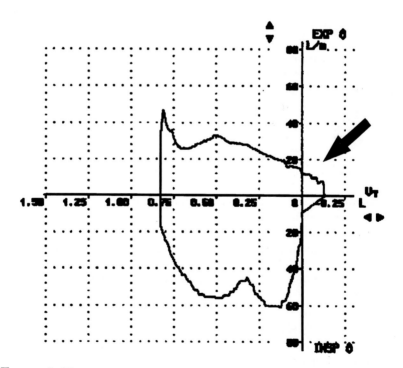

FIGURE 3.15 Example of a flow-volume loop demonstrating interrupted expiratory flow at the arrow. Flow is in liters per minute, and pulmonary volume is in liters.

flow-volume loop monitoring may also allow for the detection of endo-tracheal tube movement into an incorrect position (130) and dynamic pulmonary hyperinflation before significant morbidity.

Monitoring the Adequacy of Ventilation

With lung protective strategies and permissive hypercapnea, accurate continual assessment of $PaCO_2$ is optimal. Traditionally, $PaCO_2$ is esti-mated by end-tidal carbon dioxide ($ETCO_2$) intraoperatively. Multiple authors have challenged the accuracy of $ETCO_2$ monitoring during ab-normal patient positioning and in the presence of shunts (131, 132). Fur-ther, Yam et al. (133) described a large discrepancy between $PaCO_2$ and $ETCO_2$ during OLV because of changes in shunt and dead space. A more accurate method may be to use transcutaneous carbon dioxide moni-toring, which Tobias (134) demonstrated is more accurate than $ETCO_2$ during OLV to estimate $PaCO_2$.

SUMMARY

There is an increasing need to effectively manage OLV in patients with significant pulmonary disease. Knowledge of pulmonary ventilation and perfusion physiology, improvements in the ability to prevent and treat hypoxia, and comprehension of traditional and novel ventilatory techniques may promote improved perioperative outcomes.

References

1. Benumof JL, ed: Anesthesia for Thoracic Surgery, 2nd ed. Philadel-phia: Saunders, 1995.
2. Westbrook PR, Stubbs SE, Sessler AD, et al.: Effects of anesthesia and muscle paralysis on respiratory mechanics in normal man. J Appl Physiol 1973; 34:81–6.
3. Nunn JF: Effects of anaesthesia on respiration. Br J Anaesth 1990; 65:54–62.
4. Wahba RWM: Perioperative functional residual capacity. Can J Anaesth 1991; 38:384–400.
5. Lim TPK, Luft UCL: Alterations in lung compliance and functional residual capacity with posture. J Appl Physiol 1959; 14:164–6.
6. Lumb AB, Nunn JF: Respiratory function and ribcage contribution to ventilation in body positions commonly used during anesthe-sia. Anesth Analg 1991; 73:422–6.

7. Larsson A, Malmkivist G, Werner O: Variations in lung volume and compliance during pulmonary surgery. Br J Anaesth 1987; 59:585–91.
8. Dechman GS, Chartrand DA, Ruiz-Neto PP, et al.: The effect of changing end-expiratory pressure on respiratory system mechanics in open- and closed-chest, anesthetized, paralyzed patients. Anesth Analg 1995; 81:279–86.
9. Dechman G, Lauzon A-M, Bates JHT: Mechanical behavior of the canine respiratory system at very low lung volumes. Respir Physiol 1994; 95:119–29.
10. Kinglstedt C, Hedenstierna G, Baehrendtz S, et al.: Ventilation-perfusion relationships and atelectasis formation in the supine and lateral positions during conventional mechanical and differential ventilation. Acta Anaesthesiol Scand 1990; 34:421–99.
11. West JB: Respiratory Physiology: The Essentials, 5th ed. Baltimore: Williams & Wilkins, 1995.
12. Wantabe, S, Noguchi E, Yamada S, et al.: Sequential changes of arterial oxygen tension in the supine position during one-lung ventilation. Anesth Analg 2000; 90:28–34.
13. Bardoczky GI, Szegedi LL, d'Hollander AA, et al.: Two-lung and one-lung ventilation in patients with chronic obstructive pulmonary disease: the effects of position and F102. Anesth Analg 2000; 90:35–41.
14. Hakim TS, Lisbona R, Dean GW: Gravity-independent inequality in pulmonary blood flow in humans. J Appl Physiol 1987; 63:1114–21.
15. Glenny RW: Blood flow distribution in the lung. Chest 1998; 114:8S–16S.
16. Mure M, Domino KB, Robertson T, et al.: Pulmonary blood flow does not redistribute in dogs with reposition from supine to left lateral position. Anesthesiology 1998; 89:483–92.
17. Guenoun, T, Journois D, Silleran-Chassany J, et al.: Prediction of arterial oxyten tension during one-lung ventilation: analysis of preoperative and intraoperative variables. J Cardiothorac Vasc Anesth 2002; 16:199–203.
18. Katz JA, Laverne RG, Fairley HB, et al.: Pulmonary oxygen exchange during endobronchial anesthesia: effect of tidal volume and PEEP. Anesthesiology 1982; 56:164–72.
19. Hurford WE, Kolker AC, Strauss HW: The use of ventilation/perfusion lung scans to predict oxygenation during one-lung anesthesia. Anesthesiology 1987; 67:841–44.
20. Dunn PF: Physiology of the Lateral Decubitus Position and One-Lung Ventilation. Thorac Anesth Int Anesthesiol Clin 2000; 38:25–53.
21. Slinger P, Suissa S, Triolet W: Predicting arterial oxygenation during one-lung anaesthesia. Can J Anaesth 1992; 39:1030–5.
22. Cardus J, Burgos F, Diaz O, et al.: Increase in pulmonary ventilation-

perfusion inequality with age in healthy individuals. Am J Respir Crit Care Med 1997; 156:648–53.

23. Carveri I, Zoia MC, Fanfulla F, et al.: Reference values of arterial oxygen tension in the middle-aged and elderly. Am J Respir Crit Care Med 1995; 152:934–41.

24. Malmvist G, Fletcher R, Nordstrom L, et al.: Effects of lung surgery and one-lung ventilation on pulmonary pressure venous admixture and immediate postoperative lung function. Br J Anaesth 1989; 63:696–701.

25. Kerr JH, Crampton Smith A, Prys-Roberts C, et al.: Observations during endobronchial anaesthesia. II: oxygenation. Br J Anaesth 1974; 46:84–92.

26. Severinghaus JW, Naifeh KH: Accuracy of response of six pulse oximeters to profound hypoxemia. Anesthesiology 1987; 67:551–8.

27. Dumas JP, Bardou M, Goirand F, Dumas M: Hypoxic pulmonary vasoconstriction. Gen Pharmacol 1999; 33:289–97.

28. Leach RM, Treacher DF: Clinical aspects of hypoxic pulmonary vasoconstriction. Physiol 1995; 80:865–75.

29. Cutaia M. Rounds S: Hypoxic pulmonary vasoconstriction. Physiologic significance, mechanism, and clinical relevance. Chest 1990; 97:706–18.

30. Madden JA, Vadula MS, Kurup VP: Effects of hypoxia and other vasoactive agents on pulmonary and cerebral artery smooth muscle cells. Am J Physiol 1992; 263:L384–93.

31. Marshall JM, Metcalfe JD: Effects of systemic hypoxia on the distribution of cardiac output in the rat. J Physiol 1990; 426:335–53.

32. Farhi LE. Sheehan DW: Pulmonary circulation and systemic circulation: similar problems, different solutions. Adv Exp Med Biol 1990; 277:579–86.

33. Benumof JL: One-lung ventilation and hypoxic pulmonary vasoconstriction segment. Anesth Analg 1985; 64:821–33.

34. Marshall BE, Marshall C, Benumof J, et al.: Hypoxic pulmonary vasoconstriction in dogs: effects of lung segment size and oxygen tension. J Appl Physiol 1981; 51:1543–51.

35. Zasslow MA, Benumof JL, Trousdale FR: Hypoxic pulmonary vasoconstriction and the size of the hypoxic compartment. J Appl Physiol 1982; 53:626–30.

36. Domino KB, Wetstein L, Glasser SA: Influence of mixed venous oxygen tension (PvO_2) on blood flow to atelectatic lung. Anesthesiology 1983; 59:428–34.

37. Liu J, Ding Y, White PF, et al.: Effects of ketorolac on postoperative analgesia and ventilatory function after laparoscopic cholecystectomy. Anesth Analg 1993; 76:1061–6.

38. Naeije R, Brimioulle S: Physiology in medicine: importance of hy-

poxic pulmonary vasoconstriction in maintaining arterial oxygenation during acute respiratory failure. Crit Care 2001; 5:67–71.

39. Lennon PF, Murray PA: Attenuated hypoxic pulmonary vasoconstriction during isoflurane anesthesia is abolished by cyclooxygenase inhibition in chronically instrumented dogs. Anesthesiology 1996; 84:404–14.

40. Kjaeve J, Bjertnaes LJ: Interaction of verapamil and halogenated inhalational anesthetics on hypoxic pulmonary vasoconstriction. Acta Anaesth Scand 1989; 33:193–8.

41. Dumas JP, Bardou M, Goirand F: Hypoxic pulmonary vasoconstriction. Gen Pharmacol 1999; 33:289–97.

42. Wilkins MR, Zhao L, Al-Tubuly R: The regulation of pulmonary vascular tone. Br J Clin Pharmacol 1996; 42:127–31.

43. Archer S, Michelakis E: The mechanism(s) of hypoxic pulmonary vasoconstriction: potassium channels, redox O_2 sensors, and controversies. News Physiol Sci 2002; 17:131–7.

44. Minami T, Inoue H, Ogawa J, Shohtsu A: Effect of Ca-antagonists on pulmonary blood flow during single-lung ventilation in the dog. Jpn J Thorac Dis 1993; 31:1207–14.

45. Robertson TP, Hague D, Aaronson PI, Ward JP: Voltage-independent calcium entry in hypoxic pulmonary vasoconstriction of intrapulmonary arteries of the rat. J Physiol 2000; 525(pt 3):669–80.

46. Domino KB, Eisenstein BL, Tran T: Increased pulmonary perfusion worsens ventilation-perfusion matching. Anesthesiology 1993; 79:817–26.

47. Benumof JL: Intermittent hypoxia increases lobar hypoxic pulmonary vasoconstriction. Anesthesiology 1983; 58:399–404.

48. Chen L, Miller FL, Williams JJ, et al.: Hypoxic pulmonary vasoconstriction is not potentiated by repeated intermittent hypoxia in closed chest dogs. Anesthesiology 1985; 63:608–10.

49. Hambraeus-Jonzon K, Bindslev L, Millgard AJ, et al.: Hypoxic pulmonary vasoconstriction in human lungs. Anesthesiology 1997; 8:308–15.

50. Chen L, Miller FL, Malmkvist G, et al.: Intravenous PGF2α infusion does not enhance hypoxic pulmonary vasoconstriction during canine one-lung hypoxia. Anesthesiology 1988; 68:226–33.

51. Amira T, Matsuura M, Shiramatso T, et al.: Synthesis of prostaglandins, TXA_2 and PGI_2, during one-lung anesthesia. Prostaglandins 1987; 34:668–84.

52. Loeckinger A, Keller C, Lindner KH, et al.: Pulmonary gas exchange in coronary artery surgery patients during sevoflurane and isoflurane anesthesia. Anesth Analg 2002; 94:1107–12.

53. Choi JH, Rooke GA, Wu SC, et al.: Reduction in post-intubation

respiratory resistance by isoflurane and albuterol. Can J Anaesth 1997; 44:717–22.

54. Bjertnaes LJ: Hypoxia-induced vasoconstriction in isolated perfused lungs exposed to injectable or inhalational anesthetics. Acta Anaesth Scand 1977; 21:133–47.

55. Marshall C, Lindgren L, Marshall BF: Effects of halothane, enflurane, and isoflurane on hypoxic pulmonary vasoconstriction in rat lung in vitro. Anesthesiology 1984; 60:304–8.

56. Mathers J, Benumof JL, Wahrenbrock EA: General anesthetics and regional hypoxic pulmonary vasoconstriction. Anesthesiology 1977; 46:111–4.

57. Spies C, Zaune U, Pauli MH, et al.: A comparison of enflurane and propofol in thoracic surgery. Anaesthesist 1991; 40:14–8.

58. Liu R, Ueda M, Okazaki N, et al.: Role of potassium channels in isoflurane and sevoflurane-induced attenuation of hypoxic pulmonary vasoconstriction in isolated perfused rabbit lungs. Anesthesiology 2001; 95:939–46.

59. Loer SA, Scheeren TWL, Tarnow J: Desflurane inhibits hypoxic pulmonary vasoconstriction in isolated rabbit lungs. Anesthesiology 1995; 83:552–6.

60. Nakayama M, Murray PA: Ketamine preserves and propofol potentiates hypoxic pulmonary vasoconstriction compared with the conscious state in chronically instrumented dogs. Anesthesiology 1999; 91:760–71.

61. Van Keer L, Van Aken H, Vandermeersch E, et al.: Propofol does not inhibit hypoxic pulmonary vasoconstriction in humans. J Clin Anesth 1989; 1:284–8.

62. Hurtig JB, Tait AR, Loh L, et al.: Reduction of hypoxic pulmonary vasoconstriction by nitrous oxide administration in the isolated perfused cat lung. Can Anaesth Soc J 1977; 24:540–9.

63. Bindslev L, Cannon D, Sykes MK: Reversal of nitrous oxide-induced depression of hypoxic pulmonary vasoconstriction by lignocaine hydrochloride during collapse and ventilation hypoxia of the left lower lobe. Br J Anaesth 1986; 58:451–6.

64. Zhang C, Davies MF, Guo TZ, et al.: The analgesic action of nitrous oxide is dependent on the release of norepinephrine in the dorsal horn of the spinal cord. Anesthesiology 1999; 91:1401–7.

65. Ebert TJ, Kampine JP: Nitrous oxide augments sympathetic outflow: direct evidence from human peroneal nerve recordings. Anesth Analg 1989; 69:444–9.

66. Bjertnaes L, Hauge A, Kriz M: Hypoxia-induced pulmonary vasoconstriction: effects of fentanyl following different routes of administration. Acta Anaesthesiol Scand 1980; 24:53–7.

67. Ellmauer S, Dick W, Otto S, et al.: Different opioids in patients at

cardiovascular risk: Comparison of central and peripheral hemodynamic adverse effects [in German]. Anaesthesist 1994; 43:743–9.

68. Gibbs JM, Johnson H: Lack of effect of morphine and buprenorphine on hypoxic pulmonary vasoconstriction in the isolated perfused cat lung and the perfused lobe of the dog lung. Br J Anaesth 1978; 50:1197–201.

69. Benumof JL, Augustine SD, Gibbons JA: Halothane and isoflurane only slightly impair arterial oxygenation during one-lung ventilation in patients undergoing thoracotomy. Anesthesiology 1987; 67:910–5.

70. Slinger P, Scott WA: Arterial oxygenation during one-lung ventilation: a comparison of enflurane and isoflurane. Anesthesiology 1995; 82:940–6.

71. Karzai W, Haberstroh J, Preibe HJ: Effects of desflurane and propofol on arterial oxygenation during one-lung ventilation in the pig. Acta Anaesthesiol Scand 1998; 42:648–52.

72. Kellow NH, Scott AD, White SA, et al.: Comparison of the effects of propofol and isoflurane anesthesia on right ventricular function and shunt fraction during thoracic surgery. Br J Anaesth 1995; 75:578–82.

73. Shimizu T, Abe K, Kinouchi K, et al.: Arterial oxygenation during one-lung ventilation. Can J Anaesth 1997; 44:1162–6.

74. Abe K, Shimizu T, Tacashina M, Shiozaki H, Yoshiya I: The effects of propofol, isoflurane, sevoflurane on oxygenation and shunt fraction during one lung ventilation. Anesth Analg 1998; 87:1164–9.

75. Speicher A, Jessberger J, Braun R, et al.: Postoperative pulmonary function after lung surgery: total intravenous anesthesia with propofol in comparison to balanced anesthesia with isoflurane [in German]. Anaesthesist 1995; 44:265–73.

76. Pagel PS, Fu JJL, Damask MC, et al.: Desflurane and isoflurane produce similar alterations in systemic and pulmonary hemodynamics and arterial oxygenation in patients undergoing one-lung ventilation during thoracotomy. Anesth Analg 1998; 87:800–7.

77. Beck DH, Doepfmer UR, Sinemus C, et al.: Effects of sevoflurane and propofol on pulmonary shunt fraction during one-lung ventilation for thoracic surgery. Br J Anaesth 2001; 86:38–43.

78. Yondov D, Kounev, V, Ivanov O, et al.: A comparative study of the effect of halothane, isoflurane and propofol on partial arterial oxygen pressure during one-lung ventilation in thoracic surgery. Folia Med (Plovdiv) 1999; 41:45–51.

79. Rees DK, Gaines GY III: One-lung anesthesia: a comparison of pulmonary gas exchange during anesthesia with ketamine or enflurane. Anesth Analg 1984; 63:521–5.

80. Colley PS, Cheney FW: Sodium nitroprusside increases QS/QT in doges in regional atelectasis. Anesthesiology 1977; 47:338–41.

81. Hill AB, Sykes MK, Reves A: Hypoxic pulmonary vasoconstriction response in dogs during and after infusion of sodium nitroprusside. Anesthesiology 1979; 50:484–8.

82. D'Oliveira M, Sykes MK, Chakrabarti MK, et al.: Depression of hypoxic pulmonary vasoconstriction by sodium nitroprusside and nitroglycerine. Br J Anaesth 1981; 53:11–8.

83. Miller JR, Benumof JL, Trousdale FR: Combined effects of sodium nitroprusside and propranolol on hypoxic pulmonary vasoconstriction. Anesthesiology 1982; 57:267–71.

84. Friedlander M, Sandler A, Kavanagh B, et al.: Is hypoxic pulmonary vasoconstriction important during single lung ventilation in the lateral decubitus position? Can J Anaesth 1994; 41:26–30.

85. Scherer RW, Vigfusson G, Hultsch E, et al.: Prostaglandin F2α improves oxygen tension and reduces venous admixture during one-lung ventilation in anesthetized paralyzed dogs. Anesthesiology 1985; 62:23–8.

86. Gardaz JP, McFarlane PA, Sykes M: Mechanisms by which dopamine alters blood flow distribution during lobar collapse in dogs. J Appl Physiol 1986; 60:959–64.

87. McFarlane PA, Mortimer AJ, Ryder WA, et al.: Effects of dopamine and dobutamine on the distribution of pulmonary blood flow during lobar ventilation in hypoxia and lobar collapse in dogs. Eur J Clin Invest 1985; 15:53–9.

88. Ichinose F, Zapol WM, Sapirstein A, Ullrich R, Tager AM, Coggins K, Jones R, Bloch KD: Attenuation of hypoxic pulmonary vasoconstriction by endotoxemia requires 5-lipoxygenase in mice. Circ Res 2001; 88:832–8.

89. Van DV, Eiserich JP, Shigenaga MK, Cross CE: Reactive nitrogen species and tyrosine nitration in the respiratory tract: epiphenomena or a pathobiologic mechanism of disease? Am J Respir Crit Care Med 1999; 160:1–9.

90. Chabot F, Mitchell JA, Gutteridge JM, Evans TW: Reactive oxygen species in acute lung injury. Eur Respir J 1998; 11:745–57.

91. Baboolal HA, Ichinose F, Ullrich R, et al.: Reactive oxygen species scavengers attenuate endotoxin-induced impairment of hypoxic pulmonary vasoconstriction in mice. Anesthesiology 2002; 97:1227–33.

92. Ishikawa S, Nakazawa K, Makita R: Progressive changes in arterial oxygenation during one-lung anaesthesia are related to the response to compression of the non-dependent lung. Br J Anesth 2003; 90:21–6.

93. Del Barrio E, Varela G, Sastre JA, et al.: Inhalation administration of nitric oxide during selective pulmonary ventilation decreased the intrapulmonary shunt. Rev Esp Anestesiol Reanim 1999; 46:247–51.

94. Fradj K, Samain E, Delefosse D, et al.: Placebo-controlled study of

inhaled nitric oxide to treat hypoxaemia during one-lung ventilation. Br J Anaesth 1999; 82:208–12.

95. Rocca GD, Passariello M, Coccia C, et al.: Inhaled nitric oxide administration during one-lung ventilation in patients undergoing thoracic surgery. J Cardiothorac Vasc Anesth 2001; 15:218–23.

96. Sticher J, Scholz S, Böning O, et al.: Small-dose nitric oxide improves oxygenation during one-lung ventilation: an experimental study. Anesth Analg 2002; 95:1557–62.

97. Ullrich R, Bloch KD, Ichinose F, Steudel W, Zapol WM: Hypoxic pulmonary blood flow redistribution and arterial oxygenation in endotoxin-challenged NOS_2-deficient mice. J Clin Invest 1999; 104:1421–9.

98. Lowson SM: Inhaled alternatives to nitric oxide. Anesthesiology 2002; 96:1504–13.

99. Haché M, Denault AN, Bélisle S, et al.: Inhaled prostacyclin (PDI_2) is an effective addition to the treatment of pulmonary hypertension and hypoxia in the operating room and intensive care unit. Can J Anesth 2001; 48:924–9.

100. DeWet C, et al.: Anesth Analg 2003; 96:SCA1–141.

101. Sutcliffe N, McCluskey A: Simple apparatus for continuous nebulisation of prostacyclin. Anaesthesia 2000; 55:405.

102. Jolliet P, Bulpa P, Ritz M, et al.: Additive beneficial effects of the prone position, nitric oxide, and almitrine bismesylate on gas exchange and oxygen transport in acute respiratory distress syndrome. Crit Care Med 1997; 25:786–94.

103. Moutafis M, Liu N, Dalibon N, et al.: The effects of inhaled nitric oxide and its combination with intravenous almitrine on PaO_2 during one-lung ventilation in patients undergoing thoracoscopic procedures. Anesth Analg 1997; 85:1130–5.

104. Moutafis M, Dalibon N, Liu N, et al.: The effects of intravenous almitrine on oxygenation and hemodynamics during one-lung ventilation. Anesth Analg 2002; 94:830–4.

105. B'chir A, Mebazaa A, Losser MR, Romieu M, Payen D: Intravenous almitrine bismesylate reversibly induces lactic acidosis and hepatic dysfunction in patients with acute lung injury. Anesthesiology 1998; 89:823–30.

106. Bouche P, Lacomblez L, Leger JM, et al.: Peripheral neuropathies during treatment with almitrine: report of 46 cases. J Neurol 1989; 236:29–33.

107. Bailey J, Mikhail M, Haddy S, Thangathurai D: Problems with CPAP during one-lung ventilation in thoracoscopic surgery.

108. Bardoczy GI, Yernault JC, Engleman E, et al.: Intrinsic positive end-expiratory pressure during one-lung ventilation using double-lumen endobronchial tube. Chest 1996; 110:180–4.

109. Yokota K, Toriumi T, Sari A, et al.: Auto–positive end-expiratory pressure during one-lung ventilation for thoracic surgery. Anesth Analg 1996; 82:1007–10.
110. Tsuno K, Miura K, Takeya M, Kolobow T, Morioka T: Histopathologic pulmonary changes from mechanical ventilation at high peak airway pressures. Am Rev Respir Dis 1991; 143:1115–20.
111. Tremblay L, Valenza F, Ribeiro SP, Li J, Slutsky AS: Injurious ventilatory strategies increase cytokines and c-*fos* mRNA expression in an isolated rat lung model. J Clin Invest 1997; 99:944–52.
112. Parker JC, Hernandez LA, Peevy KJ: Mechanisms of ventilator-induced lung injury. Crit Care Med 1993; 21:131–43.
113. Dreyfuss D, Basset G, Soler P, Saumon G: Intermittent positive-pressure hyperventilation with high inflation pressures produces pulmonary microvascular injury in rats. Am Rev Respir Dis 1985; 132:880–4.
114. Webb HH, Tierney DF: Experimental pulmonary edema due to intermittent positive pressure ventilation with high inflation pressures: protection by positive end-expiratory pressure. Am Rev Respir Dis 1974; 110:556–65.
115. Kolobow T, Moretti MP, Fumagalli R, et al.: Severe impairment in lung function induced by high peak airway pressure during mechanical ventilation: an experimental study. Am Rev Respir Dis 1987; 135:312–15.
116. Hickling KG, Walsh I, Henderson S, Jackson R: Low mortality rate in adult respiratory distress syndrome using low-volume, pressure-limited ventilation with permissive hypercapnea: a prospective study. Crit Care Med 1994; 22:1568–78.
117. Amato MBP, Barbas CSV, Medeiros DM, et al.: Effect of a protective-ventilation strategy on mortality in the acute respiratory distress syndrome. N Engl J Med 1998; 338:347–54.
118. Acute Respiratory Distress Syndrome Network: Ventilation with lower tidal volumes as compared with traditional tidal volumes for acute lung injury and the acute respiratory distress syndrome. N Engl J Med 2000; 342:1301–8.
119. Takeuchi M, Goddon S, Dolhnikoff M, et al.: Set positive end-expiratory pressure during protective ventilation affects lung injury. Anesthesiology 2002; 97:682–92.
120. Williams EA, Evans TW, Goldstraw P: Acute lung injury following lung resection: is one lung anaesthesia to blame? Thorax 1996; 51:114–6.
121. Slinger PD, Hickey DR: The interaction between applied peep and auto-PEEP during one-lung ventilation. J Cardiothorac Vasc Anesth 1998; 12:133–6.
122. Slinger PD, Kruger M, McRae K, et al.: Relation of the static com-

pliance curve and positive end-expiratory pressure to oxygenation during one-lung ventilation. Anesthesiology 2001; 95:1096–102.

123. De Abreu MG, Heintz M, Heller A, et al.: One-lung ventilation with high tidal volume and zero positive end-expiratory pressure is injurious in the isolated rabbit lung model. Anesth Analg 2003; 96:220–8.

124. Tuxen D, Williams T, Scheinkestel C, et al.: Use of a measure of pulmonary hyperinflation to control the level of mechanical ventilation in patients with acute severe asthma. Am Rev Respir Dis 1992; 146:1136–42.

125. Zollinger A, Zaugg M, Wedeer W, et al.: Video-assisted thoracoscopic volume reduction surgery inpatients with diffuse pulmonary emphysema: gas exchange and anesthesiological management. Anesth Analg 1997; 84:845–51.

126. Sticher J, Müller M, Scholz S, et al.: Controlled hypercapnea during one-lung ventilation in patients undergoing pulmonary resection. Acta Anaesthesiol Scand 2001; 45:842–7.

127. Campbell RS, Davis BR: Pressure-controlled versus volume-controlled ventilation: does it matter? Respir Care 2002; 47:416–24.

128. Tugrul M, Camci E, Karadeniz H, et al.: Comparison of volume-controlled with pressure-controlled ventilation during one-lung anaesthesia. Br J Anaesth 1997; 79:306–10.

129. Bardoczky GI, d'Hollander A: Continuous monitoring of the flow-volume loops and compliance during anaesthesia. J Clin Monit 1992; 8:251–2.

130. Bardoczky GI, Levarlet M, Engelman E, et al.: Continuous spirometry for detection of double-lumen endobronchial tube displacement. Br J Anaesth 1993; 70:499–502.

131. Grenier B, Verchere E, Mesli A, et al.: Capnography monitoring during neurosurgery: reliability in relation to various intraoperative positions. Anesth Analg 1999; 88:43–8.

132. Short JA, Paris ST, Booker PD, et al.: Arterial to end-tidal carbon dioxide tension difference in children with congenital heart disease. Br J Anaesth 2001; 86:349–53.

133. Yam PC, Innes PA, Jackson M, et al.: Variation in the arterial to end-tidal PCO_2 difference during one-lung thoracic anaesthesia. Br J Anaesth 1994; 72:21–4.

134. Tobias JD: Noninvasive carbon dioxide monitoring during one-lung ventilation: end-tidal versus transcutaneous techniques. J Cardiothorac Vasc Anesth 2003; 17:306–8.

Erin A. Sullivan, MD

Anesthesia for New Thoracic Endoscopic
4 | Procedures

Thoracoscopy was first described in 1910 by the Swedish surgeon H.C. Jacobeus (1) as a technique for the diagnosis and treatment of pulmonary tuberculosis and drainage of pleural effusions. In its infancy, thoracoscopy was used for only brief procedures that were performed under local anesthesia, and the patient was maintained on spontaneous ventilation. An artificial pneumothorax was created via a small lateral thoracotomy incision, through which the thoracoscope was inserted for visualization of the chest cavity.

The development of advanced techniques in both thoracic surgery and thoracic anesthesiology revolutionized the treatment of patients with intrathoracic pathology. The discovery of endobronchial blockers, lung isolation techniques, controlled ventilation, neuromuscular-blocking agents, double-lumen endotracheal tubes, fiberoptic bronchoscopy, and advances in pain management techniques contributed significantly to this advancement. During the early 1990s, video-assisted thoracoscopic surgery (VATS) debuted as the premier minimally invasive technique for more complex operations on the lungs and mediastinum. Sophisticated fiberoptic video equipment, endoscopic stapling devices, lasers, and ultrasonic probes have helped to make VATS the preferred diagnostic and therapeutic approach for the management of pleural disease, lung biopsy, recurrent pneumothorax, and sympathectomy. Today, VATS is a common technique for the diagnosis of indeterminate pulmonary nodules as well as anterior and posterior

Progress in Thoracic Anesthesia, edited by Peter Slinger,
Lippincott Williams & Wilkins, Baltimore © 2004.

mediastinal masses, management of early empyema, evacuation of clotted hemothoraces, and for lung cancer and lung volume reduction surgery. The most recent advances are occurring in the areas of minimally invasive surgery for esophageal, cardiac, and vascular disease, particularly among the pediatric patient population. Despite the versatility of this technique, however, VATS is still considered to be an investigational approach for thymectomy.

RATIONALE FOR VATS

Thoracic surgical procedures are performed more frequently using a minimally invasive technique. Compared to the more invasive conventional technique of posterolateral thoracotomy, VATS offers many potential advantages. The patient population scheduled for thoracic surgical procedures often has numerous comorbidities, such as cardiac disease, severe pulmonary disease, renal disease, peripheral vascular disease, and diabetes mellitus. Aggressive surgical intervention in this patient population leads to a high rate of perioperative morbidity and mortality.

Compared with conventional posterolateral thoracotomy, VATS may promote a more favorable patient outcome. Studies have demonstrated improvement in postoperative pulmonary function, a reduced length of stay in both the intensive care unit and the hospital, and a decreased rate of early perioperative morbidity and mortality (1–6). In addition, Landreneau et al. (7) reported that patients experienced less chronic pain following a VATS procedure. An earlier functional recovery from surgery (8) coupled with a reduction in the overall cost of patient care make VATS an attractive technique for the diagnosis and treatment of intrathoracic pathology.

INDICATIONS FOR VATS

Video-assisted thoracoscopic surgery encompasses a wide range of diagnostic and therapeutic surgical procedures, ranging from lung and pleural biopsy to lung resection and minimally invasive cardiovascular surgery. Some indications for VATS are listed in Table 4.1 (9–14). The success of VATS in the adult population and the ongoing refinement of surgical instruments have paved the way for use of this technique in the pediatric population (15, 16). In 1995, Vakamundi et al. (17) described a new technique for one-lung ventilation in children that made possible video-assisted thoracoscopic ligation of patent ductus arteriosus possible.

TABLE 4.1   Indications for Video-Assisted Thoracoscopy

Diagnostic
    Lung and pleural biopsy
    Biopsy and staging of esophageal lesions
    Mediastinal masses
    Pericardial biopsy, pericardial effusions
Therapeutic
    Decortication, pleurodesis
    Drainage of pleural effusions
    Lung resection
        Lobectomy
        Pneumonectomy
        Lung volume reduction surgery
    Esophageal diseases
        Esophagectomy
        Achalasia
        Zenker diverticulum
    Mediastinal masses
        Thymectomy
        Chylothorax
    Cardiovascular surgery
        Pericardial window, pericardial stripping
        Internal mammary artery dissection
        Patent ductus arteriosus ligation
        Transmyocardial laser revascularization
    Sympathectomy
    Anterior thoracic spine surgery

VATS: THE PROCEDURE

Unlike the simple thoracoscopy that was performed by Jacobeus (1) during the early 1900s, VATS is performed in specially equipped operating suites. The procedure usually requires general anesthesia and single-lung ventilation. After the patient is placed in the lateral decubitus position, small plastic or metal ports are introduced through incisions that are made in the lateral chest wall. These ports provide the surgeon with an access for the introduction of light and video sources as well as surgical instruments and suction. On rare occasions, the surgeon may choose to insufflate carbon dioxide intrapleurally to enhance collapse of the nondependent lung and to improve visualization of the operative field. Carbon dioxide insufflation may be performed safely during single-lung ventilation without hemodynamic compromise as long as insufflation pressures (<10 mm Hg) and flows (1–2 L/min) are held to a minimum.

COMPLICATIONS OF VATS

Even under ideal circumstances, certain situations can prevent a planned VATS from being successful. The type and rate of complications for VATS vary depending on the procedure itself, the preexisting condition of the patient, and the experience of the surgical team. The incidence of conversion to open posterolateral thoracotomy is reported as ranging from 1% to 5% (18, 19). The most common indications for conversion of VATS to an open thoracotomy are listed in Table 4.2.

Complications of thoracoscopy may be further classified into those that occur intraoperatively and those that occur postoperatively. The most common intraoperative complications relate to placement of a double-lumen endotracheal tube (traumatic insertion, malposition, and inadvertent inclusion into the surgical site), single-lung ventilation (hypoxemia, hypercapnea, impaired hypoxic pulmonary vasoconstriction, and re-expansion pulmonary edema), and hemodynamic instability (hypoxemia, hypercapnea, intrathoracic instrumentation, mediastinal shifting, and blood loss) (20). Postoperative complications of VATS include persistent air leak, "down lung" syndrome, infection, hemorrhage, tumor seeding, chronic pain, and cardiac dysrhythmias (18, 19, 21).

ANESTHETIC CONSIDERATIONS FOR VATS

Preoperative Evaluation

The preoperative assessment and treatment of patients scheduled for thoracic surgery has been thoroughly described in Chapter 1. Because patients scheduled for VATS often present with similar comorbidities and indications for surgery as those scheduled for open thoracotomy, and because currently there is no reliable means to predict whether a VATS will be converted to an open procedure, one would conclude that the preoperative evaluation of these groups of patients would be simi-

TABLE 4.2   Common Indications for Conversion of Video-Assisted Thoracoscopic Surgery to Thoracotomy

Pleural adhesions
Inability to locate the lesion
Size of the lesion
Inadequate single-lung ventilation
Excessive bleeding
Inadvertent perforation of a major vessel or the pericardium
Inadequate pulmonary resection

lar (22). The anesthesiologist should review the patient's history and perform a physical examination; review the pertinent laboratory studies, including hematology, serum chemistry, and coagulation studies; review the patient's chest radiograph and any other special radiologic imaging studies; and review the electrocardiogram and results of other applicable cardiac studies, such as echocardiography, stress tests, and cardiac catheterization. Finally, the anesthesiologist should review the patient's pulmonary function studies and use this information to assess the impact of the surgical procedure on the patient's postoperative pulmonary function. Options for pain management, including intercostal nerve block, intravenous patient-controlled analgesia, thoracic paravertebral block, and thoracic epidural anesthesia, should be discussed with the patient. Many anesthesiologists do not use thoracic epidural anesthesia for most VATS procedures, but this mode of pain management should be offered to the patient preoperatively (in the event that the VATS is converted to an open thoracotomy). In this circumstance, the thoracic epidural catheter may be placed after the patient is awake in the postanesthesia care unit.

Intraoperative Management

Many of the same principles that apply to intraoperative treatment of the patient undergoing open thoracotomy also apply to VATS, which is most commonly performed using a general anesthetic technique with controlled ventilation and a bronchial-blocking device to provide effective lung isolation. Standard monitors, including an electrocardiogram, pulse oximetry, noninvasive blood pressure cuff, and capnography, are employed. Some studies have reported the use of only noninvasive monitoring during VATS; however, these studies have involved relatively healthy patients undergoing simple procedures (4). Depending on the patient's preexisting comorbidities as well as the complexity of the procedure, it may be appropriate to use invasive monitors, such as an arterial line, central venous pressure line, or pulmonary artery catheter. It is important to realize that the data obtained from pulmonary arterial catheter monitoring during thoracoscopy may be negatively impacted by hypoxic pulmonary vasoconstriction, single-lung ventilation, surgical manipulation, and catheter position (23, 24). Transesophageal echocardiography may also be an extremely useful and accurate intraoperative monitor for the assessment of cardiac filling and function during those VATS procedures that do not involve esophageal resection.

Although VATS can be performed using local, regional, or general anesthesia, this is, as previously stated, highly dependent on the severity of the patient's cardiopulmonary status as well as the complexity of the surgical procedure itself (25, 26). Various regional anesthetic techniques have been successfully used either alone or in combination: thoracic paravertebral blocks, intercostal nerve blocks plus ipsilateral stellate ganglion block, thoracic epidural anesthesia, and field blocks (27). Regional anesthetic techniques employed in the absence of general anesthesia require careful patient selection for VATS of brief duration. Patients who are uncooperative or have a potentially difficult airway should not be considered for VATS using regional anesthesia alone. Potential complications resulting from this anesthetic approach include failure of the regional technique to produce satisfactory surgical conditions, hypoxemia and hypercapnia as a result of paradoxic respirations, and hemodynamic compromise secondary to the creation of an open pneumothorax and mediastinal shift. All these complications require conversion to general anesthesia, sometimes on an emergent basis.

Most anesthesiologists use a general anesthetic technique with controlled ventilation and a bronchial-blocking device for their patients undergoing VATS. Effective lung isolation and deflation of the operative lung is essential for success of the VATS procedure, because the surgeon must work within the confines of a closed thoracic cavity. To facilitate satisfactory operative lung deflation, it may be helpful to ventilate the patient with oxygen before lung isolation rather than with an air/oxygen mixture, particularly if the patient has poor pulmonary elastic recoil or chronic obstructive pulmonary disease. Tidal volumes should be adjusted to 5–7 mL/kg to minimize mediastinal shifting, which may further inhibit the surgeon's ability to successfully perform VATS. Since the application of continuous positive airway pressure to the operative lung might be detrimental to the success of VATS, it is recommended that small increments of positive end-expiratory pressure be applied to the nonoperative lung if the patient's oxygenation is compromised during single-lung ventilation. (Details of lung separation are discussed in Chapters 2 and 3). Other helpful hints for lung isolation during VATS include using a double-lumen endotracheal tube whenever possible and having a fiberoptic bronchoscope available throughout the procedure.

Depending on the surgical procedure and the likelihood of conversion to an open thoracotomy, a regional anesthetic technique, such as thoracic epidural anesthesia, may be combined with the general anesthetic. Selection of specific anesthetic agents should be individualized and based on the preexisting condition of the patient as well as the anticipated length of the procedure. The goal for a general anesthetic approach is to provide satisfactory intraoperative anesthesia as well as analgesia using agents that will facilitate tracheal extubation at the conclusion of surgery and minimize the occurrence of postoperative respiratory depression (28).

Postoperative Management

Postoperative management of patients undergoing VATS is similar to that of patients undergoing thoracotomy. Although thoracoscopy is reported to be less painful and to cause less respiratory dysfunction compared with open thoracotomy, one must maintain a vigilant approach regarding postoperative pain management and pulmonary therapy.

The degree of postoperative pain experienced by patients having VATS is highly variable and dependent on the surgical procedure that is performed. Procedures involving uncomplicated thoracoscopic pulmonary resection tend to produce pain that is limited to the intercostal port insertion sites as well as the chest tubes. In many instances, this pain may be effectively managed with intravenous patient-controlled analgesia (ie, morphine, hydromorphone), intravenous nonsteroidal medications (unless otherwise contraindicated), or oral analgesic medications. At the other end of the pain spectrum are those procedures involving the pleura, such as pleural stripping or instillation of pleural sclerosing agents to minimize the reoccurrence of spontaneous pneumothorax or pleural effusions. These procedures are extremely painful and require more aggressive modalities of pain management, such as thoracic epidural analgesia. Inadequate pain management for these patients will ultimately lead to postoperative respiratory failure, particularly in those with limited pulmonary reserve.

It is just as important to provide satisfactory postoperative pulmonary therapy for patients who have had a thoracoscopic procedure as it is for those who have had thoracotomy. Judicious and appropriate use of bronchodilators, chest physiotherapy, and incentive spirometry as well as early patient ambulation will help to minimize the risk of operative morbidity and promote a timely functional recovery.

SUMMARY

Video-assisted thoracoscopic surgery is a widely used method to achieve a minimally invasive approach for an increasing variety of thoracic surgical procedures. It may reduce the risk of operative morbidity, length of hospital stay, time to functional recovery from surgery, and the overall health care costs. Anesthesiologists are challenged to provide effective care for patients undergoing VATS. A thorough preoperative evaluation of the patient's preexisting medical condition is necessary to provide optimal patient preparation. A discussion of the various options for multimodal pain management should be included during the preoperative evaluation, particularly if there is a strong possibility of the VATS being converted to an open thoracotomy. Anesthesiologists should anticipate the potential complications of VATS and be prepared to provide appropriate interventions to minimize the chance of an adverse patient outcome. The ultimate goal for the anesthesiologist is to provide an anesthetic regimen that achieves optimal surgical conditions, ameliorates hemodynamic changes during single-lung ventilation, facilitates early extubation, and provides superior analgesia.

References

1. Jacobeus HC: Ueber die Moglichkeit die Zystoskopie bei untershung seroser hohlungen auzwedenden. Munchen Med Wochenschr 1910; 57:2090–2.
2. Hazelrigg SR, Nunchuck SK, Landreneau RJ, et al.: Cost analysis for thoracoscopy: thoracoscopic wedge resection. Ann Thorac Surg 1993; 56:633–5.
3. Ferson PF, Landreneau RJ, Dowling RD, et al.: Comparison of open versus thoracoscopic lung biopsy for diffuse infiltrative pulmonary disease. J Thorac Cardiovasc Surg 1993; 106:194–9.
4. Lewis RJ, Caccavale RJ, Sisler GE, et al.: One-hundred consecutive patients undergoing video-assisted thoracic operations. Ann Thorac Surg 1992; 54:421–6.
5. Waller DA, Forty J, Morritt G: Video-assisted thoracoscopic surgery versus thoracotomy for spontaneous pneumothorax. Ann Thorac Surg 1994; 58:372–7.
6. Giudicelli R, Thomas P, Lonjon T, et al.: Video-assisted minithoracotomy versus muscle-sparing thoracotomy for performing lobectomy. Ann Thorac Surg 1994; 58:712–8.
7. Landreneau RJ, Keenan RJ, Hazelrigg SR, et al.: Prevalence of chronic pain after pulmonary resection by thoracotomy or video-assisted thoracic surgery. J Thorac Cardiovasc Surg 1994; 107:1079–86.
8. Rubin JW, Finney NR, Borders BM, et al.: Intrathoracic biopsies, pulmonary wedge excision, and management of pleural disease: is video-assisted closed chest surgery the approach of choice? Am Surg 1994; 60:860–3.
9. Walker WS, Craig SR: Video-assisted thoracoscopic pulmonary surgery—current status and potential evolution. Eur J Cardiothorac Surg 1996; 10:161–7.
10. McAfee PC, Regan JR, Zdeblick T, et al.: The incidence of complications in endoscopic anterior thoracolumbar spinal reconstructive surgery: a prospective multicenter study comprising the first 100 consecutive cases. Spine 1995; 20:1624–32.
11. Milano A, Pietrabissa A, Bortolotti U: Transmyocardial laser

revascularization using a thoracoscopic approach. Am J Cardiol 1997; 80:538–9.

12. Luketich JD, Fernando HC, Christie NA, et al.: Outcomes after minimally invasive esophagomyotomy. Ann Thor Surg 2001; 72:1909–13.

13. Roviaro G, Federico V, Nucca O, et al.: Videothoracoscopic approach to primary mediastinal pathology. Chest 2000; 117:1179–83.

14. Reisfeld R, Nguyen R, Pnini A: Endoscopic thoracic sympathectomy for hyperhidrosis: experience with both cauterization and clamping methods. Surg Laparosc Endosc Percutan Tech 2002; 12:255–67.

15. Rodgers BM, Moazam F, Talbert JL: Thoracoscopy in children. Ann Surg 1979; 189:176–80.

16. Rodgers BM, Talbert JL: Thoracoscopy for the diagnosis of intrathoracic lesions in children. J Pediatr Surg 1976; 11:703–8.

17. Vakamundi M, Shenoy V, Haldr J, et al.: New technique for one-lung ventilation during video-assisted thoracoscopic surgical interruption of patent ductus arteriosus in children. Thorac Cardiovasc Surg 1995; 110:273–4.

18. Inderbitzi RG, Grillet MP: Risk and hazards of video-thoracoscopic surgery: a collective review. Eur J Cardiothorac Surg 1996; 10:483–9.

19. Krasna MJ, Deshmukh S, McLaughlin JS: Complications of thoracoscopy. Ann Thorac Surg 1996; 61:1066–9.

20. Shibutani HC: Pulmonary resection. In: Youngberg JA, ed: Cardiac, Vascular, and Thoracic Anesthesia. New York: Churchill Livingstone, 2000:639–59.

21. Dieter RA JR, Kuzycz GB: Complications and contraindications of thoracoscopy. Int Surg 1997; 82:232–9.

22. Horswell JL: Anesthetic techniques for thoracoscopy. Ann Thorac Surg 1993; 56:624–9.

23. Nadeau S, Noble W: Misinterpretation of pressure measurements from the pulmonary artery catheter. Can Anaesth Soc J 1986; 33:352–63.

24. Tuman K, Carroll G, Ivankovich A: Pitfalls in interpretation of the pulmonary artery catheter data. J Cardiothorac Anesth 1989; 3:625–41.

25. Plummer S, Hartley M, Vaughan R: Anaesthesia for telescopic procedures in the thorax. Br J Anaesth 1998; 80:223–34.

26. Nezu K, Kushibe K, Tojo T, et al.: Thoracoscopic wedge resection of blebs under local anesthesia with sedation for treatment of a spontaneous pneumothorax. Chest 1997; 111:230–5.

27. Mulder D: Pain management principles and anesthesia techniques for thoracoscopy. Ann Thorac Surg 1993; 56:630–2.

28. Weiss S, Aukburg S: Thoracic anesthesia. In: Longnecker D, Tinker J, Morgan G eds: Principles and Practice of Anesthesiology. 2nd ed. St. Louis; Mosby–Year Book, 1998.

Karen McRae, MDCM, FRCPC
Shaf Keshavjee, MD, MSc, FRCSC, FACS

The Future of Lung
5 Transplantation

HISTORICAL PERSPECTIVE

The history of lung transplantation is one of surgical and immunological innovation, beginning with many decades of using animal models to confirm the prospect of pulmonary engraftment. In 1963, Hardy et al. (1) implanted the first human single-lung allograft after left pneumonectomy for an obstructing bronchial malignancy in a recipient with advanced emphysema. Available immunosuppression consisted of azathioprine, prednisone, and cobalt radiation therapy directed to the mediastinum. Despite good early lung function, the patient survived only 18 days. Isolated lung transplants were attempted during the next two decades, with more than 40 patients receiving transplants worldwide and having a mean survival of 8.5 days and a longest survival of 10 months (2). Durable human lung transplantation was achieved by a combination of improvements in surgical technique and introduction of the first calcineurin-inhibitor, cyclosporine, to augment immunosuppression. Successful heart-lung transplantation was accomplished by the Shumway group at Stanford University in 1981 (3), and a single-lung transplant was accomplished by the Cooper et al. (4) at the University of Toronto in 1983. Double-lung, and then bilateral lung, transplantation was pioneered by the Patterson and Cooper group at the University of Toronto between 1986 and 1990 (5, 6). Early double-lung transplantation involved anastomosis of the trachea, main pulmonary artery, and left atrium, and like the first single-lung transplants, they were made possible by the use of omental wrapping to

Progress in Thoracic Anesthesia, edited by Peter Slinger,
Lippincott Williams & Wilkins, Baltimore © 2004.

facilitate an adequate blood supply for healing of the airway anastomosis. Bilateral sequential lung transplantation with anastomoses of each main bronchus and pulmonary artery offers a reduced incidence of airway dehiscence without need for laparotomy. The resulting operation remains the standard of care to this day for bilateral lung replacement.

CURRENT PRACTICE

Current transplant practice has been shaped by the needs of an ever-growing group of patients awaiting organ transplant. An interdisciplinary team approach is required for patient and donor selection, choice of operation, perioperative care, and recognition as well as treatment of pulmonary rejection and infection. Improved patient outcome has resulted in pulmonary transplantation becoming an accepted therapy for suitable recipients with end-stage pulmonary disease that is unresponsive to medical therapy. Consequently, the recipient list is expanding, but the number of donors is relatively static—a phenomenon occurring for all solid-organ transplants. Whereas numbers of patients listed, numbers of donors per capita, and numbers of transplants performed vary considerably by region, the importance of the situation is illustrated by the historical and current numbers of donors and potential recipients in the province of Ontario (Figure 5.1). Despite unchanging numbers of donors, the number of lung transplants in Toronto is increasing (Figure 5.2) as lung-preservation strategies have improved and donor selection criteria have been extended.

The indications for transplant are shown in Table 5.1 and represent a diverse group of diseases. Considerable variation is found between centers regarding the indications for transplant, the number of high-risk recipients, and the type of operation chosen—all of which undoubtedly influence outcomes. The International Society for Heart and Lung Transplantation (ISHLT) maintains a database of recipients of pulmonary transplantation; to date, more than 15,000 lung transplants have been registered, with more than 1,500 per year. Recipient demographic and survival data published by this organization are important benchmarks for transplant programs (7).

Extended Recipients

International guidelines for the selection of lung transplant candidates exist(8), but patients exceeding these recommendations have been transplanted with success. Examples of higher-risk, extended recipients include patients older than the suggested age limits, those infected with

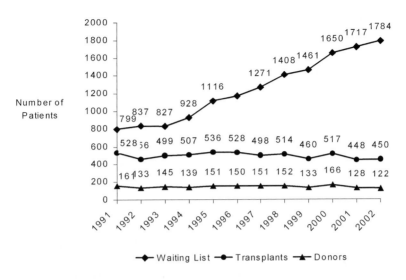

FIGURE 5.1 Number of patients listed for organ transplantation, number of patients transplanted, and number of cadaveric organ donors per year in the province of Ontario, Canada, 1991–2002.

multiresistant organisms, those undergoing retransplantation, and patients with coronary artery disease but with favorable anatomy and preserved myocardial function who are amenable to simultaneous lung transplant and coronary artery bypass.

Respiratory failure that has progressed to the point of requiring intubation and ventilation incurs significant perioperative risk be-

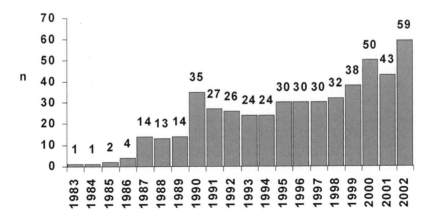

FIGURE 5.2 Number of patients transplanted by the Toronto Lung Transplant Program.

TABLE 5.1   Indications for lung transplantation in the first
516 patients in the Toronto Lung Transplant Program

Etiology	Patients (%)
Chronic obstructive pulmonary disease	36
Cystic fibrosis	24
Idiopathic pulmonary fibrosis	19
Primary pulmonary hypertension	6
Eisenmenger's syndrome	3
Retransplant	3
Malignancy	1
Other	5

cause of the patient's potential for preoperative infection and the loss of muscle function related to minimal mobility. The ability of the recipient to remain mobile is considered to be an important prognosticator of postoperative survival. Until recently, mechanical ventilation was considered in Toronto to be an absolute contraindication to lung transplant; currently selected patients who are already listed for transplant and who have required ventilation may be considered. The most extreme example of preoperative respiratory support are rare patients in whom advanced mechanical ventilation techniques no longer provide adequate oxygenation and who are placed on extracorporeal membrane oxygenation (ECMO) while awaiting transplantation (9). These patients are predicted to incur correspondingly high perioperative risk because of a propensity to sepsis, inflammation, and coagulopathy.

Neoplastic disease is usually a contraindication to lung transplantation, but certain pulmonary malignancies may represent a new indication for the procedure. In Toronto, two patients have received transplants for advanced bronchoalveolar carcinoma (BAC) and one for metastatic uterine leiomyoma, all of whom had progressed to life-threatening respiratory compromise (Figure 5.3). A recent international survey examined the outcome of transplantation in recipients with pulmonary malignancy. Despite recurrence of tumor in most patients, survival was 60% at 5 years for 26 patients transplanted for known BAC, which is better than the ISHLT survival data for lung transplant recipients as a whole. The disease progressed slowly even in the presence of immunosuppression. Occasionally, a bronchial carcinoma is an incidental finding in the explanted native lungs of a recipient. Forty-three patients were identified as having incidental carcinoma; these patients had a 5-year survival rate of a mere 20%. All patients with disease more advanced than stage 1A had rapid progression leading to death (10).

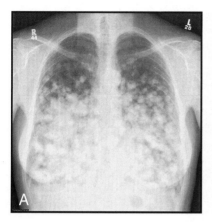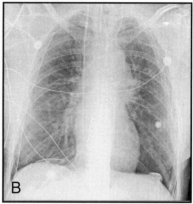

FIGURE 5.3   Transplantation for malignancy. Chest radiographs of a 42-year-old woman (A) before and (B) after lung transplant for metastatic uterine leiyoma causing hypoxia and severe breathlessness are shown. At 34 months after bilateral lung transplantation, this patient remained well and recurrence free.

Extended recipients most often do not meet one of the traditional selection criteria but otherwise are good candidates. It is desirable not to exclude these patients from transplantation. It must be recognized, however, that they might suffer greater perioperative morbidity and mortality and that their inclusion further increases the list of recipients waiting for transplant.

Choice of Operation

The choice of transplant operation can vary between transplant centers, in some cases being related to the surgeon's familiarity with a procedure and to survival rates in that center. The regional organ allocation system can also influence the transplant being performed, particularly those systems that offer lungs based on waiting time on a regional list. In Canada, the transplant surgeon will chose the most appropriate recipient based on the rate of clinical deterioration and then determine whether to do a bilateral or single transplant when both lungs are available. Ideally, the choice of operation is intended to optimize the outcome for the individual patient while allowing as many patients as possible to receive a transplant from a single donor (Figure 5.4). In Toronto, bilateral lung transplant is favored over single-lung transplant whenever possible, particularly for younger patents, with more than 80% of our patients receiving two lungs. Recently, reports have confirmed a survival advantage for some groups with bilateral transplantation (11).

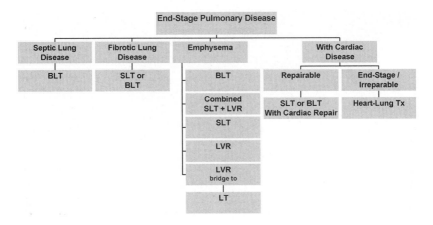

FIGURE 5.4 The Toronto surgical algorithm for end-stage lung disease.

Heart-lung transplant should be performed only when end-stage or irreparable cardiac disease is coexistent with pulmonary failure; this type of operation represents only 3% of cases in Toronto.

Treatment options, either complimentary or alternative, to a transplant should ideally be available within the transplant center. Patients with primary pulmonary hypertension should be evaluated for response to intravenous prostaglandins and other pulmonary vasodilators. Hyperinflated patients with chronic obstructive pulmonary disease may be anatomically suitable for lung volume reduction, for some as a definitive treatment and for others as a bridge to transplant. Unilateral lung volume reduction can also be combined with a single-lung transplant as a combined procedure (12).

Current Outcomes

As larger numbers of patients have been transplanted and the follow-up period of early patients approaches 20 years, trends in outcome are becoming more apparent (13). In the overall Toronto patient group, the 1-, 3-, 5-, and 10-year survival rates are 76%, 65%, 55%, and 35%, respectively. Both early and late survival are dependent on the etiology of native lung disease (Figure 5.5). It is notable that some groups have consistent longevity, particularly those transplanted for cystic fibrosis who are not infected with the pan-resistant organism *Burkolderia cepacia*, 80% of whom are alive after 5 years. Even patients with primary pulmonary hypertension (considered a high-risk group) have a 5-year survival of 50%.

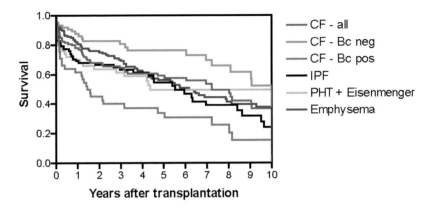

FIGURE 5.5 Patient survival after lung transplantation in the Toronto Lung Transplant Program. Classification is by etiology of lung disease. Bc neg = *Burkolderia cepacia* negative; Bc pos = *Burkolderia cepacia* positive; CF = cystic fibrosis; IPF = idiopathic pulmonary fibrosis; PHT = pulmonary hypertension.

Sepsis is the predominant cause of death in the first posttransplant year, and the risk of sepsis remains throughout the transplant patient's lifetime (Figure 5.6). Early deaths from primary graft failure are the result of ischemia reperfusion injury, which can be regarded as the end result of a series of insults to the lung beginning at the time of brain death

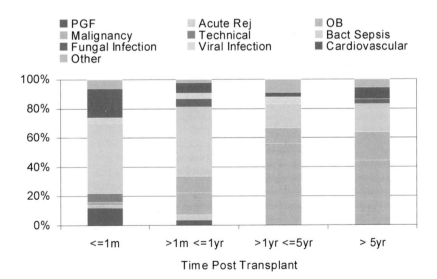

FIGURE 5.6 Cause of patient death after lung transplantation in the Toronto Lung Transplant Program. Classification is by duration of survival. OB = obliterative bronchiolitis; PGF = primary graft failure.

of the donor (Figure 5.7). Lung injury induced by ischemia-reperfusion is characterized by nonspecific alveolar damage, pulmonary edema, and hypoxemia within 72 hours of lung transplantation. The Toronto Lung Transplant Program has developed a protocol for donor management, lung preservation, and recipient care, with a goal of minimizing lung injury, that has recently been described (14). Use of high-dose steroids in donors is widely accepted, despite the lack of a randomized study, to result in an increased proportion of lung being suitable for transplantation (15). In Toronto, a dextran-containing preservative solution of extracellular composition (Perfadex; Vitrolife) is used with improved postoperative lung function compared to historical controls (16). Surgical technique has been modified to include a period of slow reperfusion (14). Little hard evidence exists for the effects of anesthetic or analgesic technique on transplant outcome. Detrimental pulmonary and neurological outcomes from the use of cardiopulmonary bypass for lung replacement have been postulated but have not been definitively proven (17, 18). Mechanical ventilation is essential both during and immediately after lung transplantation, but it can worsen pre-existing lung injury. A recent study in a rat model of lung transplantation demonstrated that injurious ventilation with high tidal volume and low positive end-expiratory pressure (PEEP) significantly worsened lung function after reperfusion than a protective ventilation strategy (19), but this has not yet been examined in a clinical setting. Routine use of 20 ppm of nitric oxide in the ventilation gas mixture was recently shown

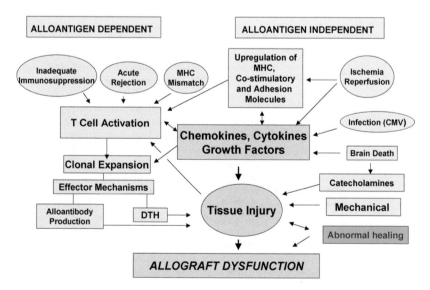

FIGURE 5.7 Transplant-related lung injury.

not to improve lung function in a blinded, controlled, randomized study (20). Although the prophylactic use of nitric oxide is not justified, it is certainly appears to be helpful in managing patients with established ischemia-reperfusion injury. Primary graft failure from ischemia-reperfusion can be so severe that it necessitates ECMO to support the patient until the injury improves. This degree of injury carries a high mortality, although a survival rate of 50% to 60% is reported in contemporary series of ECMO-supported patients and is increased when ECMO is initiated early after identification of the injury (21, 22). In addition, ECMO has been used in an elective manner in certain centers to provide support during transplantation for pulmonary hypertension instead of cardiopulmonary bypass. The ECMO support is weaned promptly, and the reported perioperative mortality rate is 5.9% (9).

The ultimate desired outcome of lung transplantation is increased survival and quality of the life for the patient. Most late deaths in transplant recipients result from obliterative bronchiolitis, which is chronic graft dysfunction from chronic rejection, or from the increased susceptibility to infection and neoplasm from lifelong immunosuppression (Figure 5.6). The morbidity caused by immunosuppressive agents remains substantial. The nephrotoxicity of cyclosporine contributes to the failing health of many lung transplant recipients and their dependence on health care facilities. Major strides are being made in the development of improved immunosuppressive regimens; however, recent progress and future trends in transplant immunology are beyond the scope of this chapter.

NEW DIRECTIONS

Innovations in lung transplantation are directed toward expanding the lung donor pool and improving both short- and long-term allograft function in recipients. This includes optimizing and standardizing the care of organ donors, developing tools for pretransplant allograft assessment, and intervention to extend graft preservation time, improve graft function, and minimize perioperative injury. Extended donors are increasingly accepted in high-volume transplant centers, and innovative surgeries and immunological strategies are being explored in a limited number of centers. Repair strategies and xenotransplantation remain experimental, however, and have not yet been applied to human practice.

Extended donors

Historically, approximately 10% to 20% of donors were considered to be suitable for lung donation using traditional criteria (17). Notably, use of lungs from donors varies considerably between centers both within the United States and internationally, with usage rates of 7% to 50% being described (23). Parameters used to assess donor lungs include donor history, serial arterial blood gas tensions, chest radiographic appearance, bronchoscopic findings, and direct physical examination findings of lung parenchyma at the time of retrieval (24). A systematic classification of donor lungs to distinguish extended donors from those who are truly unacceptable under most circumstances is proposed in Table 5.2. Initially, intensive management of extended donors with strict fluid management, bronchoscopic removal of retained secretions, antibiotic therapy, and alteration of ventilation settings to include pressure support and increased PEEP was reported to increase the donor pool with-

TABLE 5.2   Classification of donor selection criteria suggested by the Toronto Lung Transplant Group

Selection criteria	Standard criteria (ideal donors)	Extended criteria (extended donors)	Contraindications (marginal donors)
ABO compatibility	Identical	Compatible	Incompatible
Donor history			
Age	<55 years old	>55 years old	
Smoking history	<20 pack-years	>20 pack-years	
Chest trauma	No trauma	Localized trauma	Extensive lung trauma
Duration of mechanical ventilation	<48 hours	>48 hours	
History of asthma	No	Yes	
History of cancer	No (except low-grade skin cancer and carcinoma in situ)	Primary central nervous tumors	History of cancer
Sputum gram stain	Negative	Positive	
Oxygenation[a]	>300 mm Hg	<300 mm Hg	
Chest radiography	Clear	Localized abnormality	Diffuse infiltrates
Bronchoscopy	Clear	Secretions in main airways	Persistent pus/signs of aspiration

[a]Last blood gas performed in the operating room with an FIO_2 of 100% and positive end-expiratory pressure of 5 cm H_2O.
From de Perrot et al. (14).

out compromising recipient results (25). Recent re-evaluation of the use of 51% extended donors in 128 lung transplant recipients in the Toronto Lung Transplant Program revealed that although many extended donor lungs resulted in good early function, extended donor use did result in increased early mortality compared with ideal donors. In particular, risk may be incurred with the combination of extended donors and extended (higher-risk) recipients (26).

The irreversible loss of brain stem activity leads to progressive deterioration in organ function. Strategies to stabilize donors are being more widely applied. Correction of anemia, acidosis, and electrolyte disturbances as well as adjustment of fluids and inotropes to maintain adequate systemic perfusion with low to moderate filling pressures are generally accepted. Much of the experimental and human evidence related to the benefit of metabolic resuscitation with the administration of insulin, arginine vasopressin, and triiodothyronine has focused on effects on donor hearts, but improved hemodynamic stability of the multiorgan donor may well improve lung allograft function. After brain stem death, hypotension caused by vasodilation often occurs, which can be related to vasopressin deficiency even in the absence of signs of diabetes insipidus. A continuous infusion of low-dose vasopressin can increase systemic blood pressure and allow weaning of catecholamine vasopressors (27). A retrospective analysis of more than 10,000 brain-dead donors in the United States suggested that an increased number of organs per donor were successfully transplanted from the 701 donors who received hormonal resuscitation (28). Of transplanted organs, the smallest increase was seen in lungs, and allograft outcome was not reported. A randomized, prospective study would be required to distinguish the effect of metabolic resuscitation from those of other donor interventions.

The deleterious effects of brain stem death on donor lung function are well described and contribute to the enhanced inflammatory response in the allograft (17, 24, 29). The donor's mode of death may be important; increased hydrostatic pressure across the pulmonary capillary has been attributed to the surge of sympathetic activity with acute neurological injury. Traumatic brain injury may influence recipient outcome. In a study of long-term follow-up of 500 lung recipients, patients who received lungs from donors with traumatic brain death developed a significantly increased incidence of obliterative bronchiolitis, although increased mortality was not seen (30).

In the future, objective parameters describing not only the functional state of the lung within the donor but also the inflammatory state at the time of retrieval will be sought. Analysis by enzyme-linked immunosorbent assay for cytokines in pre- and postreperfusion allograft biopsy specimens has revealed a significant correlation between the level of the chemokine interleukin (IL)-8 and the incidence of primary graft failure after reperfusion (29). Rapid reverse transcription-polymerase chain reaction techniques for analysis of proinflammatory cytokines and adhesion molecules are being developed; the hope is that methods can be developed to assess parenchymal lung biopsy specimens of the allograft with sufficient rapidity to allow a clinical decision regarding whether to proceed with the transplant. A favorable profile of inflammatory markers may permit the use of donor lungs that otherwise would be rejected for transplant. What remains to be determined are those markers that are most prognostic. The concentration of nitric oxide in exhaled breath can be measured and is associated with airway inflammation. A preliminary clinical report has suggested that higher levels of exhaled nitric oxide before reperfusion of the allograft lung is associated with a favorable postoperative course (31). This effect, however, has not been reproduced in larger series of patients or from analysis of exhaled breath of the lung within the donor.

Donor Operations: Lobar, Split-Lung, and Living Donor Lung Transplantation

Fewer donors are available from the extremes of body size. Small recipients, both children and adults of small stature, are therefore at a disadvantage when waiting for size-matched organs. Lobar transplantation was born from the need to downsize available adult lung grafts to accommodate small patients who are critically ill. Oversized donor lungs can be reduced by peripheral parenchymal resection, but transplantation of single adult lobes into small recipients allows for greater size mismatches (32). Couetil et al. (33) in Paris further extended the use of cadaveric lobes by the partitioning of single left donor lung, with implantation of the lower lobe into the recipient's left hemithorax and the upper lobe into the right. The right donor lung could then be used for a single-lung transplant in another recipient.

In lobar transplant, the recipient operation is notable for the need to retain adequate lengths of bronchial and vascular pedicles to avoid anastomotic tension when ventilation is resumed. Anastomosis of the lobar structures to the recipient's hilum present technical challenges (Figure 5.8). Lobar grafts are likely to have a smaller pulmonary vasculature capacity and, therefore, are assumed to be more prone to reperfusion pulmonary edema should the lobe be exposed to the entire cardiac output. Additionally, recipients are critically ill and of small stature; therefore, lobar transplants are most often performed on cardiopulmonary bypass. A minimum of 48 hours of mechanical ventilation with nitric oxide and moderate PEEP are recommended by some

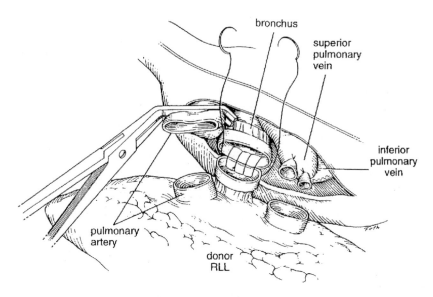

bronchus

superior
pulmonary
vein

inferior
pulmonary
vein

pulmonary
artery

donor
RLL

Right lower lobe *(RLL)* implantation: bronchial anastomosis.

FIGURE 5.8   Right lower lobe implantation and pulmonary venous anastomosis. [From Starnes et al. (32).]

groups to minimize pulmonary artery pressure, decrease atelectasis, and optimize expansion of undersized lobes (34, 35). This is not universally practiced, however, and it is unclear if this approach influences outcome when the graft size is well matched to the recipient thorax.

At the University of Southern California, the use of living donors was explored as a supply of lobar allografts (32). Transplantation of the lobes of living donors provides predictability in the timing and location of donor and recipient operations. Therefore, the procedure can be scheduled urgently, and ischemic time can be minimized. The living donor lung lobe has not been subjected to the deleterious effects of brain death or extended mechanical ventilation. An immunological advantage may exist when first-degree relatives are donors. Most recipients are children or young adults with cystic fibrosis who undergo bilateral pneumonectomy and receive one donor's right lower and a second donor's left lower lobe. Several family members may need to be considered before suitable donors of compatible ABO blood type are identified. Donors are required to be in excellent physical health, and it is preferable that the donors are taller than the recipient. Donor lobectomy differs from standard lobectomy in that a cuff of lobar bronchus, artery, and vein must be removed to allow successful implantation into the recipient (34). Intrapericardial dissection of the inferior pulmonary vein results in a left atrial suture line that potentially predisposes the donor to atrial arrhythmia and pericarditis (35). Development of the interlobar fissure and an oblique bronchotomy may increase the incidence of prolonged air leaks (34, 35). Prostaglandin E_1 is administered to the donor to dilate the pulmonary vascular bed; systemic vasodilation also occurs. Intravenous steroids and heparin are given; the latter may increase the risk of hemorrhage.

The University of South California group recently reported recipient outcome in 128 living donor lobar transplants with survival rates for the first 5 years, which do not differ from those of the patients included in the ISHLT registry. Survival has been better in children than in adults (34). These results may reflect the particular expertise developed at this center for living donor transplantation (36).

To our knowledge, no living lung donor deaths have been reported, but complication rates vary considerably, ranging from 20% to as high as 61.3%. Reported complications include prolonged air leak, empyema, hemorrhage, pericarditis, and pulmonary artery thrombosis (34, 35). The process of enlisting living donors presents serious ethical challenges. Many donors are the parents of the seriously ill child or young adult recipient, although siblings, aunt and uncles, spouses, and other persons who are emotionally related to the recipient have undergone thoracotomy for donor lobectomy. Donor informed consent must be assured, with emphasis on an understanding of potential complications and an opportunity to discuss options and to make their decision in a confidential setting that minimizes coercion. In the Toronto Lung Transplant Program, a living related program was initiated in 2001. Only pediatric patients with a rapidly deteriorating condition have been considered. Our policy is that recipients are listed for deceased donor transplant while living donor assessment is ongoing, with living related transplant proceeding only should the recipient become critically ill. To date, all evaluated patients have been successfully transplanted with cadaveric whole-lung or lobar transplants, obviating the need to resort to living donors.

Recently, Date et al. (37) described a series of living donor lobar lung transplants performed at Okayama University Hospital in high-risk recipients. The cases are remarkable for the diverse etiology of recipient pulmonary failure, with pulmonary hypertension being the predominant indication and both restrictive and obstructive diseases being represented, and for the critical state of the recipients, with both inotrope- and ventilator-dependant patients. Because of extreme need, the size requirements for donors were liberalized. No perioperative deaths occurred, and early- and intermediate-term results were good. The authors emphasized the potential for living related transplant in countries with restrictive brain-death laws and very low rates of organ donation (37).

In conclusion, consistent clinical success in medium to large case series of lobar lung transplants has been reported by a few transplant centers. These operations remain technically challenging, and widespread practice has not yet occurred.

Induction of Tolerance

Tolerance is a state of unresponsiveness by lymphoid cells to a particular antigen as a result of their interaction with that antigen. The induction of lifelong, donor-specific tolerance would eliminate the need for immunosuppressive drugs. This has been achieved in rodent models of experimental transplantation, but it has not proved to be possible nor do we know if it is possible in large animals or in human transplantation. The potential for partial tolerance to reduce the need for and morbidity from lifelong immunosuppression is being explored in select transplant centers.

The immunological mechanisms by which tolerance may be induced and the potential for tolerance in thoracic transplantation were recently reviewed (38). Two strategies are under active investigation to produce tolerization in recipient T cells, the predominant effector cell of the cellular immune response. The first, mixed chimerism, implies the coexistence in a recipient of hematopoietic populations of both recipient and donor origin and is induced by the transplantation of stem cells into a conditioned host. This form of tolerance is dependant on the presence of donor dendridic cells in the recipient thymus, in which donor-reactive T cells are eliminated intrathymically through a process know as clonal deletion. To ensure the continuous presence of these hematopoietic cells in the thymus, a bone marrow transplant of donor stem cells is required at the time of solid-organ transplant. Because mature, reactive recipient T cells exist in the adult recipient, elimination of these cells is required before a cohort of tolerant T cells can be created. Until recently, pre-existing recipient T cells were globally destroyed, either by myeloablation with total-body irradiation and cytotoxic drugs or by depletion with cytotoxic antibodies, before to transplant. More recently, nonmyeloablative protocols have been explored, in which bone marrow transplant is performed with costimulatory blockade (a considerably less toxic regimen), and have resulted in the specific elimination of donor-reactive T cells (38). Another clinical approach recently reported is telerogenic immunosuppression, in which the recipient is depleted of T cells with cytotoxic antibody for a few hours before transplant and a regimen of minimal immunosuppression is initiated after transplant, just enough to prevent irreversible immune damage to the graft. The cohort of recipient T cells that subsequently develop are partially tolerant. Early reports in abdominal transplantation are encouraging (39). Use of this approach in thoracic transplantation remains to be explored. A significant drawback of all these preconditioning regimens is the considerable implementation time that is required before transplant.

Non-Heart-Beating Donors

The unrestricted use of lungs from non-heart-beating donors (ie, cadavers) might provide a large pool of organs (40). The lungs of patients who suffered cardiac arrest and in whom prompt resuscitation efforts were unsuccessful are unique among "solid" organs in their tolerance to a warm ischemic state. During resuscitation, the conducting airways and alveoli are filled with gas having a high oxygen fraction, and the pulmonary vasculature blood has an oxygen saturation of 70% to 100%. The alveolar capillary membrane is normally oxygenated by diffusion, and the supporting framework of the lung has a low metabolic rate.

Compared with traditional organ procurement, the greatest challenge in non-heart-beating donation is the lack of control over the timing of the cessation of circulation. Organ integrity must be preserved for a considerable period of time while consent for donation from a third party, most often grieving family members, is obtained, while blood typing and serological studies are performed to rule out contraindication to transplant, and while a suitable recipient is located. To allow for this period of delay, cooling the lungs to slow metabolism and ex vivo perfusion to maintain viability have been proposed. The physiological potential of these techniques were thoroughly explored in animal models, but the barrier to human application was recognized to be ethical and organizational. Steen et al. (41), at the University of Lund, mounted a dedicated campaign to explore the feasibility and acceptability of human donation from cadavers in Sweden. A broad public information program was mounted to inform the Swedish population of the issues regarding organ donation in general and non-heart-beating donation in particular. A multidisciplinary focus group determined that surgery on the recently deceased body would not be acceptable within the first hour after death, but if lung cooling could be performed discreetly in that time frame, then it would be acceptable. Patient advance directives could then be verified or family consent obtained in that time period. In response to this decision, the technique of topical lung cooling via intrapleural catheters and ex vivo perfusion was established in experimental models.

The first transplant from a non-heart-beating donor was performed on October 6, 2000, in Sweden. A right single-lung transplant was performed on a 54-year-old woman suffering from end-stage emphysema. The donor had died from cardiac arrest 12.5 hours before reperfusion of the lung. The donor was heparinized after declaration of death; the next of kin were informed of his death and consented to topical cooling and lung donation for transplant. Fifty-five minutes after the declaration of death, pleural cannulae were inserted, and topical cooling commenced using an infusion of extracellular composition (Perfadex) into the pleural cavities (Figure 5.9). The lungs were excised 3 hours after death and rewarmed by perfusion with a lung function assessment solution mixed with red blood cells to achieve a hematocrit of 10% to 20% while blood gas and hemodynamic data were collected over a 1-hour period. The lungs were then cooled and preserved for 8 hours before implantation of the single lung. The recipient had an uneventful recovery from a pulmonary perspective (41).

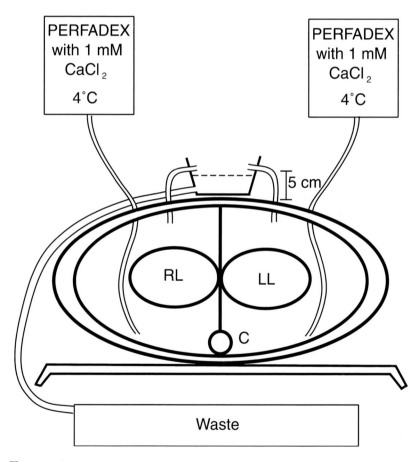

FIGURE 5.9 Topical cooling of lungs via pleural catheters in the non-heart-beating donors. [From Steen et al. (41).]

This case illustrates the technical feasibility of human lung transplantation from a non-heart-beating donor. This remains the only reported case despite well-prepared medical teams and a well-informed population in Sweden. It is unlikely that all societies would be as accepting of the process. Donation from those without a heartbeat may have a role to play other clinical scenarios, such as in cases of patients with severe neurological injury who die in the intensive care unit never having met the criteria for brain death. When informed of the patient's prognosis, family members may provide permission for donation of organs on the patient's death.

Ex Vivo Evaluation

Ex vivo evaluation techniques pioneered for non-heart-beating donors have the potential to extend lung preservation time, to permit evaluation of lung function, and to provide a period of lung allograft isolation for application of repair strategies. Steen et al. (40) described a large animal model of ex vivo perfusion and ventilation. After death, porcine lungs are topically cooled for 6 hours. The heart-lung block is excised, placed in a reservoir, and then cannulated and perfused with a colloid/crystalloid solution mixed with blood of venous gas tensions (Figure 5.10). Ventilation is resumed gradually after the lungs were rewarmed by increasing the perfusate temperature. Steen et al. (40, 41) described functional assessment comprising several measurements. Serial arterial gas tensions are measured with a variety of inspired oxygen levels. Arterial to end-tidal carbon dioxide gradients were determined to reflect the presence of respiratory deadspace to assess for vascular thromboembolic obstruction. Pulmonary vascular resistance was measured; vascular response to the introduction of nitric oxide in the ventilation gas mixture can be assessed (41). All measurements can be used to determine suitability of the lung for transplant (Figure 5.11).

Potential future assessment and therapeutic strategies may be directed toward the inflammatory state of the donor lung. This could include analysis of parenchymal lung samples for inflammatory markers in biopsy specimens taken from the lung before retrieval, during cold ischemic storage, or even during an ex vivo perfusion stage. A period of graft perfusion could allow washout of inflammatory mediators and activated neutrophils. Extracellular lung water could be removed by modification of the osmotic pressure of the perfusate. Antibiotic therapy could be commenced.

Gene therapy is discussed in the following section, but a general limitation on its application has been vector-mediated inflammation. During a period of ex vivo perfusion, gene therapy could be delivered

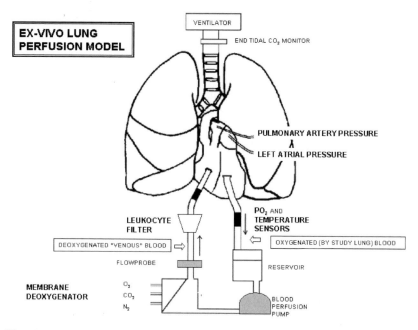

FIGURE 5.10   Ex vivo lung perfusion model. [Courtesy *of* Dr. Stig Steen.]

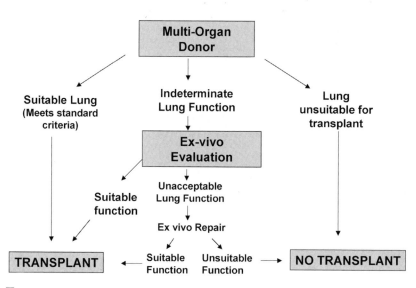

FIGURE 5.11   Proposed algorithm for ex vivo evaluation of donor lung function.

transbronchially or intravascularly to the isolated lung, without exposure to other donor organs. Expression of the transfected gene increases with time (42, 43). Immunological preparation of the recipient with a preconditioning regimen for acquired tolerance was previously described and would be facilitated by a period of ex vivo perfusion.

Increased lung preservation time would allow more specific tissue typing and better immunological matching of the donor and recipient. Lymphocytotoxic cross-matching is performed in a specialized laboratory; lymphocytes are extracted from the spleen of the donor and are cross-matched with recipient serum. Most heart and lung transplant centers will only perform a retrospective cross-match for logistical reasons, including both laboratory availability and time constraints. The role of a positive cross-match in predicting worse outcomes is not as clearly established in lung transplantation as it has been in cardiac transplantation (44).

Currently, most transplant centers do not prospectively match human leukocyte antigen (HLA), both because of the time required and because the likelihood of matching ABO blood group, lung volume, and a majority of the six HLA loci when considering that the local recipient pool is small. Extended preservation would permit the time to consider a larger recipient pool for a closer HLA match. The effects of HLA matching of lung transplants on long-term outcome are not clear; to date, studies have been limited by small numbers of recipients who had four or more matches with their donor (44).

Finally, if lung preservation time could be lengthened, then lung transplants could be reliably scheduled during the day. The effects of sleep depravation and fatigue on medical staff are increasingly recognized. It is conceivable that the quality of medical care would improve when the health care team was not obligated to operate at night, often after many hours of donor management.

Modification of Organs for Transplantation: Gene Therapy and Regenerative Strategies

Gene Therapy

Use of gene therapy in the transplantation setting is enhanced, because immunosuppressive therapy allows effective and repeated transfection even with the current generation of viral vectors. Multiple strategies have been used experimentally to transfect donor lungs. Genes have been administered to the donor before lung retrieval, on the back table during the cold ischemic time, or to the recipient after reperfusion. They have been delivered intravascularly, intramuscularly, or transtracheally in a naked form or with the help of a vector, either viral or nonviral (14, 43).

Transfection of the donor lung is possible through the transtracheal route using a second-generation adenoviral vector without contaminating other organs, such as the heart, liver, or kidneys (44). Because the transfection rate is significantly decreased at cold temperature, this mode of administration is useful in that it allows for efficient transfection before retrieving and cooling the lungs. Interleukin-10 is an anti-inflammatory cytokine that exerts anti-inflammatory and immunosuppressive effects on a large variety of cells, including macrophages, lymphocytes, and neutrophils, and it has been shown to be beneficial in various models of ischemia-reperfusion injury. Transtracheal administration of the gene coding for human IL-10 to the donor 12 to 24 hours before lung retrieval reduces ischemia-reperfusion injury and improves lung function in a single-lung rat transplant model (45). Similar experiments in large animal models with endoscopic delivery of adenoviral-mediated human IL-10 gene to the donor, are ongoing. Once optimal gene delivery to large animals can be achieved, human lung protection from ischemia-reperfusion and immunological injury by gene therapy may be possible.

As research continues to improve our understanding of the mechanisms of injury related to lung preservation and as the genes that control these processes are identified, gene-based therapy may provide the tools to modify organs to withstand the stresses of the transplant process. Staining techniques have been developed to examine the fate of cells within the lung allograft after reperfusion, under a variety of experimental conditions (Figure 5.12). In a rat model of single-lung transplant, lungs reperfused after 6 to 12 hours of ischemia had approximately 30% dead cells, almost all of which had undergone apoptosis (programmed cell death). Necrosis accounted for a small number of the dead cells. After 18 to 24 hours of ischemia, a similar percentage of cells in the graft were dead. Few, however, were apoptotic. Most were necrotic. The percentage of necrotic cells was inversely correlated to posttransplant graft function, specifically oxygenation (46, 47). In downregulating the inflammatory response, IL-10 can inhibit apoptosis. Lungs that were transfected with IL-10 gene and transplanted after 24 hours ischemia showed increased apoptosis and less necrosis than lungs that did not receive gene transfection. Although the total number of cells dying as a result of the transplant process did not change, the pattern of cell death was shifted by gene transfection to a less tissue-damaging mode (apoptosis rather than necrosis) (47). Microarray analysis of allograft tissue shows differences in the patterns of gene expression upregulated depending on reperfusion conditions (Figure 5.13). Identification of the specific genes involved in ischemia-reperfusion injury in lung transplantation is an area of active investigation (48).

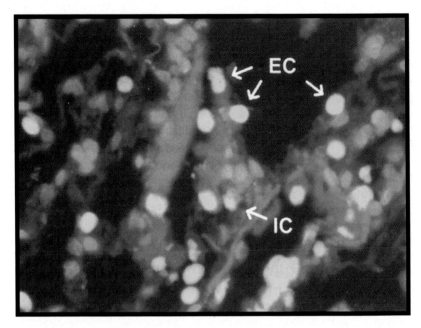

FIGURE 5.12   Human lung allograft biopsy 2 hours after reperfusion after in situ labeling of DNA fragments (TUNEL assay). Fluorescent cells are apoptotic and are identified as epithelial lining calls (EC) and interstitial cells (IC).

Regenerative Approaches to Lung Disease

Clearly, the current approach to end-stage lung disease is lung replacement or transplantation. The ultimate goal, however, would be to repair the organs before they are damaged so severely that transplantation becomes necessary. Repair might take the form of replacing defective genes or upregulating reparative genes (as used in the IL-10 gene therapeutic strategy described above). Cell-based therapies, such as replacing defective cells using stem cells or using carrier cells to carry replacement genes, are other strategies now emerging. These exciting strategies could potentially be applied to the native lungs to treat the underlying disease or to the transplanted lung to treat injury either from the donor or from the transplant process itself.

Xenotransplantation

Humans are most immunologically compatible with primates. For economic and ethical reasons, pigs have emerged as the most likely species to support clinical xenotransplantation. Pigs may also pose the least

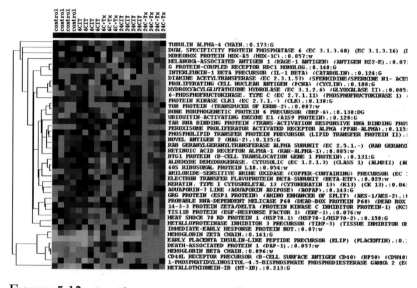

FIGURE 5.13 Specific gene expression profile associated with ischemia-reperfusion injury in a rat lung transplant model. The microarray representation of genes is shown for grafts with reperfusion after 6 hours of ischemia (left side of column) versus 24 hours of ischemia (right side of column). The patterns of gene upregulation for the two ischemic time periods are distinct.

risk of infection to humans. Lungs are highly susceptible to xenogenic injury and have lagged behind other organs in experimental xeno-transplantation, which has primarily involved implantation of pig organs into primates (49).

Hyperacute rejection results in the rapid loss graft function after implantation. Basic mechanisms of hyperacute xenograft rejection include binding of preformed circulating antibodies against foreign antigens in the graft. These antibodies initiate complement deposition, endothelial activation and apoptosis, as well as thrombosis and ischemic necrosis of the graft parenchyma. Naturally occurring antibodies in primates and humans directed against Galactose α-1,3-galactose epitopes (ie, anti-Gal antibodies) are prime initiators of hyperacute rejection of pig organs. Experimental strategies to diminish this response include depletion of antibodies in the recipient by plasmapheresis, depletion of complement, or use of organs from transgenic pigs that express human complement regulatory protein or from galactosyl transferase-knockout pigs that lack the gene that encodes the enzyme responsible for the production of Gal oligosaccharides. Despite increased resistance to hyperimmune rejection, these interventions have extended pig-to-primate organs to survive, at most, for months—or, in the case of lungs, for hours (50).

When hyperacute rejection is controlled, xenografts succumb to acute humoral xenograft rejection, which is also antibody mediated but independent of complement. High-affinity elicited (T-cell dependant) antibodies, predominantly immunoglobulin M, are deposited on graft endothelium, causing progressive inflammatory destruction (49). Even if antibody responses are successfully eliminated, it remains to be seen if T cell–mediated cellular response can be controlled with immunosuppression. Preliminary animal data suggest that T-cell responses might be controllable with regimens now approaching clinical practicability. Physiological barriers to xenotransplantation include incompatibilities between porcine and primate coagulation factors, with the resulting procoagulant state being prone to intragraft thrombosis and disseminated intravascular coagulation (49). Recently, von Willebrand factor shed by porcine lung xenografts has been shown to trigger antibody-mediated aggregation of primate platelets and is postulated to play an important role in the pathogenesis of pulmonary xenograft dysfunction (51).

At present, xenotransplantation remains firmly in the realm of basic science investigation. The lung appears to be particularly susceptible to xenograft rejection. Experimental strategies that have been moderately successful in other organs have been less so in lungs. A comprehensive approach, including genetically modified donor organs, recipient antibody depletion or tolerance induction, and multitargeted drug therapy likely is required for any possibility of clinical success (49). In addition to formidable technical and immunological barriers, ethical concerns specific to xenotransplantation include the obvious sacrifice of animals to extend human life and the infectious risk to society at large; these concerns must be explored before implementation of any clinical program.

SUMMARY

It has been only 20 years since the first successful lung transplant was performed in humans. During the past two decades, lung transplantation has evolved from a heroic, high-risk, experimental endeavor to a relatively routine clinical procedure that has improved the survival and quality of life of many patients with end-stage lung disease. Many patients do suffer short- and long-term morbidity, and survival for lung transplant remains the least among solid-organ transplant groups. By necessity, this relatively young field is closely associated with ongoing advances in the basic science investigation of lung transplantation. The future of lung transplantation likely will involve improved use of donor organs, with increasing safety and improved outcomes for a wider spectrum of patients with end-stage lung disease. An improved understanding of the overall process will allow effective exploration of emerging technologies, such as gene therapy and regenerative strategies, which show promise to modify organs to improve both early and late outcomes.

ACKNOWLEDGMENTS

The authors wish to thank Dr. Marc de Perrot and Dr. Tom Waddell for their helpful suggestions concerning this review.

References

1. Hardy JD, Webb WB, Dalton ML, Walker GR: Lung homotransplantations in man: report of the initial case. JAMA 1963; 186:1065–74.
2. Derom F, Barbier F, Ringoir S, Versieck J, Rolly G, Berzsenyi G, Vermeire P, Vrints L: Ten-month survival after lung homotransplantation in man. J Thorac Cardiovasc Surg 1971; 61:835–46.
3. Reitz BA, Wallwork JL, Hunt SA, Pennock JL, Billingham ME, Oyer PE, Stinson EB, Shumway NE: Heart-lung transplantation: successful therapy for patients with pulmonary vascular disease. N Engl J Med 1982; 306:557–64.
4. Cooper JD, Pearson FG, Patterson GA, Todd TR, Ginsberg RJ, Goldberg M, DeMajo WA: Technique of successful lung transplantation in humans. J Thorac Cardiovasc Surg 1987; 93:173–81.
5. Patterson GA, Cooper JD, Goldman B, Weisel RD, Pearson FG, Waters PF, Todd TR, Scully H, Goldberg M, Ginsberg RJ: Technique of successful clinical double-lung transplantation. Ann Thorac Surg 1988; 45:626–33.
6. Pasque MK, Cooper JD, Kaiser LR, Haydock DA, Triantafillou A, Trulock EP: Improved technique for bilateral lung transplantation: rationale and initial clinical experience. Ann Thorac Surg 1990; 49:785–91.
7. Trulock EP, Edwards LB, Taylor DO, Boucek MM, Mohacsi PJ, Keck BM, Hertz MI: The registry of the international society for heart and lung transplantation: twentieth official adult lung and heart-lung transplant report—2003. J Heart Lung Transplant 2003; 22:625–35.
8. Maurer JR, Frost AE, Estenne M, Higenbottam T, Glanville AR: International guidelines for the selection of lung transplant candidates. J Heart Lung Transplant 1998; 17:703–9.
9. Pereszlenyi A, Lang G, Steltzer H, Hetz H, Kocher A, Neuhauser P,

Wisser W, Klepetko W: Bilateral lung transplantation with intra- and postoperatively prolonged ECMO support in patients with pulmonary hypertension. Eur J Cardiothorac Surg 2002; 21:858–63.

10. De Perrot M, Chernenko S, Waddell TK, Shargall Y, Pierre A, Singer L, Hutcheon, Keshavjee S: Impact of bronchogenic carcinoma in patients undergoing lung transplantation. Results of an international survey. J Heart Lung Transplant 2003; 22(suppl 1):S212.

11. Cassivi SD, Meyers BF, Battafarano RJ, Guthrie TJ, Trulock EP, Lynch JP, Cooper JD, Patterson GA. Thirteen-year experience in lung transplantation for emphysema. Ann Thorac Surg 2002; 74:1663–9.

12. Todd TR, Perron J, Winton TL, Keshavjee SH: Simultaneous single-lung transplantation and lung volume reduction. Ann Thorac Surg 1997; 63:1468–70.

13. De Perrot M, Chaparro C, McRae K, Waddell TK, Hadjiliadis D, Singer LG, Pierre AF, Hutcheon M, Keshavjee S: Twenty-year experience of lung transplantation at a single center: Influence of recipient diagnosis on long-term survival. J Thorac Cardiovasc Surg (in press).

14. De Perrot M, Liu M, Waddell TK, Keshavjee S: Ischemia-reperfusion-induced lung injury. Am J Respir Crit Care Med 2003; 167:490–511.

15. Follette DM, Rudich SM, Babcock WD: Improved oxygenation and increased lung donor recovery with high-dose steroid administration after brain death. J Heart Lung Transplant 1998; 17:423–9.

16. Fischer S, Matte-Martin A, de Perrot M, Waddell TK, Sekine Y, Hutcheon M, Keshavjee S: Low-potassium dextran solution improves early graft function in clinical lung transplantation. J Thorac Cardiovasc Surg 2001; 121:594–6.

17. McRae KM: Pulmonary transplantation. Curr Opin Anaesthesiol 2000; 13:53–9.

18. McRae K: Con: lung transplantation should not be routinely performed with cardiopulmonary bypass. J Cardiothorac Vasc Anesth 2000; 14:746–50.

19. De Perrot M, Imai Y, Volgyesi GA, Waddell TK, Liu M, Mullen JB, McRae K, Zhang H, Slutsky AS, Ranieri VM, Keshavjee S: Effect of ventilator-induced lung injury on the development of reperfusion injury in a rat lung transplant model. J Thorac Cardiovasc Surg 2002; 124:1137–44.

20. Meade MO, Granton JT, Matte-Martyn A, McRae K, Weaver B, Cripps P, Keshavjee SH: Toronto Lung Transplant Program: a randomized trial of inhaled nitric oxide to prevent ischemia-reperfusion injury after lung transplantation. Am J Respir Crit Care Med 2003; 167:1483–9.

21. Nguyen DQ, Kulick DM, Bolman RM III, Dunitz JM, Hertz MI,

Park SJ: Temporary ECMO support following lung and heart-lung transplantation. J Heart Lung Transplant 2000; 19:313–6.

22. Meyers BF, Sundt TM III, Henry S, Trulock EP, Guthrie T, Cooper JD, Patterson GA: Selective use of extracorporeal membrane oxygenation is warranted after lung transplantation. J Thorac Cardiovasc Surg 2000; 120:20–6.

23. Rosengard BR, Feng S, Alfrey EJ, Zaroff JG, Emond JC, Henry ML, Garrity ER, Roberts JP, Wynn JJ, Metzger RA, Freeman RB, Port FK, Merion RM, Love RB, Busuttil RW, Delmonico FL: Report of the Crystal City meeting to maximize the use of organs recovered from the cadaver donor. Am J Transplant 2002; 2:701–11.

24. De Perrot M, Keshavjee S: Lung preservation. Chest Surg Clin N Am 2002; 13:443–62.

25. Gabbay E, Williams TJ, Griffiths AP, MacFarlane LM, Kotsimbos TC, Esmore DS, Snell GI: Maximizing the utilization of donor organs offered for lung transplantation. Am J Respir Crit Care Med 1999; 160:265–71.

26. Pierre AF, Sekine Y, Hutcheon MA, Waddell TK, Keshavjee SH: Marginal donor lungs: a reassessment. J Thorac Cardiovasc Surg 2002; 123:421–7.

27. Chen JM, Cullinane S, Spanier TA, Artrip JH, John R, Edwards NM, Oz MC, Landry DW: Vasopressin deficiency and pressor hypersensitivity in hemodynamically unstable organ donors. Circulation 1999; 100:II-244–6.

28. Rosendale JD, Kauffman HM, McBride MA, Chabalewski FL, Zaroff JG, Garrity ER, Delmonico FL, Rosengard BR: Aggressive pharmacologic donor management results in more transplanted organs. Transplantation 2003; 75:482–7.

29. De Perrot M, Sekine Y, Fischer S, Waddell TK, McRae K, Liu M, Wigle DA, Keshavjee S: Interleukin-8 release during early reperfusion predicts graft function in human lung transplantation. Am J Respir Crit Care Med 2002; 165:211–5.

30. Ciccone AM, Stewart KC, Meyers BF, Guthrie TJ, Battafarano RJ, Trulock EP, Cooper JD, Patterson GA: Does donor cause of death affect the outcome of lung transplantation. J Thorac Cardiovasc Surg 202; 123:429–36.

31. Marczin N, Riedel B, Gal J, Polak J, Yacoub M: Exhaled nitric oxide during lung transplantation. Lancet 1997; 350:1681–2.

32. Starnes VA, Barr ML, Cohen RG: Lobar transplantation. Indications, technique, and outcome. J Thorac Cardiovasc Surg 1994; 108:403–10.

33. Couetil JP, Tolan MJ, Loulmet DF, Guinvarch A, Chevalier PG, Achkar A, Birmbaum P, Carpentier AF: Pulmonary bipartitioning and lobar transplantation: a new approach to donor organ shortage. J Thorac Cardiovasc Surg 1997; 113:529–37.

34. Barr ML, Baker CJ, Schenkel FA, Bowdish ME, Bremner RM, Cohen RG, Barbers RG, Woo MS, Horn MV, Wells WJ, Starnes VA: Living donor lung transplantation: selection, technique, and outcome. Transplant Proc 2001; 33:3527–32.
35. Battafarano RJ, Anderson RC, Meyers BF, Guthrie TJ, Schuller D, Cooper JD, Patterson GA: Perioperative complications after living donor lobectomy. J Thorac Cardiovasc Surg 2000; 120:909–15.
36. Bowdish ME, Barr ML, Starnes VA: Living lobar transplantation. Chest Surg Clin N Am 2003; 13:505–24.
37. Date H, Aoe M, Nagahiro I, Sano Y, Andou A, Matsubara H, Goto K, Tedoriya T, Shimizu N: Living-donor lobar lung transplantation for various lung diseases. J Thorac Cardiovasc Surg 2003; 126:476–81.
38. Wekerle T: Transplantation tolerance induced by mixed chimerism. J Heart Lung Transplant 2001; 20:816–23.
39. Starzl TE, Murase N, Abu-Elmagd, Gray EA, Shapiro R, et al: Telerogenic immunosuppression for organ transplantation. Lancet 2003; 361:1502–10.
40. Steen S, Liao Q, Wierup PN, Bolys R, Pierre L, Sjoberg T: Transplantation of lungs from non-heart-beating donors after functional assessment ex vivo. Ann Thorac Surg 2003; 76:244–52.
41. Steen S, Sjoberg T, Pierre L, Liao Q, Eriksson L, Algotsson L: Transplantation of lungs from a non-heart-beating donor. Lancet 2001; 357:825–9.
42. De Perrot M, Fischer S, Liu M, Imai Y, Martins S, Sakiyama S, Tabata T, Bai XH, Waddell TK, Davidson BL, Keshavjee S: Impact of human interleukin-10 on vector-induced inflammation and early graft function in rat lung transplantation. Am J Respir Cell Mol Biol 2003; 28:616–25.
43. Cassivi SD, Liu M, Boehler A, Tanswell AK, Slutsky AS, Keshavjee S: Transgene expression after adenovirus mediated retransfection of rat lungs is increased and prolonged by transplant immunosuppression. J Thorac Cardiovasc Surg 1999; 117:1–7.
44. Aigner C, Seebacher G, Klepetko W: Donor selection. Chest Surg Clin N Am 2003; 13:429–42.
45. Fischer S, Liu M, MacLean AA, de Perrot M, Ho M, Cardella JA, Zhang XM, Bai XH, Suga M, Imai Y, Keshavjee S: In vivo transtracheal adenovirus-mediated transfer of human interleukin-10 gene to donor lungs ameliorates ischemia-reperfusion injury and improves early posttransplant graft function in the rat. Hum Gene Ther 2001; 12:1513–26.
46. Fischer S, de Perrot M, Liu M, MacLean AA, Cardella JA, Imai Y, Suga M, Keshavjee S: Dynamic changes in apoptosis and necrotic

cell death correlate with severity of ischemia-reperfusion injury in lung transplantation. J Thorac Cardiovasc Surg 2003; 126:1174–80.

47. Fischer S, de Perrot M, Liu M, MacLean AA, Cardella JA, Imai Y, Suga M, Keshavjee S: Interleukin-10 gene transfection of donor lungs ameliorates posttransplant cell death by a switch from cellular necrosis to apoptosis. J Thorac Cardiovasc Surg 2003; 126:1174–80.

48. Yamane M, Quadri SM, Segall L, Dutly A, Waddell TK, Liu M, Keshavjee S: Specific gene expression profile associated with ischemia-reperfusion injury during lung transplantation identified by CDNA microarray. J Heart Lung Transplant 2003; 22:S187.

49. Waddell TK, Peterson MD: Xenotransplantation. Chest Surg Clin N Am 2003; 13:559–76.

50. Cooper DKC: Clinical xenotransplantation—how close are we. Lancet 2003; 362:557–9.

51. Lau CL, Cantu E III, Gonzalez-Stawinski GV, Holzknecht ZE, Nichols TC, Posther KE, Rayborn CA, Platt JL, Parker W, Davis RD: The role of antibodies and von Willebrand factor in discordant pulmonary xenotransplantation. Am J Transplant 2003; 3:1065–75.

Jay B. Brodsky, MD
Stephen T. Kee, MD

6 | Airway Stents

INTRODUCTION

Prosthetic stents are used to provide structural support for stenotic blood vessels, airways, and ducts. Because the placement of a stent is a relatively noninvasive procedure, they have become a popular alternative to painful surgery for a wide variety of diseases. A metallic or silicone-based endobronchial stent can open a stenotic central airway (eg, trachea, carina, main bronchi) and provide immediate symptomatic relief.

The current status of airway stenting, the medical indications for stenting, and the anesthetic considerations for patients undergoing an airway stenting procedure are reviewed.

PREOPERATIVE EVALUATION

Central airway strictures can result from a great variety of benign and malignant processes (Table 6.1). The nature of the lesion and whether it is expected to be temporary (infection or inflammation) or permanent (malignancy) will usually dictate the appropriate treatment.

The effects of the obstruction on ventilation depend on several factors, each of which must be evaluated before proceeding with the stenting procedure. Factors include the cause, size, and location of the stenosis as well as the phase of ventilation at which obstruction to airflow occurs.

Progress in Thoracic Anesthesia, edited by Peter Slinger,
Lippincott Williams & Wilkins, Baltimore © 2004.

Table 6.1 Causes of Central Airway Obstruction

Malignant (primary or metastatic)
  Intraluminal (obstruction)
  Extraluminal (compression)
Benign
  Congenital
    Vascular
      Vascular rings
      Dilated aorta
    Enlarged thymus or thyroid gland
    Tracheogenic cyst
    Tracheal stenosis or malacia
  Acquired
    Traumatic
      Complication of tracheal intubation/tracheostomy
      Burn/smoke injury
      Airway hematoma
    Anastomotic
      Lung transplantation
      Sleeve resection of trachea or bronchus
    Inflammatory
      Wegener's granulomatosis
      Relapsing polychondritis
      Amyloidosis
    Infectious
      Tuberculosis
      Papillomas
      Rhinoscleroma
      Viral tracheobronchitis
      Bacterial tracheitis
    Other
      Aortic aneurysm
      Retrosternal goiter
      Lymphadenopathy
      Mediastinal fibrosis

    The reduction in intraluminal size is significant. Respiratory symptoms first become apparent with exercise when tracheal internal diameter (ID) is decreased from the normal 15.0 to 20.0 mm to approximately 8.0 mm (1) (Figure 6.1) Inspiratory stridor occurs at rest, when the tracheal diameter is further reduced to between 5.0 and 6.0 mm (2, 3).

    Important preprocedural information is obtained from imaging studies. A plain-film chest radiograph will not accurately demonstrate the exact location, size, and extent of an upper airway obstruction (4, 5). Conventional chest computed tomography (CT), magnetic resonance studies, and contrast cinetracheobronchography (6–8) have been used in the past but have now been replaced by virtual bronchoscopy using helical CT with three-dimensional multiplanar reconstruction (9, 10).

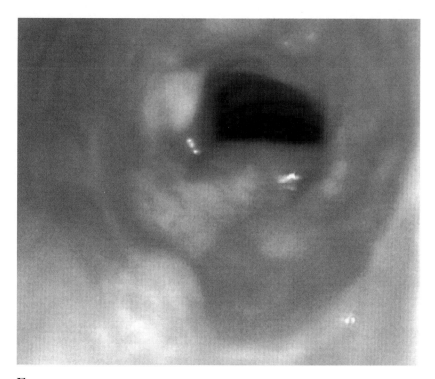

FIGURE 6.1   Bronchoscopic view of a high tracheal obstruction. The airway is narrowed approximately 50%. The patient was symptomatic at rest.

The combined modality is more accurate than thin-section axial chest CT for demonstrating the site and degree of tracheal and main bronchi stenosis (11, 12).

The normal diameter of the airway is first determined using an uninvolved airway segment, and then the length of the stricture is measured. If tracheomalacia is suspected, imaging studies are performed at maximum expiration and maximum inspiration to identify the extent of airway narrowing during each phase of ventilation. Measurements give the interventional radiologist important information regarding which type, what size, and what length of stent will be needed. For the anesthesiologist, imaging studies also can be used to determine what size endotracheal tube (ETT) to use, how far the ETT can be safely advanced down a proximally obstructed trachea, or whether an ETT can be used at all (13).

The most important nonimaging diagnostic study is the dynamic flow-volume loop, which measures forced expiratory and inspiratory vital capacity (14). It can help to differentiate between an intrathoracic and an extrathoracic obstruction. It can also demonstrate whether resistance to airflow is the same during both inspiration and expiration (fixed obstruction) or whether airflow changes with each phase of ventilation (variable obstruction) (15, 16).

The extrathoracic central airway (upper trachea) is surrounded by atmospheric pressure, whereas intrathoracic central airways (lower trachea and main bronchi) are surrounded by pleural pressure. The difference between intra-airway pressure and external pressure is transmural pressure. If external pressure exceeds intra-airway pressure (positive transmural pressure), the airway will collapse. A negative transmural pressure will open the airway.

The nature of the obstruction (ie, whether it is fixed or variable) determines the changes in transmural pressure during inspiration and expiration (17). With a fixed lesion, no changes occur during either phase of ventilation, so the airway remains obstructed during both inspiration and expiration. The flow-volume loop of a fixed extrathoracic obstruction is similar to that of a fixed intrathoracic obstruction. A plateau is observed with limitation of airflow during both inspiration and expiration. For a variable obstruction, a reduction in inspiratory or expiratory airflow will depend on the location of the lesion (18, 19).

With a variable extrathoracic lesion, the degree of obstruction increases during inspiration. The pressure inside the trachea falls on forced inspiration, resulting in a greater transmural pressure at the site of the lesion, which worsens the obstruction. On expiration, intratracheal pressure rises, which reverses the transmural pressure gradient, thus lessening the degree of obstruction and improving flow. The flow-volume loop demonstrates flow limitation during inspiration.

With a variable intrathoracic obstruction, airflow is limited during expiration. The rise in pleural pressure on forced expiration may exceed the rise in intratracheal pressure, thus reducing the size of the airway at the site of the stenosis. Pleural pressure becomes markedly negative during forced inspiration, which lessens the obstruction by reversing the transmural pressure, which improves airflow.

ANESTHETIC MANAGEMENT

The patient with a airway obstruction may initially present as an airway emergency (20). The anesthesiologist may be faced with a critically ill patient who has significant medical comorbidities. Associated medical conditions frequently include chronic obstructive airway disease and pulmonary infection, the problems of advanced neoplastic disease, superior vena cava syndrome, and myocardial disease (21). Each of these conditions influences anesthetic management.

Sedative premedication should only be considered for the very anxious patient, because hypoventilation and further airway compromise must be avoided. Patients should never be medicated or left alone in an unmonitored environment.

All patients being considered for a tracheobronchial stent must have a complete endoscopic evaluation of their airway before placement of the stent to determine the exact site and length of the stenosis, its distance below the vocal cords, and its relationship to bifurcations (eg, the tracheal carina and lobar bronchi). The general anesthetic principles for rigid and fiberoptic bronchoscopic (FOB) procedures apply (22, 23).

During bronchoscopy cardiovascular instability (hypertension or hypotension) is not uncommon.(24) "Light" anesthesia, hypoxia, and hypercapnia all contribute to arrhythmias. Anticholingerics, midazolam, and/or propofol are given to reduce these problems (25–27). The anticholinergics will counter any vagotonic effects from other drugs (eg, remifentanil) and reflex bradycardia from stimulation by the bronchoscope. Anticholingerics also may help to reduce airway secretions that impair the effectiveness of topical anesthesia. A dry airway decreases the need for frequent suctioning during the procedure.

Many patients are oxygen dependent at rest and must be fully preoxygenated before the start of anesthesia. In patients with very severe tracheal obstruction, a helium/oxygen mixture may have some benefit (28, 29). The low density of such a mixture markedly increases inspiratory and expiratory flow, reduces work of breathing and respiratory acidosis, and relieves dyspnea in some patients.

TRACHEAL INTUBATION

Fiberoptic bronchoscopy-assisted procedures can be performed under local anesthesia with intravenous sedation. Local anesthesia with sedation is a poor choice if patient movement or coughing can jeopardize the procedure (30).

Most stenting procedures require general anesthesia. The method of achieving airway control will depend on the patient's disease. Often, the stricture will be too distal to benefit from an elective tracheostomy or transtracheal jet ventilation, so endotracheal intubation must be accomplished.

For a fixed obstruction, a conventional intravenous anesthetic induction with a muscle relaxant usually is appropriate. For patients with a variable intrathoracic obstruction (eg, those with a large anterior mediastinal mass), an inhalational anesthetic induction can avoid the use of muscle relaxants for tracheal intubation. The special anesthetic considerations for management of airway compression from an anterior mediastinal mass are reviewed elsewhere (31, 32). Sevoflurane, with its rapid onset and minimal airway irritation, is the current agent of choice for an inhalational anesthetic induction in these patients (33, 34).

The ETT must be carefully advanced down the trachea to avoid aggravation of an intraluminal obstruction and bleeding. Optimally, the distal tip of the ETT is positioned at least 1 cm above the stenotic segment for the interventional radiologist to perform the stenting procedure. Fiberoptic bronchoscopy-assisted intubation and visual placement of the ETT should be considered for mid or high tracheal lesions. An FOB can be advanced directly through a laryngeal mask airway (LMA) for lesions in the proximal trachea that prevent the use of an ETT (35).

After the trachea is intubated, the airway distal to the ETT must be shared with the endoscopist and the interventional radiologist. Total airway obstruction can occur at any time during the procedure. A rigid bronchoscope—and someone familiar with its use—must always be readily available to establish a patent airway.

Muscle paralysis is required during dilations and stent placement. A short-acting agent should be used. We prefer succinylcholine, either given as an infusion or in small, divided doses. Mivacurium is an acceptable alternative. Paralysis must be fully reversed before tracheal extubation is attempted.

TECHNIQUE

General anesthesia is administered either by a total intravenous anesthesia technique or by a combination of intravenous and inhalational agents.

All inhalational anesthetics have bronchodilatory effects that can be helpful, especially in patients with reactive airway disease. The major benefit of the intravenous agents (barbiturates, propofol, opioids, and ketamine) is that they allow continued maintenance of anesthesia during suctioning, bronchial dilation, and stenting, during which ventilation with an inhalational agent must be interrupted (36).

We use an inhalational agent (isoflurane or sevoflurane) with 100% oxygen initially and then convert to a total intravenous anesthesia technique (propofol and remifentanil) during airway manipulation and stenting. Minimal pain is experienced by the patient following stent insertion, and postoperative respiratory depression is dangerous. Thus, longer-acting opioids should be avoided.

VENTILATION

For procedures performed through an ETT, ventilation is assisted by hand during the procedure. For procedures performed with rigid bronchoscopy, ventilation can be accomplished in several ways. Positive-pressure ventilation can be performed through a side-arm adapter attached to the anesthetic breathing system (37). Occlusion of the proximal end of the bronchoscope with an eyepiece allows controlled ventilation through the lumen of the bronchoscope. A gas leak always occurs, so very high oxygen flow is required. In addition, ventilation must be interrupted whenever the eyepiece is removed.

The Sanders technique employs the Venturi principle to allow positive-pressure ventilation through an open, rigid bronchoscope (38, 39). Intermittent bursts of high-pressure oxygen are delivered through a cannula attached to the proximal end of the bronchoscope. Ventilation can continue uninterrupted when the eyepiece of the rigid bronchoscope is removed (40).

Oxygenation can be maintained and ventilation can proceed uninterrupted by using jet ventilation through either a rigid bronchoscope or an FOB (41, 42). For patients with severe proximal tracheal stenosis with or without an ETT, jet ventilation through a cannula as small as 2.0-mm ID can provide adequate ventilation. An adequate expiratory passage must be present (43–45). The thin cannula does not obstruct the visual field. An LMA can be a conduit for an ETT or small-bore catheter for jet ventilation.(46–48).

Cardiopulmonary bypass is sometimes recommended. This is not practical, however, especially in the cramped radiology suite where stenting procedures are performed (49, 50).

RECOVERY AND COMPLICATIONS

Airway patency may actually worsen as the patient recovers from anesthesia. Edema in the upper airway can manifest once the bronchoscope is removed. Coughing will further increase bleeding.

If a rigid bronchoscope has been used, it should be replaced with an ETT. At the completion of the procedure, the patient must be fully awake before the ETT is removed. If the patient is not breathing adequately or the airway has been traumatized, the trachea should remain intubated. Before extubation, a tube exchanger can be placed in the trachea to be used as a guide if reintubation becomes necessary (51).

The patient may make minimal efforts at breathing immediately following the procedure, and he or she may be unable to cough and clear secretions as well as blood from the airway. It is not uncommon for the patient to experience respiratory distress, hypoxemia, hypercapnia, dysrhythmias, and cardiovascular instability during emergence from anesthesia. Carbon dioxide retention can cause obtundation, which further delays recovery. Ventilatory support, either by mask or by ETT, may be needed. Positive-pressure hyperventilation and vigorous airway suctioning can be life-saving.

Patients must receive mask oxygen following airway extubation, during transport, and while in the postanesthesia care unit (52). Postprocedural stridor may require treatment with humidified oxygen, nebulized epinephrine, steroids, and reintubation of the trachea.

During or after stent placement, a marked resistance to ventilation can occur at any time because of a misplaced or dislodged stent, fragmented tumor material, or blood clot (53, 54).

Massive hemorrhage or airway perforation, which may require emergency thoracotomy, is always a possibility. For procedures with a high likelihood of serious complications, an operating room should be available and prepared even when the actual stenting procedure is to be performed in the radiology suite.

AIRWAY STENTS

History

The first airway endoluminal prostheses were silicone-rubber stents, such as the Montgomery T-tube, that were inserted through a tracheostomy stoma to treat subglottic stenosis (55). Straight silicone tubes were then adapted for more distal tracheal strictures (56, 57). In 1986, Wallace et al. (58) reported their initial experience with metallic airway stents (58). Since then, a variety of rigid silicone stents as well as self-expanding and balloon-expandable metallic stents have been used in the treatment of central airway stenosis (59).

Indications

Stenting is an appropriate approach to palliative management of both extraluminal airway compression and intraluminal obstructions from benign and malignant diseases (60–64). The widest application of endobronchial stenting is for airway obstruction from tumors (65) (Fig. 6.2)

Complications following lung transplantation (eg, bronchial stenosis at the suture site, dehiscence, granulation tissue accumulation, bronchomalacia) are common (66, 67). Posttransplant problems are managed by a combination of debridement, laser ablation, cryotherapy, balloon dilation, and airway stent placement (68–71).

Stents are useful for airway strictures following prolonged tracheal intubation or injury (72), for suture-line stenosis following pulmonary resection (73), to close esophageal-airway fistulae (74, 75), and for the

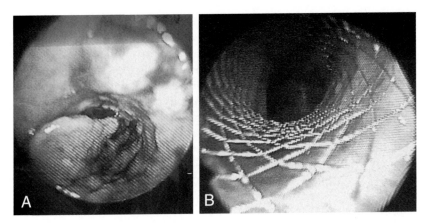

FIGURE 6.2 (A) Bronchoscopic view of intraluminal tumor growth causing tracheal obstruction. (B) Deployment of an expandable-mesh metallic stent results in complete opening of the stenotic area.

numerous other causes of central airway obstruction not readily amenable to other therapies (76–80).

Stents have been used to treat congenital airway stenosis in patients as young as 7 days (47, 81). Ventilatory-dependent children can be extubated following the stenting procedure, but their long-term outlook is unknown (82). Stenting in children presents an interesting challenge, because as the child grows, the diameter of the stent must be increased. Either a self-expanding or a balloon-expandable stent can be used. The patient must be followed by intermittent spirometry or chest CT, and the stent may need to be dilated at periodic intervals.

Benefits

Following recovery from anesthesia, a stent can provide immediate symptomatic relief of life-threatening dyspnea. Mean forced vital capacity, mean peak expiratory flow, mean forced expiratory volume in 1 second (FEV_1), and arterial partial pressure of oxygen all improve after stent placement (83–85). Many patients requiring ventilatory support can be weaned from their ventilator and have their trachea extubated immediately (86–88).

In lung transplant recipients with bronchial stenosis and bronchomalacia, stent placement improves lung function and reduces pulmonary infection rates for up to 1 year after insertion (89).

Stenting is not curative. Even so, the immediate palliation of symptoms results in improved quality of life in patients who are terminally ill (90, 91). If the patient survives long enough, tumor or granulation tissue will reaccumulate, and restenosis may occur (92, 93).

Currently, the only surgical treatments for emphysema are lung volume reduction procedures (94–96). In an in vitro study of excised human lungs, placement of small, expandable metallic stents from segmental bronchi into adjacent lung parenchyma resulted in highly significant increases in FEV_1 (97). The creation of these extra-anatomic bronchopleural passages resulted in reduced dynamic hyperinflation with improved expiratory flow. In the future, stenting of small bronchi may have therapeutic applications for patients with severe emphysema.

Types of Stents

The two types of stents, silicone and metallic, are compared in Table 6.2.

Silicone Stents

Straight T-shaped and bifurcated Y-shaped silicone stents are available. Straight stents are flanged on both ends to prevent dislodgment. Selection of the correct size and length is critical. The stent must be long enough to enable its flanges to anchor it within the stricture but also short enough not to compromise a lobar bronchus distally or the trachea

TABLE 6.2   Comparison of Metallic and Silicone
Airway Stents

Metallic stents	Silicone stents
Wire mesh (open or coated)	Solid
Uncoated mesh allows cilia activity	No cilia clearance
	More atelectasis and infection
Flexible	Rigid
No bifurcated stents available	Bifurcated stents
Expandable	Nonexpandable
Balloon expandable (bronchi)	
Self-expanding stents (trachea)	
Thin wall	Thick wall
Wider internal lumen	Narrow internal lumen
Not easily displaced (considered permanent)	Easily displaced (considered temporary)
Indications	Indications
Tumor	Infection
Infection	Inflammation
Topical or general anesthesia	General anesthesia only
Fiberoptic or rigid	Rigid bronchoscope only

proximally. Stent diameter must be of sufficient size to maintain the caliber of the airway.

Because the walls of a silicone stent are relatively thick, placement results in a smaller internal airway diameter than results with a metallic stent. Before placement, the stricture must be dilated, whereas a metallic stent can be inserted first and the stricture subsequently dilated (98). Balloon dilation of a tight bronchial stricture is illustrated in Figure 6.3.

Silicone stents are inserted with a rigid bronchoscope under general anesthesia. The stent is mounted on the rigid bronchoscope, which is advanced across the stricture. The bronchoscope is then withdrawn, leaving the stent in place. In a patient with a tracheal stoma, a T-shaped tube stent can be inserted that extends up to the vocal cords and down to the carina.

Currently, only silicone stents can accommodate a bifurcation. When placed at the carina, a silicone stent can maintain the patency of the distal trachea and both mainstem bronchi (99). For obstructions of the carina, a Y-shaped tube is placed, with forceps being used to advance a limb into each bronchus.

Silicone stents interfere with ciliary clearance and are easily occluded with mucous plugs. Periodic bronchoscopic examination and debridement may be necessary, because granulation tissue and tumor can grow at either end of the stent.

Early silicone stents were easily dislodged, but current versions have rows of studs on the external surface to decrease migration. The

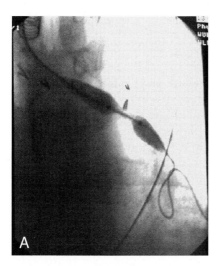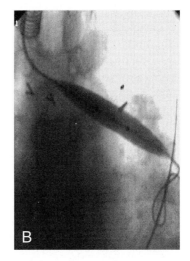

FIGURE 6.3 (A) A balloon dilator is placed across the stenotic segment. (B) and the stricture is dilated before stent placement.

anesthesiologist must be aware that a previously placed silicone stent, especially in the trachea, can be displaced during tracheal intubation.

Silicone stents are indicated for temporary strictures caused by inflammation and infection, because they can be removed when the stenosing disease subsides (100, 101). In patients with benign airway disease, follow-up bronchoscopy is performed at 6-month intervals. The stent is removed, and the airway is inspected. If airway patency is maintained at that time, the stent may not need to be reinserted.

Metallic Stents

Although metallic stents can be placed under topical anesthesia with sedation (102, 103), an immobile patient is essential for airway measurement, dilation, and accurate stent positioning. Therefore, general anesthesia is a better choice.

Metal stents are expandable. They are easier to insert and have a lower inner-to-outer diameter ratio (and, hence, wider internal lumens) than silicone stents. They adapt to anatomical contours, and their flexibility allows them to conform to tortuous airways better than rigid silicone stents. They are engineered to exert constant, gentle radial pressure to maintain airway patency while reducing the risk of trauma. Modern metallic stents are magnetic resonance imaging compatible.

Metallic stents can be either uncovered or covered by a polyethylene membrane. For benign strictures, an uncovered stent is usually used; for neoplastic strictures, a covered stent is deployed in an attempt to reduce tumor in-growth. Covered stents are also used to occlude tracheobronchial fistulae. Uncovered wire-metallic stents have extremely thin walls with gaps between the wires so that ciliary movement is not impaired and drainage of sputum is not interrupted (104).

Metallic stents are much less likely than silicone stents to become displaced. This is both an advantage and their major disadvantage. Once deployed, metallic stents are considered to be permanent. Over a period of weeks, the stent is incorporated into the airway wall, and its mesh becomes covered with mucosa. Newer metallic stents, such as the Ultraflex™ nitinol stent (Boston Scientific, Natick, MA), can be removed, but only before the stent is completely epithelialized (105).

Bronchoscopy is first performed to identify the position of the stricture, and radiopaque markers are placed on the patient's skin to mark the obstruction. A guidewire with a soft tip is advanced down either a bronchoscope or an ETT past the obstruction and into the distal airway. At this point, the stenosis is either dilated or the lesion immediately stented (Figure 6.4).

The most difficult lesions to treat are those at the tracheal carina. Only preformed, bifurcated silicone stents are currently available for

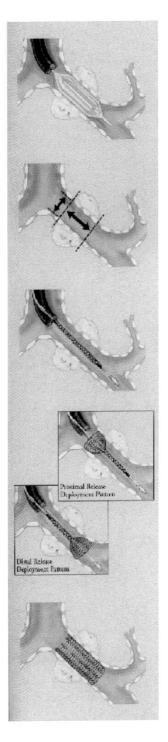

FIGURE 6.4 The sequence of steps for placement of an expandable metallic airway stent. The length and diameter of the stricture is determined by bronchoscopy, fluoroscopy, or chest computed tomography. A balloon dilator is then used to dilate the stricture until the lumen of the airway is wide enough to allow a bronchoscope to pass. An appropriately sized stent is chosen; it must be long enough to bridge the stricture. The expanded stent diameter should be approximately the same as the normal airway lumen. Under fluoroscopic or bronchoscopic guidance, the stent is positioned by a guidewire across the stricture. The stent is then deployed. Complete deployment of the stent is confirmed by bronchoscopy and fluoroscopy. Illustrations are of the Ultraflex™ Tracheobronchial Stent System. [Used by permission of Boston Scientific Corporation, Natick, MA.]

this use. Creation of a bronchial carina using two metallic stents is illustrated in Figure 6.5. A tracheal carina can be reconstructed by placing one stent in the distal trachea and two others in the proximal portions of each main bronchus (106).

Intraluminal tumor or granulation tissue can eventually grow at either end of the stent or between the interstices of the uncovered wire mesh (98). Newer stents are more malleable and can be re-expanded by balloon dilation if restenosis occurs (107, 108). If the patient survives, serial bronchoscopy, laser tissue ablation, and restenting procedures may be necessary.

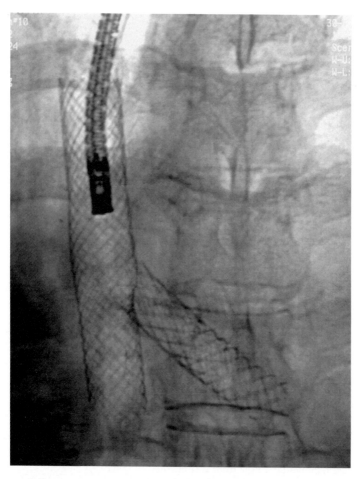

FIGURE 6.5 A carina can be created using two metallic stents. One stent is deployed in the left main bronchus and another in the left upper-lobe bronchus.

COMPLICATIONS

Stent displacement with airway obstruction, airway laceration, and massive hemoptysis can occur early after stent placement, with potentially fatal consequences if aggressive treatment is not provided (109).

To assess stent function, periodic follow-up evaluations are performed with either chest CT or FOB (110). For stent displacement or fracture, endoscopic removal of the stent is attempted (111). The longer a metallic stent is in place, the more difficult it is to remove.

Airway laceration, mucus impaction, granulation tissue formation, and development of esophago-airway fistulae are potential long-term complications (112–116). An esophageal fistula can be treated with a double-stenting technique (ie, placing one covered stent in the airway and another in the esophagus) (117).

CONCLUSION

Airway stenting often is the only available treatment for strictures of the central airways refractory to other treatments, for recurrent or unresectable tumors, for extrinsic airway compression, and for tracheobronchial malacia (118).

Successful management of these patients is dependent on a multidisciplinary team approach that involves a thoracic surgeon or pulmonologist, an interventional radiologist, and an anesthesiologist (119, 120). Plans must be thoroughly discussed and coordinated before the actual procedure is performed (121).

The interventional radiologist and the surgeon must decide which stent (metallic or silicone, covered or uncovered) to use, where to place the stent, and what the long-term implications are for the patient. Anesthetic management depends on the nature and site of the airway lesion and the specific needs of the interventional radiologist.

References

1. Al-Bazzaz F, Grillo H, Kazemi H: Responses to exercise in upper airway obstruction. Am Rev Respir Dis 1975; 111:631–40.
2. Geffin B, Grillo HC, Cooper JD, Pontoppidan H: Stenosis following tracheostomy for respiratory care. JAMA 1971; 216:1984–8.
3. Lavelle TF Jr, Rotman HH, Weg JG: Isoflow-volume curves in the diagnosis of upper airway obstruction. Am Rev Respir Dis 1978; 117:845–52.

4. Demedts M, Melissant C, Buyse B, et al.: Correlation between functional, radiological and anatomical abnormalities in upper airway obstruction (UAO) due to tracheal stenosis. Acta Otorhinolaryngol Belg 1995; 49:331–9.
5. Taichman DB, Tino G, Aronchick J, et al.: Diffuse airway narrowing from carcinoma metastatic to the bronchial submucosa: identification by chest CT. Chest 1998; 114:1217–20.
6. Weber AL: Radiologic evaluation of the trachea. Chest Surg Clin N Am 1996; 6:637–73.
7. Callanan V, Gillmore K, Field S: The use of magnetic resonance imaging to assess tracheal stenosis following percutaneous dilatational tracheostomy. J Laryngol Otol 1997; 111:953–7.
8. Burden RJ, Shann F, Butt W, et al.: Tracheobronchial malacia and stenosis in children in intensive case: bronchograms help to predict outcome. Thorax 1999; 54:511–7.
9. Zwischenberger JB, Wittich GR, van Sonnenberg E, et al.: Airway simulation to guide stent placement for tracheobronchial obstruction in lung cancer. Ann Thorac Surg 1997; 64:1619–25.
10. Grenier PA, Beigelman-Aubry C, Fetita C, et al.: New frontiers in CT imaging of airway disease. Eur Radiol 2002; 12:1022–44.
11. Whyte RI, Quint LE, Kazerooni EA, et al.: Helical computed tomography for the evaluation of tracheal stenosis. Ann Thorac Surg 1995; 60:27–30.
12. Quint LE, Whyte RI, Kazerooni EA, et al.: Stenosis of the central airways: evaluation by using helical CT with multiplanar reconstructions. Radiology 1995; 194:871–7.
13. Graeber GM, Shriver CD, Albus RA, et al.: The use of computer tomography in the evaluation of mediastinal masses. J Thorac Cardiovasc Surg 1986; 91:662–6.
14. Vander Els NJ, Sorhage F, Bach AM, Straus DJ, White DA: Abnormal flow volume loops in patients with intrathoracic Hodgkin's disease. Chest 2000; 117:1256–61.
15. Miller RD, Hyatt RE: Obstructing lesions of the larynx and trachea: clinical and physiologic characteristics. Mayo Clin Proc 1969; 44:145–61.
16. Davidson FF Jr, Burke GW III: Physiologic differentiation of upper and lower airway obstruction. Ann Otol Rhinol Laryngol 1977; 86:630–2.
17. Gamsu G, Borson DB, Webb WR, Cunningham JH: Structure and function in tracheal stenosis. Am Rev Respir Dis 1980; 121:519–31.
18. Acres JC, Kryger MH: Clinical significance of pulmonary function tests: upper airway obstruction. Chest 1981; 80:207–11.
19. Lunn WW, Sheller JR: Flow volume loops in the evaluation of upper airway obstruction. Otolaryngol Clin North Am 1995; 28:721–9.

20. Spinelli P, Cerrai FG, Spinelli A: Palliation of tracheobronchial malignant obstruction with metal stents in emergency conditions. Minerva Chir 1998; 53:373–6.
21. Conacher ID: Anaesthesia and tracheobronchial stenting for central airway obstruction in adults. Br J Anaesth 2003; 90:367–74.
22. Plummer S, Hartley M, Vaughan RS: Anaesthesia for telescopic procedures in the thorax. Br J Anaesth 1998; 80:223–34.
23. Benjamin B: Anesthesia for pediatric airway endoscopy. Otolaryngol Clin North Am 2000; 33:29–47.
24. Davies L, Mister R, Spence DP, et al.: Cardiovascular consequences of fibreoptic bronchoscopy. Eur Respir J 1997; 10:695–8.
25. Williams T, Brooks T, Ward C: The role of atropine premedication in fiberoptic bronchoscopy using intravenous midazolam sedation. Chest 1998; 113:1394–8.
26. Cowl CT, Prakash UB, Kruger BR: The role of anticholinergics in bronchoscopy. A randomized clinical trial. Chest 2000; 118:188–92.
27. Gronnebech H, Johansson G, Smedebol M, Valentin N: Glycopyrrolate vs. atropine during anaesthesia for laryngoscopy and bronchoscopy. Acta Anaesthesiol Scand 1993; 37:454–7.
28. Milner QJW, Abdy S, Allen JG: Management of severe tracheal obstruction with helium/oxygen and a laryngeal mask airway. Anaesthesia 1997; 52:1087–9.
29. Jolliet P, Tassaux D: Helium-oxygen ventilation. Respir Care Clin N Am 2002; 8:295–307.
30. Conacher ID, Paes ML, McMahon CC: Anesthetic management of laser surgery for central airways obstruction. J Cardiothorac Vasc Anesth 1998; 12:1–5.
31. Pullerits J, Holzman R: Anaesthesia for patients with mediastinal masses. Can J Anaesth 1989; 36:681–8.
32. Narang S, Harte BH, Body SC: Anesthesia for patients with a mediastinal mass. Anesthesiol Clin North Am 2001; 19:559–79.
33. Watters MP, McKenzie JM: Inhalational induction with sevoflurane in an adult with severe complex central airways obstruction. Anaesth Intensive Care 1997; 25:704–6.
34. Teh J, Platt H: Inhalational induction with sevoflurane in central airway obstruction. Anaesth Intensive Care 1998; 26:458–9.
35. Okada S, Ishimori S, Satoh M, Satoh S: Bronchoscopic treatment for upper tracheal lesions with a laryngeal mask. Kyobu Geka 2002; 55:198–202.
36. Choudhury M, Saxena N: Total intravenous anaesthesia for tracheobronchial stenting in children. Anaesth Intensive Care 2002; 30:376–9.
37. Carden E, Burns WW, McDevitt NB, Carson T: A comparison of Venturi and side-arm ventilation in anesthesia for bronchoscopy. Can Anaesth Soc J 1973; 20:569–74.

38. Smith CO, Shroff PF, Steele JD: General anesthesia for bronchoscopy. The use of the Sanders bronchoscopic attachment. Ann Thorac Surg 1969; 8:348–54.
39. Vourc'h G, Fischler M, Michon F, et al.: High frequency jet ventilation v. manual jet ventilation during bronchoscopy in patients with tracheobronchial stenosis. Br J Anaesth 1983; 55:969–72.
40. Blomquist S, Algotsson L, Karlsson SE: Anaesthesia for resection of tumours in the trachea and central bronchi using the Nd-Yag-laser technique. Acta Anaesthesiol Scand 1990; 34:506–10.
41. Giunta F, Chiaranda M, Manani G, Giron GP: Clinical uses of high frequency jet ventilation in anaesthesia. Br J Anaesth 1989; 63(suppl):102S-6S.
42. Hautmann H, Bauer M, Pfeifer KJ, Huber RM: Flexible bronchoscopy: a safe method for metal stent implantation in bronchial disease. Ann Thorac Surg 2000; 69:398–401.
43. Baraka AS, Siddik SS, Taha SK, et al.: Low frequency jet ventilation for stent insertion in a patient with tracheal stenosis. Can J Anaesth 2001; 48:701–4.
44. El-Baz N, Jensik R, Faber LP: One-lung high-frequency ventilation for tracheoplasty and bronchoplasty: a new technique. Ann Thorac Surg 1982; 34:564–70.
45. Hautmann H, Gamarra F, Henke M, et al.: High frequency jet ventilation in interventional fiberoptic bronchoscopy. Anesth Analg 2000; 90:1436–40.
46. Catala JC, Pedrajas FG, Carrera J, et al.: Placement of an endotracheal device via the laryngeal mask airway in a patient with tracheal stenosis. Anesthesiology 1996; 84:239–40.
47. Filler RM, Forte V, Chait P: Tracheobronchial stenting for the treatment of airway obstruction. J Pediatr Surg 1998; 33:304–11.
48. Van de Putte P, Martsens P: Anaesthetic management for placement of a stent for high tracheal stenosis. Anaesth Intensive Care 1994; 22:619–21.
49. Ishikawa S, Yoshida I, Otani Y, et al.: Intratracheal stent intubation under extracorporeal lung assist. Surg Today 1995; 25:995–7.
50. Scherhag A, Hafner D, Dick W, Mann V: High-frequency jet ventilation for placing tracheal stents—a case report. Anaesthesiol Reanim 1999; 24:164–6.
51. Arndt GA, Ghani GA: A modification of an Eschmann endotracheal tube changer for insufflation. Anesthesiology 1988; 69:282–3.
52. Peacock AJ, Benson-Mitchell R, Godfrey R: Effect of fiberoptic bronchoscopy on pulmonary function. Thorax 1990; 45:38–41.
53. Tzabar Y: Intraoperative tracheal obstruction by tumour fragments. Anaesthesia 1995; 50:249–50.

Airway Stents | 139

54. Phillips MJ: Stenting therapy for stenosing airway diseases. Respirology 1998; 3:215–9.
55. Guha A, Mostafa SM, Kendall JB: The Montgomery T-tube: anaesthetic problems and solutions. Br J Anaesth 2001; 87:787–90.
56. Cooper J, Pearson F, Patterson G: Use of silicone stents in the management of airway problems. Ann Thorac Surg 1989; 47:371–8.
57. Bollinger CT, Probst R, Tschopp K, et al.: Silicone stents in the management of inoperable tracheobronchial stenosis. Indications and limitations. Chest 1993; 104:1653–9.
58. Wallace M, Charnsangavej C, Ogawa K: Tracheo-bronchial tree: expandable metallic stents used in experimental and clinical applications, work in progress. Radiology 1986; 158:309–12.
59. O'Sullivan GJ, Kee ST, Semba CP, Dake MD: Techniques in stenting the tracheobronchial tree. Techniques in Interventional Radiology 1999; 2:219–31.
60. Edell ES, Cortese DA, McDougall JC: Ancillary therapies in the management of lung cancer: photodynamic therapy, laser therapy, and endobronchial prosthetic devices. Mayo Clin Proc 1993; 68:685–90.
61. Stephens KE Jr, Wood DE: Bronchoscopic management of central airway obstruction. J Thorac Cardiovasc Surg 2000; 119:289–96.
62. Lee P, Kupeli E, Mehta AC: Therapeutic bronchoscopy in lung cancer. Laser therapy, electrocautery, brachytherapy, stents, and photodynamic therapy. Clin Chest Med 2002; 23:241–56.
63. Simoff MJ: Endobronchial management of advanced lung cancer. Cancer Control 2001; 8:337–43.
64. Madden BP, Datta S, Charokopos N: Experience with Ultraflex expandable metallic stents in the management of endobronchial pathology. Ann Thorac Surg 2002; 73:938–44.
65. Wilson GE, Walshaw MJ, Hind CR: Treatment of large airway obstruction in lung cancer using expandable metal stents inserted under direct vision via the fiberoptic bronchoscope. Thorax 1996; 51:248–52.
66. Lonchyna VA, Arcidi JM Jr, Garrity ER Jr, et al.: Refractory post-transplant airway strictures: successful management with wire stents. Eur J Cardiothorac Surg 1999; 15:842–9.
67. Orons PD, Amesur NB, Dauber JH, et al.: Balloon dilation and endobronchial stent placement for bronchial strictures after lung transplantation. J Vasc Interv Radiol 2000; 11:89–99.
68. Susanto I, Peters JI, Levine SM, et al.: Use of balloon-expandable metallic stents in the management of bronchial stenosis and bronchomalacia after lung transplantation. Chest 1998; 114:1330–5.
69. Martinez-Ballarin JI, Diaz-Jimenez JP, Castro MJ, Moya JA.: Silicone stents in the management of benign tracheobronchial

stenosis. Tolerance and early results in 63 patients. Chest 1996; 109:626–9.

70. Chhajed PN, Malouf MA, Tamm M, et al.: Interventional bronchoscopy for the management of airway complications following lung transplantation. Chest 2001; 120:1894–9.

71. Mulligan MS: Endoscopic management of airway complications after lung transplantation. Chest Surg Clin N Am 2001; 11:907–15.

72. Kovitz KL, Foroozesh MB, Goyos JM, Rubio ER: Endoscopic management of obstruction due to an acquired bronchial web. Can Respir J 2002; 9:189–92.

73. Tsang V, Goldstraw P: Endobronchial stenting for anastomotic stenosis after sleeve resection. Ann Thorac Surg 1989; 48:568–71.

74. Wood DE. Airway stenting. Chest Surg Clin N Am 2001; 11:841–60.

75. Yamamoto R, Tada H, Kishi A, et al.: Double stent for malignant combined esophago-airway lesions. Jpn J Thorac Cardiovasc Surg 2002; 50:1–5.

76. Araujo CE, Rubio ER, Ie SR, et al.: Airway obstruction due to bilateral giant pulmonary artery aneurysms. South Med J 2002; 95:366–8.

77. Nagappan R, Parkin G, Wright CA, et al.: Adult long-segment tracheal stenosis attributable to complete tracheal rings masquerading as asthma. Crit Care Med 2002; 30:238–40.

78. Fitzmauric BG, Brodsky JB, Kee ST, et al.: Anesthetic management of a patient with relapsing polychondritis. J Cardiothorac Vasc Anesth 1999; 13:309–11.

79. Kim S, Gotway MB, Webb WR, et al.: Tracheal compression by the stomach following gastric pull-up: diagnosis with CT and treatment with expandable metallic stent placement. Chest 2002; 121:998–1001.

80. Chan KP, Eng P, Hsu AA, et al.: Rigid bronchoscopy and stenting for esophageal cancer causing airway obstruction. Chest 2002; 122:1069–72.

81. Maeda K, Yasufuku M, Yamamoto T: A new approach to the treatment of congenital tracheal stenosis: Balloon tracheoplasty and expandable metallic stenting. J Pediatr Surg 2001; 36:1646–9.

82. Kumar P, Roy A, Penny DJ, et al.: Airway obstruction and ventilator dependency in young children with congenital cardiac defects: a role for self-expanding metal stents. Intensive Care Med 2002; 28:190–5.

83. Gelb AF, Zamel N, Colchen A, et al.: Physiologic studies of tracheobronchial stents in airway obstruction. Am Rev Respir Dis 1992; 146:1088–90.

84. Eisner MD, Gordon RL, Webb WR, et al.: Pulmonary function im-

proves after expandable metal stent placement for benign airway disease. Chest 1999; 115:1006–11.

85. Gotway MB, Golden JA, LaBerge JM, et al.: Benign tracheobronchial stenoses: changes in short-term and long-term pulmonary function testing after expandable metallic stent placement. J Comput Assist Tomogr 2002; 26:564–72.

86. Zannini P, Melloni G, Chiesa G, Carretta A: Self-expanding stents in the treatment of tracheobronchial obstruction. Chest 1994; 106:86–90.

87. Shafer JP, Allen JN: The use of expandable metal stents to facilitate extubation in patients with large airway obstruction. Chest 1998; 114:1378–82.

88. Scheinhorn DJ, Chao DC, Stearn-Hassenpflug M: Approach to patients with long-term weaning failure. Respir Care Clin N Am 2000; 6:437–61.

89. Burns KE, Orons PD, Dauber JH, et al.: Endobronchial metallic stent placement for airway complications after lung transplantation: longitudinal results. Ann Thorac Surg 2002; 74:1934–41.

90. Jack CI, Lye M, Wilson G, Hind CR: The use of expandable metal stents for large airway obstruction in older patients. J Am Geriatr Soc 1995; 43:543–5.

91. Vonk-Noordegraaf A, Postmus PE, Sutedja TG: Tracheobronchial stenting in the terminal care of cancer patients with central airways obstruction. Chest 2001; 120:1811–4.

92. Tanigawa N, Sawada S, Okuda Y, et al.: Symptomatic improvement in dyspnea following tracheobronchial metallic stenting for malignant airway obstruction. Acta Radiol 2000; 41:425–8.

93. De Mello-Filho FV, Antonio SM, Carrau RL: Endoscopically placed expandable metal tracheal stents for the management of complicated tracheal stenosis. Am J Otolaryngol 2003; 24:34–40.

94. Gelb AF, Brenner M, McKenna RJ Jr, et al.: Lung function 12 months following emphysema resection. Chest 1996; 110:1407–15.

95. Sciurba FC, Rogers RM, Keenan RJ, et al.: Improvement in pulmonary function and elastic recoil after lung-reduction surgery for diffuse emphysema. N Engl J Med 1996; 334:1095–9.

96. Koebe HG, Kugler C, Dienemann H: Evidence-based medicine: lung volume reduction surgery (LVRS). Thorac Cardiovasc Surg 2002; 50:315–22.

97 Lausberg HF, Chino K, Patterson GA, et al.: Bronchial fenestration improves expiratory flow in emphysematous human lungs. Ann Thorac Surg 2003; 75:393–7.

98. Tojo T, Iioka S, Kitamura S, et al.: Management of malignant tracheobronchial stenosis with metal stents and Dumon stents. Ann Thorac Surg 1996; 61:1074–8.

99. Shiraishi T, Okabayashi K, Kuwahara M, et al.: Y-shaped tracheo-bronchial stent for carinal and distal tracheal stenosis. Surg Today 1998; 28:328–31.

100. Schmidt B, Olze H, Borges AC, et al.: Endotracheal balloon dilation and stent implantation in benign stenosis. Ann Thorac Surg 2001; 71:1630–4.

101. Wan IY, Lee TW, Lam HC, et al.: Tracheobronchial stenting for tuberculous airway stenosis. Chest 2002; 122:370–4.

102. Coolen D, Slabbynck H, Galdermans D, et al.: Insertion of a self-expandable endotracheal metal stent using topical anaesthesia and a fibreoptic bronchoscope: a comfortable way to offer palliation. Thorax 1994; 49:87–8.

103. Spinelli P, Meroni E, Cerrai FG: Self-expanding tracheobronchial stents using flexible bronchoscopy. Preliminary clinical experience. Surg Endosc 1994; 8:411–3.

104. Slonim SM, Razavi M, Kee S, et al.: Transbronchial Palmaz stent placement for tracheobronchial stenosis. J Vasc Interv Radiol 1998; 9:153–60.

105. Miyazawa T, Yamakido M, Ikeda S, et al.: Implantation of Ultraflex nitinol stents in malignant tracheobronchial stenosis. Chest 2000; 118:959–65.

106. Lo CP, Soo TB, Hsu AA, Eng PC: Treatment of severe carinal stenosis with overlapping metallic endoprosthesis. Ann Thorac Surg 2001; 71:1335–6.

107. Nesbitt JC, Carrasco H: Expandable stents. Chest Surg Clin N Am 1996; 6:305–28.

108. Noppen M, Schlesser M, Meysman M, et al.: Bronchoscopic balloon dilation in the combined management of postintubation stenosis of the trachea in adults. Chest 1997; 112:1136–40.

109. Stotz WH, Berkowitz ID, Hoehner JC, Tunkel DE: Fatal complication from a balloon-expandable tracheal stent in a child: a case report. Pediatr Crit Care Med 2003; 4:115–7.

110. Ferretti GR, Kocier M, Calaque O, et al.: Follow-up after stent insertion in the tracheobronchial tree; role of helical computed tomography in comparison with fiberoptic bronchoscopy. Eur Radiol 2003; 13:1172–8.

111. Zakaluzny SA, Lane JD, Mair EA: Complications of tracheobronchial airway stents. Otolaryngol Head Neck Surg 2003; 128:478–88.

112. Alfaro J, Varela G, De-Minguel E, et al.: Successful management of a tracheo-innominate artery fistula following placement of a wire self-expandable tracheal Gianturco stent. Eur J Cardiothorac Surg 1993; 7:615–6.

113. Niwa H, Masaoka A, Yamakawa Y, et al.: Esophageal tracheo-

bronchoplasty for membranous laceration caused by Dumon stent. Eur J Cardiothorac Surg 1995; 9:213–5.

114. Puma F, Farabi R, Urbani M, et al.: Long term safety and tolerance of silicone and self-expandable airway stents. Ann Thorac Surg 2000; 69:1030–40.

115. Kim H: Stenting therapy for stenosing airway disease. Respirology 1998; 3:221–8.

116. Burningham AR, Wax MK, Andersen PE, et al.: Metallic tracheal stents: complications associated with long-term use in the upper airway. Ann Otol Rhinol Laryngol 2002; 111; 285–90.

117. Urschel JD: Delayed massive hemoptysis after expandable bronchial stent placement. J Laparoendosc Adv Surg Tech A 1999; 9:155–8.

118. Riker AI, Vigneswaran WT: Management of tracheobronchial strictures and fistulas: a report and review of the literature. Int Surg 2002; 87:114–9.

119. Watkinson AF, Francis S, Torrie P, Platts AD: The role of anaesthesia in interventional radiology. Br J Radiol 2002; 75:105–6.

120. Unger M: Endobronchial therapy of neoplasms. Chest Surg Clin N Am 2003; 13:129–47.

121. Jones LM, Mair EA, Fitzpatrick TM, et al.: Multidisciplinary airway stent team: a comprehensive approach and protocol for tracheobronchial stent treatment. Ann Otol Laryngol 2000:109; 889–98.

Edda M. Tschernko, MD

Anesthesiological Considerations for Lung Volume
7 Reduction Surgery

INTRODUCTION

Chronic obstructive pulmonary disease (COPD) is the major cause of pulmonary disability in the United States and Europe (1). Specific guidelines for the diagnosis and care of patients with COPD are given by the American Thoracic Society (2). The cardinal physiologic defect in emphysema is a decrease in elastic recoil of the lung tissue. This results in the principal physiologic abnormalities of emphysema: decreased maximum expiratory airflow leading to air-trapping, hyperinflation, and severely limited exercise capacity (3, 4). The destruction of the alveolar-capillary membrane surface leads to a reduction in diffusion capacity. Emphysema is usually the result of cigarette smoking, but it can also be caused by α_1-antitrypsin deficiency (5, 6). It is a chronic, progressive disorder that ultimately leads to disability and early death.

In 1995, Cooper et al. (7) introduced lung volume reduction surgery (LVRS), a new surgical procedure leading to substantial improvement in lung function and exercise capacity in patients with end-stage emphysema. The initial unbridled enthusiasm was followed by skepticism, leading to the National Emphysema Treatment Trial (NETT), a large, randomized trial with uniform criteria for inclusion, lengthy follow-up, and a medical control group (8). However, for the anesthesiologist, LVRS is a challenging procedure requiring a profound knowledge of the pathophysiology of emphysema, anesthesia for thoracic surgery,

Progress in Thoracic Anesthesia, edited by Peter Slinger,
Lippincott Williams & Wilkins, Baltimore © 2004.

postoperative pain therapy, and ventilatory mechanics in anesthetized and awake patients suffering from end-stage emphysema.

INTRODUCTION OF LVRS FOR TREATMENT OF EMPHYSEMA

The failure of medical treatment to produce prolonged improvement of symptoms has promoted the introduction of various surgical procedures over the last 90 years. Surgical procedures such as phrenic nerve paralysis, thoracoplasty, denervation of the lung, and stabilization and fixation of the trachea, however, have produced minimal or no benefit to patients (9).

In 1957, Brantigan and Mueller (10) reported the surgical excision of lung tissue to reduce the volume of the hyperinflated lung parenchyma, and they named this procedure "lung volume reduction surgery," or LVRS. Although 75% of patients reported clinical improvement, the lack of objective documentation for benefit from the procedure and an operative mortality rate of 18% prevented widespread acceptance of the procedure.

In 1995, Cooper et al. (7) reported a modified Brantigan procedure in which lung tissue was resected from both lungs via a median sternotomy. In the initial series of 20 selected patients undergoing LVRS with this method, no operative mortality occurred, and the operation produced an 82% increase in forced expiratory volume in 1 second (FEV_1). Lung volume reduction surgery (ie, bilateral resection of 20–30% of lung volume) was associated with significant improvement of lung function, alleviation of dyspnea, and improvement of exercise tolerance in *selected* patients with severe emphysema (7).

Approximately 20% of patients, however, show no objective or subjective improvement after LVRS, and various centers report early operative mortality rates ranging from 2.5 % to 13.3 % (11–13). By now, it is generally accepted that patient selection for LVRS is of crucial importance. The NETT could identify patients with increased mortality risk (14) and patients who are likely to benefit from LVRS (15). However, generally accepted criteria for patient selection are still under investigation by the NETT, and as of this writing, final conclusions have not been made (15). Nevertheless, it seems to be undoubted by all experts that a precondition for successful conduct of LVRS is "the obvious need for highly experienced surgical, anesthetic, and critical care teams," (page 1913) as Weinmann and Hyatt put it (13). Therefore, it must be emphasized that for the anesthesiologist involved in LVRS, a profound knowledge of the pathophysiology of emphysema, anesthesia for thoracic surgery, pain therapy, and ventilatory mechanics in both

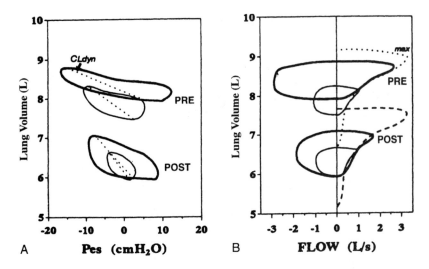

FIGURE 7.1   In one representative subject, pressure-volume (A) and flow-volume (B) relations are shown during a typical tidal breath at rest (thin lines) and during an equivalent level of exercise (thick lines) before and after volume reduction surgery. Comparisons were made at similar levels of ventilation before surgery (rest, 19.7 L/min; exercise, 37.4 L/min) and after surgery (rest, 20.4 L/min; exercise, 34.0 L/min). Dotted (presurgery) and dashed (postsurgery) lines in indicate the maximal expiratory flow-volume envelopes performed at rest. Clydyn = dynamic compliance; max = maximum. [From O'Donnell et al. (23); with permission.]

anesthetized and awake patients suffering from end-stage emphysema is mandatory.

MECHANISMS OF FUNCTIONAL IMPROVEMENT AFTER LVRS

Maximal flow in normal and diseased lungs is determined by lung elastic recoil and the characteristics of the airway. The defining characteristic of COPD is a reduction of the maximal expiratory flow (2, 16, 17). As the disease progresses, patients must breathe at a higher lung volume to achieve the flows that are necessary to meet their ventilatory requirements. Total lung capacity (TLC), which is the maximum lung volume that patients can achieve, increases because of diminished elastic recoil of the lung and remodeling of the rib cage and diaphragm. However, this adaptive response is limited. In patients with incapacitating COPD, the end-inspiratory volume approaches the TLC. Patients are dyspneic at rest and unable to increase ventilation enough during exercise to maintain normal PaO_2 and $PaCO_2$, because they are already breathing near or at the maximal flows at rest. In addition, marked abnormalities can occur in ventilation-perfusion matching.

Immediately after reintroduction of LVRS, investigators examined the mechanism of functional improvement after LVRS during rest and during exercise. Because of the pathophysiology of emphysema, the main targets of these studies were changes in ventilatory mechanics and diaphragmatic function after LVRS.

CHANGES IN LUNG FUNCTION TESTING AND VENTILATORY MECHANICS AFTER LVRS

Changes in Lung Function Testing after LVRS

Lung volume reduction surgery is known to produce marked changes in several parameters characterizing lung function testing, the most important being a significant increase in FEV_1. Table 7.1 depicts the changes that can be expected 3 to 6 months after surgery (13). Table 7.1 also shows what can be expected as an average change. Note, however, that a significant number of subjects exhibit no significant improvement in lung function testing after LVRS and that the reported surgical mortality rates range from 2.5 % to 13.3 % (11, 12).

Changes in Ventilatory Mechanics

Several investigators have shown an improvement in elastic recoil, a reduction in expiratory flow limitation, a decrease in dynamic pulmonary hyperinflation (DPH), and a decrease in work of breathing (WOB) during resting conditions after LVRS (18–22). Expiratory flow limitation becomes best visible in the pressure-volume curve of a subject, where transpulmonary pressure is shown on the *x*-axis and volume on the *y*-axis. In pa-

TABLE 7.1 Average Baseline and Postoperative Values

Test	Baseline	Postoperative
Total lung capacity	130–140% predicted	20% decrease
Residual volume	>200% predicted	30% decrease
Forced vital capacity	50–70% predicted	30–40% increase
Forced expiratory volume in 1 second	25–30% predicted	50–60% increase
Carbon monoxide diffusing capacity	30–40% predicted	No change
Six-minute walk test	700–1,200 feet	20–30% increase

From Weinmann and Hyatt (13); with permission.

tients with COPD, inspiration is not markedly altered, whereas expiration is characterized by a very flat slope of the pressure-volume curve (Figure 7.1). O'Donnell et al. (23) and Gelb et al. (19) showed very early after the reintroduction of the LVRS procedure that the slope of expiration becomes markedly steeper in the pressure-volume curve of patients after successful LVRS (Figure 7.2), indicating a significant reduction in expiratory airflow limitation. Thus, it seems to be accepted today that improvement of expiratory airflow limitation is one of the mechanism leading to functional improvement in selected patients with emphysema after LVRS.

Another issue was the time course of improvement in ventilatory mechanics after surgery. Cooper et al. (7)reported successful extubation after bilateral resection of 20% to 30% of lung volume in patients with severely respiratory limitation in the operating room). This was surprising, because an FEV_1 of 800 mL was usually considered to be a criterion of inoperability in patients scheduled for lung resection (24). Therefore, it must be suspected that ventilatory mechanics improve almost immediately after surgery. To test this hypothesis, ventilatory mechanics were assessed before and within 24 hours after surgery and at later time points. Improvement in WOB (Figure 7.2), intrinsic positive end-expiratory pressure ($PEEP_i$, a measure for DPH), and pulmonary resistance (R_L) were present as early as 24 hours after LVRS (22, 25), probably enabling successful early extubation in these patients with severe respiratory limitation. Furthermore, various investigators have

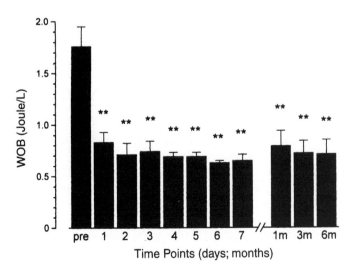

FIGURE 7.2   Changes in work of breathing (WOB) at various time points after lung volume reduction surgery. $**p < 0.001$. [From Tschernko et al. (22); with permission.]

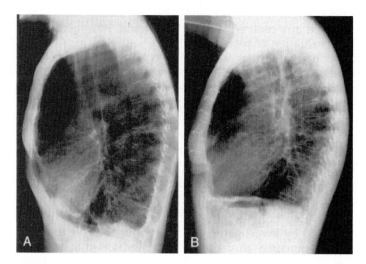

FIGURE 7.3   Lateral chest radiography. (A) The patient is shown before lung volume reduction surgery (LVRS). The thorax is barrel shaped, with high transparency of the lunge, a large retrosternal air-filled space, and a flattened-to-even, concave shape of the diaphragm. (B) The same patient 3 months after LVRS. The lung fields are less transparent, the air-filled retrosternal space is decreased significantly. Additionally, the diaphragm exhibits an almost normal, convex shape.

shown that improvement in exercise capacity was caused by improved ventilatory mechanics (26–28). In exercise tests with continuous monitoring of ventilatory mechanics, significantly decreased $PEEP_i$, WOB, and R_L were found at isowatt after LVRS (28).

CHANGES IN DIAPHRAGMATIC FUNCTION AFTER LVRS

Benditt et al. (29) found improved diaphragmatic pressure generation in patients undergoing exercise tests 3 months after LVRS. Investigations at other institutions have found similar results (22, 30). However, improved diaphragmatic pressure generation was found no earlier than 3 months after surgery (25, 31), and diaphragmatic force generation was not significantly different from preoperative values when compared as early as 1 month after LVRS (25). Thus, the improvement in diaphragmatic function likely is a late benefit of LVRS.

To date, it seems to be accepted that selected patients with end-stage emphysema benefit from LVRS by means of early improvement in ventilatory mechanics and somewhat later improvement in diaphragmatic function. However, the duration of improvement remains unclear (15).

OPTIMAL CONDUCT OF LVRS

Optimal conduct of LVRS involves patients selection, preoperative patients preparation, and anesthesia.

Patient Selection

General Criteria

General patient selection criteria and recommendations for screening procedures are given by Weinmann and Hyatt (13). However, selection criteria may vary between centers. Distinct selection criteria for LVRS candidates have already been published in 1996 by Daniel et al. (32) and are shown in Table 7.2. Most of these criteria still apply. However, it was shown in the NETT trial that patients presenting with an FEV1 below 20% have an increased perioperative risk and little benefit after LVRS. Thus, these patients are no longer regarded as suitable LVRS candidates.

Some institutions report significant (coronary artery stenosis of >70%) coronary artery disease diagnosed in 15% of their asymptomatic LVRS candidates; thus, they recommend left- and right-heart cardiac catheterization preoperatively (33). Additionally, this invasive cardiac screening seems to be justified by several case reports of myocardial infarction during and after LVRS. However, other centers recommend

TABLE 7.2   General Inclusion Criteria for Lung Volume Reduction Surgery

Diagnosis of COPD
Patient history, physical examination, lung function test, chest radiography, etc.
Smoking cessation for more than 1 month
Age < 75 years
FEV_1 between 15% and 35% of predicted
$PaCO_2$ <55 mm Hg
Prednisone dosage <20 mg/day
PAP_{sys} <50 mm Hg
No previous thoracotomy or pleurodesis
Absence of symptomatic coronary artery disease
Absence of chronic asthma or bronchitis
Commitment to preoperative and postoperative supervised pulmonary rehabilitation
for 6 weeks

Criteria from Daniel et al. (32).
COPD = chronic obstructive pulmonary disease; FEV_1 = forced expiratory volume in 1 second; $PaCO_2$ = arterial carbon dioxide pressure; PAP_{sys} = systolic pulmonary arterial pressure.

limiting cardiac screening to transthoracic echocardiography (32). In general, it is reasonable for centers with little experience to use restrictive criteria for patient selection to keep mortality and complication rates low.

Morphological Criteria

The chest radiograph should show evidence of hyperinflated lungs, large intercostal spaces, retrosternal airspace, flattened diaphragm, and high transparency of the lungs, as shown in Figure 7.3*A*. For the precise morphological evaluation, high-resolution computer tomography (CT) of the chest is essential to identify inhomogeneities within the lungs (34). By means of high-resolution CT, the target areas for resection are located. A preferable anatomical precondition for LVRS is marked inhomogeneity of the lung structure (ie, almost-normal lung tissue and severely destroyed, overdistended tissue in the same lung) (Figure 7.4*A*) Completely homogeneous distribution of the disease has proved to be an unfavorable precondition (Figure 7.4*B*). Several authors have shown that patients presenting with severe inhomogeneity are very likely to benefit after LVRS (35–37). Two reasons might account for this. First, compressed, normal lung tissue is released after removal of adjoining hyperinflated, nonfunctional, destroyed tissue; thus, ventilatory mechanics of the remaining tissue are improved. Second, surgery is easier to perform if the target areas are clearly visible. This has been recently confirmed by the NETT trial,

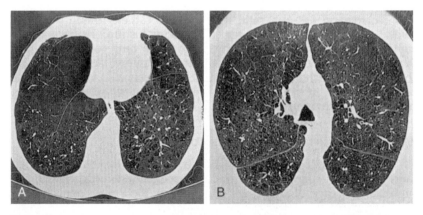

FIGURE 7.4   (A) High-resolution computed tomographic (CT) scan of a patient presenting with inhomogeneous distribution of the disease. The ventral parts of the lung are far more destroyed than the dorsal parts; thus, the functionally better parts can be easily distinguished from the destroyed parts. (B) High-resolution CT scan of a patient with homogeneous distribution of the disease, in which case it is difficult for the surgeon to decide which part should be resected.

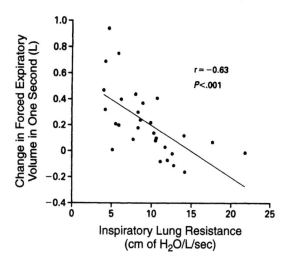

FIGURE 7.5 Inverse correlation between preoperative inspiratory lung resistance (in cm H_2O/L/sec, shown on the x-axis) and the gain in forced expiratory volume in 1 second (shown on the y-axis). [From Ingenito et al. (39); with permission.]

which has shown good benefit and low operative risk in patients with inhomogeneous distribution of emphysema (15). Patients with emphysema in the upper lobes are more likely to benefit compared to patients with lower-lobe emphysema (15). Lung perfusion scintigraphy is still routinely performed for screening LVRS candidates in many centers to rule out ventilation-perfusion mismatch. However, chest computed tomography is superior to lung perfusion scintigraphy for the evaluation of patients (38).

Functional Criteria for Patient Selection

Today, a preoperative predicted FEV_1 of less than 20 % in combination with homogenous morphology or a carbon monoxide diffusion capacity of less than 20 % of the predicted value is regarded as a contraindication for surgery. These patients were found to have significantly increased morbidity and mortality after LVRS compared to conventional medical treatment (14).

Ventilatory mechanics are severely impaired in patients suffering from emphysema, and LVRS leads to a significant improvement. Several parameters characterizing ventilatory mechanics show specific changes after LVRS. Therefore, several of these parameters were tested by investigators for their value as preoperative predictors of outcome after LVRS.

Ingenito et al. (39) hypothesized that patients with markedly elevated inspiratory resistance likely have predominantly airway disease, and, thus, are unlikely to show improvement of expiratory flow after LVRS, thereby limiting the benefit of the procedure. The investigators could prove their hypothesis by showing that preoperative inspiratory lung resistance was negatively correlated with changes in FEV_1 ($r = -0.63; p < 0.001$). In contrast, patients with elevated expiratory lung resistance showed good improvement (Figure 7.5).

Additionally, preoperative $PEEP_i$, which is a correlate of dynamic pulmonary hyperinflation, and postoperative gain in normalized predicted FEV_1 were found to be well correlated ($r = 0.69, p < 0.0002$) (40). Similar results were found for changes in dyspnea score.

Despite these and other promising findings of functional parameters predicting outcome, most parameters require more or less time-consuming and sophisticated measuring techniques; thus, they are difficult to introduce into clinical routine. Therefore, none of the evaluated parameters has gained widespread acceptance in clinical routine to date. Recently, it was shown that the capacity of the patient to perform physical work might be a parameter predicting outcome. A low exercise capacity before surgery was found to be well correlated with reduced mortality after LVRS and with better improvement in exercise capacity (15).

Pharmacological Preparation

Pharmacological Preparation

Most patients presenting for LVRS are on long-term bronchodilator therapy (β_2-adrenergic agonists), steroid therapy (inhalation or systemically), and mucolytic therapy. Additionally, these patients frequently take antibiotics. Most centers recommend that maximal bronchodilator and mucolytic therapy be optimized and continued before LVRS, including on the day of surgery. The patient must have been free of respiratory infections for at least 3 weeks before LVRS and, thus, require no antibiotic therapy preoperatively. In terms of steroid therapy, the aim is generally for a dose reduction of systemic steroids before LVRS.

Many patients are on theophylline therapy before LVRS. However, some patients experience toxic symptoms while theophylline blood levels are in the therapeutic range (41). The main side effects are nervousness, tremor, and tachycardia. Theophylline therapy should be discontinued before LVRS if the patient shows significant side effects.

Preoperative Exercise Program

Almost all centers advocate a preoperative exercise program for their patients. The optimal training program is supervised by a specialized nurse and physician and lasts for at least 6 weeks (and preferably 3 months) before surgery. Training may consist of regular walking, bicycle ergometer training, and weight lifting combined with a special diet. Leg exercise is usually better tolerated than arm exercise. An exercise program before surgery has several advantages:

1. The patient's will to cooperate can be assessed.
2. Endurance and exercise tolerance is increased, which will be helpful for early mobilization after surgery (7).
3. Maximal oxygen consumption can be increased in many subjects (42).

Psychological Preparation

Patients presenting for LVRS frequently are very anxious because of dyspnea and asthmatic crises that they have experienced in the past. Psychological factors can induce an asthma attack, which is a dangerous complication during the perioperative period. Anxiety is associated with an increase in respiratory frequency, leading to increases in dynamic pulmonary hyperinflation and dyspnea (43). Therefore, it is important that the anesthesiologist establish a good relationship with the patient before surgery. The optimal psychological preconditions are likely to be achieved when preoperative preparation, preoperative visit, insertion of the thoracic epidural, general anesthesia, and early postoperative therapy are conducted by the same physician or by a team the patient knows well. Furthermore, it might be necessary to use anxiolytic drug therapy during the pre- and perioperative periods.

Thoracic Epidural Analgesia for Patients Undergoing LVRS

Thoracic Epidural Analgesia for Patients Undergoing LVRS

By now, it is a generally accepted that thoracic epidural analgesia (TEA) is mandatory for optimal pain therapy after LVRS. The TEA is regularly inserted at the level T3–4 or T4–5 in the awake patient immediately before surgery. The spread of anesthesia and analgesia should be tested carefully before the induction of general anesthesia to avoid problems resulting from pain causing ventilatory depression during the immediate postoperative period. Usually, a local analgesic, such as bupivacaine or ropivacaine, can be used for TEA, preferably in combination with an opioid. It is important in patients with emphysema that they are properly volume loaded (1–2 mL/kg) before fully activating the TEA to avoid severe hypotension, because these patients tend to be volume depleted. Furthermore, a potent vasopressor, such as norepinephrine or phenylephrine, should be prepared before activating the TEA. To avoid marked hypotension, ropivacaine is preferred over bupivacaine as the local analgesic, because it causes less circulatory depression.

Literally all anesthesiologists who perform anesthesia for LVRS are convinced that TEA is crucial in reducing perioperative morbidity and mortality. However, no controlled studies are available to prove this theory. For ethical reasons, most anesthesiologists would not attempt to perform such a study using a placebo-control group. In patients with normal lung function undergoing lung resection, evidence indicates that sufficient postoperative analgesia with TEA can reduce morbidity and mortality (44). However, other authors emphasize that the influence of TEA on outcome after lung resection has not been proven (45). Nevertheless, use of TEA is the worldwide established means for intra- and postoperative analgesia in patients undergoing LVRS. To guarantee optimal analgesia, TEA should be kept in place and activated until all the drains are removed.

General Anesthesia for LVRS

Monitoring

Monitoring for LVRS should include six-lead electrocardiography, pulsoximetry, invasive blood-pressure monitoring, a temperature probe for continuous core temperature measurement, and a central venous catheter to assess central venous pressure. Use of a Swan-Ganz catheter is controversial. However, continuous monitoring of pulmonary arterial pressure may be helpful, because this measure can rise substantially during single-lung ventilation because of permissive hypercapnia, and, thus, cause intraoperative right ventricular decompensation.

Anesthetic drugs for LVRS

For orotracheal intubation with the double-lumen tube, the intravenous analgesic requirement can be substantially reduced if the pharynx and larynx are carefully anesthetized with a local anesthetic spray (eg, lidocaine 2%) (46). After intubation, analgesia should be carried out with TEA. However, it is important to mention that intubation in a poorly anesthetized patient with emphysema can lead to life-threatening bronchospasm (47).

Only short-acting drugs should be used for sedation and muscle paralysis during general anesthesia for LVRS, because the patient should breath spontaneously as early as possible after the procedure to avoid prolonged air leakage caused by positive-pressure ventilation. Thus, propofol is a suitable choice for sedation. If the patient is prone to bronchospasm, a volatile inhalational anesthetic, such as sevoflurane or isoflurane, may be preferred over an intravenous agent. For muscle paralysis, drugs with short duration and absence of histamine liberation, such as vecuronium or cisatracurium, are frequently chosen. For intraoperative analgesia, the TEA should be used to avoid the sedative and ventilatory depressive side effects of opioids. For intubation, fentanyl of remifentanyl seems to be most suitable.

Mechanical ventilation during LVRS

Proper mechanical ventilation for LVRS must guarantee sufficient arterial oxygenation while minimizing air-trapping (43) with the potential threat of pneumothorax. Air-trapping can be avoided by using moderate tidal volumes (<9 mL/kg during ventilation of both lungs, <5 mL/kg during single-lung ventilation), low respiratory frequencies (<12 breaths/min during ventilation of both lungs, <16 breaths/min during single-lung ventilation), and prolonged expiratory time (Ti/Te = 1/3 during double- and single-lung ventilation). If the preoperative high-resolution CT depicts a substantial side difference in the quality of lung tissue, it can be helpful for the surgeon to operate first on the more destroyed lung.

Furthermore, it is important to set an upper pressure limit (<35 cm H_2O) on the ventilator to avoid pneumothorax formation and barotrauma. The anesthesiologist should pay constant attention if the entire volume delivered to the lung during inspiration is exhaled during expiration. For this purpose, watch the flow curves of the ventilator. In most patients undergoing LVRS, the anesthesiologist will have to accept elevated values of end-tidal and $PaCO_2$ during single-lung ventilation. This permissive hypercapnia is the prize for the prevention of barotrauma during mechanical ventilation for LVRS. However, $PaCO_2$ values will be in the normal range soon after the procedure, when both lungs can be ventilated again.

Patient warming during LVRS

Sufficient patient warming can be achieved using warming blankets, heating mats, and warm infusions. Core body temperature and the peripheral temperature of the patient should be kept in the normal range. A decrease in the body heat content of the patient will ultimately lead to shivering after extubation, with increased carbon dioxide production and oxygen consumption. Frequently, it is impossible for the patients with emphysema and severe respiratory limitation to meet the increased ventilatory demands caused by shivering. Thus, postoperative shivering may require reintubation.

Early extubation after LVRS

Even with the new surgical techniques using staplers buttressed with bovine pericardium, it is difficult to avoid air leakage entirely. Air leakage can be aggravated by positive-pressure ventilation, whereas the negative intrapleural pressure generated during spontaneous breathing minimizes air leakage. Therefore, early extubation after LVRS is of special importance. Nevertheless, several conditions, as shown in Table 7.3, need to be met before the patient can be extubated. If the patient fails to meet all the criteria listed in Table 7.3, it is reasonable to stabilize the patient in a quiet environment, such as an intensive care unit or the postoperative holding area, before extubation. Usually, this will be possible in 1 or 2 hours and is not harmful for the patient. Either way, it is preferred over a premature extubation in the operating room followed by prolonged episodes of arterial hypoxemia.

SUMMARY

Patient selection is of crucial importance regarding outcome after LVRS. The anesthesiologist should be actively involved in patient selection, because he or she is in charge of the treatment during the critical perioperative period. Patient history and status as well as results derived from chest radiography, high-resolution CT, and catheterization of the right heart should be carefully taken into account during the patient selection process. In addition, careful selection and preoperative preparation of patients are important to avoid complications and to keep the success rate high. Furthermore, it must be emphasized that a profound knowledge on the part of the anesthesiologist is of crucial importance for the successful conduct of LVRS.

TABLE 7.3   Extubation Criteria after Lung Volume Reduction Surgery

Patient awake and cooperative
Patient breathing sufficiently (ie, rapid shallow breathing index [respiratory frequency per min/tidal volume in L] of <70)
Sufficient arterial oxygenation ($SaO_2 \geq 92$ while patient is breathing spontaneously ($FIO_2 \leq 0.35$)]
Patient does not suffer thoracotomy pain
Core temperature >35.5°C
No shivering
Stable hemodynamic conditions

FIO_2=fraction of inspired oxygen; SaO_2=arterial oxygen saturation.

To date, it is unclear if LVRS is superior in the long run compared to conventional medical therapy, because the decline in lung function is progressive after the procedure. Nevertheless, the NETT trial has identified those patients with excessive operative risk and those patients likely to benefit most during the early postoperative period (15).

References

1. National Heart, Lung, and Blood Institute, Division of Lung Disease Workshop Report: The definition of emphysema. Am Rev Respir Dis 1985; 132:182–5.
2. American Thoracic Society: Standards for the diagnosis and care of patients with chronic obstructive pulmonary disease (COPD) and asthma. Am Rev Respir Dis 1987; 136:225–44.
3. Potter WA, Olafsson S, Hyatt RE: Ventilatory mechanics and expiratory flow limitation during exercise in patients with obstructive lung disease. J Clin Invest 1971; 50:910–9.
4. Stubbing DC, Pengelly LD, Morse JLC, Jones NL: Pulmonary mechanics during exercise in subjects with chronic airflow obstruction. J Appl Physiol 1980; 49:511–5.
5. Carrell RW, Jeppsson JO, Laurell CB, et al.: Structure and variation of the human $á_1$-antitrypsin. Nature 1982; 298:329–34.
6. Janus ED, Phillips NT, Carrell RW.: Smoking, lung function and $á_1$-antitrypsin deficiency. Lancet 1985; i:152–4.
7. Cooper JD, Trulock EP, Triantafillou AN, et al.: Bilateral pneumectomy volume reduction for chronic obstructive pulmonary disease. J Thorac Cardiovasc Surg 1995; 109:106–19.
8. The National Emphysema Treatment Trial Research Group: Rationale and design of the National Emphysema Treatment Trial: a prospective randomized trial of lung volume reduction surgery. Chest 1999; 116:1750–61.
9. Carter MG, Gaensler EA, Kyllonen A: Pneumoperitoneum in the treatment of pulmonary emphysema. N Engl J Med 1950; 243:549–58.
10. Brantigan OC, Mueller E: Surgical Treatment of pulmonary emphysema. Am Surg 1957; 23:789–804.
11. Miller JI, Lee RB, Mansour KA: Lung volume reduction surgery: lessons learned. Ann Thorac Surg 1996; 61:1464–9.
12. Naunheim KS, Ferguson MK: The current status of lung volume reduction operations for emphysema. Ann Thorac Surg 1996; 62:601–12.
13. Weinmann GG, Hyatt R: Evaluation and research in lung volume reduction surgery. Am J Respir Crit Care Med 1996; 154:1913–8.
14. Geddes D, Davies M, Koyama H, et al.: Effect of lung-volume-

reduction surgery in patients with severe emphysema. N Engl J Med 2000; 343:239–45.

15. Drazen JM, Epstein AM: Guidance concerning surgery for emphysema. N Engl J Med 2003; 348:2134–6.
16. Babb TG, Viggiano R, Hurley B, Staats BA, Rodarte JR: Effect of mild-to-moderate airflow limitation on exercise capacity. J Appl Physiol 1991; 70:223–30.
17. Tobin MJ: Respiratory muscles in disease. Clin Chest Med 1988; 9:263–86.
18. Dueck R, Cooper S, Kapelanski D, Colt H, Clauser J: A pilot study of expiratory flow limitation and lung volume reduction surgery. Chest 1999; 116:1762–71.
19. Gelb AF, Zamel N, McKenna RJ, Brenner M: Mechanism of short-term improvement in lung function after emphysema resection. Am J Respir Crit Care Med 1996; 154:945–51.
20. Marchand E, Gayan-Ramirez G, De Leyn P, Decramer M: Physiological basis of improvement after lung volume reduction surgery for severe emphysema: where are we? Eur Respir J 1999; 13:686–96.
21. Sciurba FC, Rogers RM, Keenan RJ, Slivka WA, Gorcsan J, Ferson PF, Holbert JM, Brown ML, Landreneau RJ: Improvement in pulmonary function and elastic recoil after lung-reduction surgery for diffuse emphysema. N Engl J Med 1996; 334:1095–99.
22. Tschernko EM, Wisser W, Hofer S, et al.: Influence of lung volume reduction on ventilatory mechanics in patients suffering from severe COPD. Anesth Analg 1996; 83:996–1001.
23. O'Donnell DE, Webb KA, Bertley JC, Laurence KL, Chau MB, Conlan AA: Mechanisms of relief of exertional breathlessness following unilateral bullectomy and lung volume reduction surgery emphysema. Chest 1996; 110:18–27.
24. American College of Physicians: Preoperative pulmonary function testing. Ann Intern Med 1990; 112:793–4.
25. Tschernko EM, Wisser W, Wanke T, Rajel MA, Kritzinger M, Lahrmann H, Kontrus M, Benditte H, Klepetko W: Changes in ventilatory mechanics and diaphragmatic function after lung volume reduction surgery in patients with COPD. Thorax 1997; 52:545–50.
26. O'Donnell DE, Webb KA, Bertley JC, Laurence KL, Chau MB, Conlan AA: Mechanisms of relief of exertional breathlessness following unilateral bullectomy and lung volume reduction surgery emphysema. Chest 1996; 110:18–27.
27. Hoppin FG: Theoretical basis for improvement following reductiopneumoplasty in emphysema. Am J Respir Crit Care Med 1997; 155:520–5.
28. Tschernko EM, Gruber EM, Jaksch P, et al.: Ventilatory mechanics

and gas exchange during exercise before and after lung volume reduction surgery. Am J Respir Crit Care Med 1998; 158:1424–31.

29. Benditt JO, Wood DE, McCool D, Lewis S, Albert RK: Changes in breathing and ventilatory muscle recruitment patterns induced by lung volume reduction surgery. Am J Respir Crit Care Med 1997; 155:279–84.

30. Baydur A: Improvements in lung and respiratory muscle function following lung volume reduction surgery. Chest 1999; 116:1507–9.

31. Lahrmann H, Wild M, Wanke T, Tschernko E, Wisser W, Klepetko W, Zwick H: Neural drive to the diaphragm after lung volume reduction surgery. Chest 1999; 116:1593–1600.

32. Daniel TM, Barry BK, Chan MD, Varun Bhaskar MD, et al.: Lung volume reduction surgery: case selection, operative technique, and clinical results. Ann Surg 1996; 223:526–33.

33. Thurnheer R, Muntwyler J, Stammberger U, Bloch KE, Zollinger A, Weder W, Russi EW: Coronary artery disease in patients undergoing lung volume reduction surgery for emphysema. Chest 1997; 112:122–8.

34. Weder W, Thurnheer R, Stammberger U, Buerge M, Russi EW, Bloch KE: Radiologic emphysema morphology is associated with outcome after surgical lung volume reduction. Ann Thorac Surg 1997; 64:313–20.

35. Hamacher J, Block KE, Stammberger U, Schmid RA, Laube I, Russi EW, Weder W: Two years' outcome of lung volume reduction surgery in different morphologic emphysema types. Ann Thorac Surg 1999; 68:1792–8.

36. Rogers RM, Coxson HO, Sciurba FC, Keenan RJ, Whittall KP, Hogg JC: Preoperative severity of emphysema predictive of improvement after lung volume reduction surgery—use of CT morphometry. Chest 2000; 118:1240–7.

37. Salzman SH: Can CT measurement of emphysema severity aid patient selection for lung volume reduction surgery? Chest 2000; 118:1231–2.

38. Thurnheer R, Engel H, Weder W, Stammberger U, Laube I, Russi EW, Bloch KE: Role of lung perfusion scintigraphy in relation to chest computed tomography and pulmonary function in the evaluation of candidates for lung volume reduction surgery. Am J Respir Crit Care Med 1999; 159:301–10.

39. Ingenito EP, Evans RB, Loring SH, et al.: Relation between preoperative inspiratory lung resistance and the outcome of lung-volume-reduction surgery for emphysema. N Engl J Med 1998; 338:1181–5.

40. Tschernko EM, Kritzinger M, Gruber EM, Jantsch-Watzinger U, Jandrasits O, Mares P, Wisser W, Klepetko W, Haider W: Lung vol-

ume reduction surgery: preoperative functional predictors for postoperative outcome. Anesth Analg 1999; 88:28–33.

41. Weinberg M, Hendeles L. Methylxanthines. In: Weiss EB, Segal MS, Stein M, eds: Bronchial Asthma. Mechanisms and Therapeutics. 2nd ed. Boston: Little, Brown and Company, 1985; 57–90.

42. Hughes RL, Davison R: Limitations of exercise reconditioning in COPD. Chest 1983;83:241–9.

43. Tuxen DV, Lane S: The effects of ventilatory pattern on hyperinflation, airway pressures, and circulation in mechanical ventilation of patients with severe air-flow obstruction. Am Rev Respir Dis 1987; 136:872–9.

44. Ballantyne JC, Carr DB, de Ferranti S, et al.: The comparative effects of postoperative analgesic therapies on pulmonary outcome: cumulative meta-analyses of randomized, controlled trials. Anesth Analg 1998;86:598–612.

45. Warner DO: Preventing postoperative pulmonary complications. Anesthesiology 2000;92:1467–72.

46. Loehning RW, Waltemath CL, Bergman NA: Lidocaine and increased respiratory resistance produced by ultrasonic aerosols. Anesthesiology 1976; 44:306–10.

47. Brandus V, Joffe S, Benoit CV, Wolff WI: Bronchial spasm during general anesthesia. Can Anesth Soc J 1970; 17:269–74.

Stephen H. Pennefather, MRCP, FRCA
G.N. Russell, FRCA

Postthoracotomy Analgesia: Recent Advances and Future Directions

8

INTRODUCTION

Lung cancer is the leading cause of cancer death in Europe (1), and surgery offers the only realistic prospect of a cure. In the United States, the incidence of esophageal adenocarcinoma is rising more quickly than that of any other cancer (2). Esophageal cancer is now the eighth most common malignancy worldwide (3), and again, surgery offers the only realistic prospect of a cure. In addition, thoracotomies are increasingly utilized to provide access in patients undergoing cardiac, vascular, orthopaedic, and neurosurgical procedures. In the medium term, it is anticipated that an increasing number of patients will undergo open thoracotomy and require effective postthoracotomy analgesia. The profile of patients referred for thoracic surgery is ageing. Although increasing age is associated with increased comorbidity, recent data suggest that up to the age of 80, age itself has no significant effect on mortality (4). It is anticipated that in the future, elderly patients will form a larger proportion of the population requiring postthoracotomy analgesia.

When compared to open thoracotomy, video-assisted surgical techniques can significantly reduce postoperative pain. The perioperative morbidity and mortality for thoracoscopic lobectomy is similar to that of open lobectomies (5), as is the long-term survival (5, 6). Currently, in the United Kingdom, less than 2% of lobectomies are performed by video-assisted techniques (7). The technology is, however, developing rapidly, and

Progress in Thoracic Anesthesia, edited by Peter Slinger,
Lippincott Williams & Wilkins, Baltimore © 2004.

it is anticipated that in the future, widespread use of minimal-access surgery will simplify the provision of postthoracotomy analgesia.

Postthoracotomy pain can be very severe. The standard posterolateral thoracotomy has been described as one of the most painful iatrogenic procedures (8). Elderly patients (and their surgeons) may be reluctant to undergo thoracotomy if the postthoracotomy pain control is considered to be poor; thus, the discussion to operate is influenced by the availability of reliable and effective postthoracotomy analgesia. Effective postthoracotomy analgesia may, in addition, decrease perioperative stress (9, 10), reduce perioperative chest complications (11–13), improve outcome (11, 14), and limit chronic postthoracotomy pain (15–17).

During the past decade, significant improvements have been made in our understanding of the efficiency, safety, and limitations of the various methods for providing postthoracotomy analgesia. Changes have resulted from the adaptation and refinement of existing drugs and techniques rather than from the introduction of radically new approaches. For patients not receiving epidural analgesia, thoracic paravertebral blocks are increasingly used as part of a multimodal therapy. In the West, thoracic epidural analgesia has now replaced systemic opioids as the mainstay of postthoracotomy analgesia.

PATHOPHYSIOLOGY OF POSTTHORACOTOMY PAIN

An open thoracotomy necessitates a skin incision, division and retraction of underlying muscles, as well as retraction and, possibly, fracture of ribs. The incised pleura may be further irritated by partial surgical stripping, chest drains, and residual pleural blood. Costophrenic joints may be dislocated, and intercostal nerves are sometimes injured. Not surprisingly, postthoracotomy pain can be very severe. Inspiration stretches these injured structures, and reflex contraction of the expiratory muscles occurs to limit distraction of the injured structures. Thus, the usually passive expiration becomes active. Functional residual capacity (FRC) falls, usually to below closing capacity, and airway closure occurs, with resultant atelectasis, shunting, and hypoxemia. Deep inspiration is limited by pain, and forced expiratory flow is reduced. Sputum clearance is impaired. Effective analgesia can reverse some of these changes and improve pulmonary function after thoracotomy. There are, however, many other causes for the deterioration in pulmonary function that occurs after thoracotomy (Table 8.1). To date, it has not been possible to determine with any accuracy the relative importance of pain in the etiology of the changes in pulmonary function seen after thoracotomy.

TABLE 8.1   Causes for Deterioration in Pulmonary Function after Thoracotomy

Lung tissue resection
Hemorrhage and edema in residual lung tissue
Distortion in bronchial architecture, with resultant lobar collapse
Gastric and abdominal distension
Increased airway resistance
Impaired mucociliary clearance
Residual effects of anesthesia
Pain-related changes in lung mechanics
Diaphragmatic dysfunction

It has been widely accepted that three main mechanisms transmit the postthoracotomy pain to the sensorium (8, 18):

1. Stimuli from the chest wall and most of the pleura via the intercostal nerves.
2. Stimuli from the diaphragmatic pleura via the phrenic nerve.
3. Stimuli from the lung and mediastinum, including the mediastinal pleura via the vagus nerve.

A possible role for the sympathetic nerves, stretching of the brachial plexuses, and distraction of the shoulder has also been postulated (8, 19).

Recent work has improved our understanding of the mechanisms of postthoracotomy pain. Thoracic epidural analgesia provides excellent postthoracotomy pain relief in the dermatomes incised; however, most patients still experience ipsilateral shoulder pain, which is sometimes severe (20, 21). Blocking the phrenic nerve with lidocaine at the level of the diaphragm abolishes this shoulder pain in most patients (21). Further analysis of that study shows that patients without shoulder pain experienced almost no early postthoracotomy pain as well as a mean visual analog scale pain score of 1 (scale, 0–10 cm) 2 hours after thoracotomy.

The vagus nerve contains somatic and visceral afferent nerve fibres, and blockade of the vagus nerve has been advocated for thoracic surgery (22). However, the contribution, if any, of the vagus nerve to postthoracotomy pain is unclear. The ability of a combined phrenic nerve block and thoracic epidural to almost eliminate early postthoracotomy pain suggests that any contribution of vagal nerve block to postthoracotomy analgesia is minimal. In contrast, vagal nerve stimulation suppresses human pain (23), and it is possible that blocking the vagus nerve would increase pain by reducing vagally mediated central inhibition of pain.

Blocking the phrenic nerve at the level of the diaphragm does not prevent shoulder pain in all patients (21). The phrenic nerve supplies

sensory branches to the mediastinal pleura and to the fibrous pericardium and the parietal layer of the serous pericardium. It may be necessary to infiltrate the phrenic nerve more proximally to block the sensory branches to the pericardium and mediastinal pleura. Indirect
support for this comes from the observation that blocking the phrenic
nerve at the level of the diaphragm was not effective in preventing
shoulder pain in patients undergoing intrapericardial pneumonectomy
(21), although the presence of an accessory phrenic nerve in some patients needs to be considered.

Shoulder pain is unlikely to be the result of shoulder distraction,
because patients receiving thoracic epidural analgesia postthoracotomy
do not experience a reduction in ipsilateral shoulder pain with suprascapular nerve blockade (24). Phrenic nerve blockade may not be appropriate for many patients undergoing thoracotomy because of the associated loss of motor supply to the diaphragm. However, phrenic
nerve block may be beneficial for patients undergoing bilobectomies or
pneumonectomies, because the associated unilateral loss of diaphragmatic function may help to reduce the "pneumonectomy space."

POSTTHORACOTOMY ANALGESIC TECHNIQUES

Well-informed patients may experience less pain (25), so all patients
should receive a full and accurate account of what to expect postoperatively. Postthoracotomy analgesic strategies should be selected (Table
8.2) and adapted to suit the individual patient.

In the past, systemic opioids were the most frequently used method
of providing postthoracotomy analgesia. However, because the pain

TABLE 8.2 Factors to Consider when Choosing a Postthoracotomy Analgesic Technique

Surgical factors
  Planned procedure (eg, pneumonectomy vs pleurectomy)
  Painfulness of incision (clam shell > posterolateral > axillary muscle sparing
    > sternotomy)
  Planned access (open vs video-assisted thoracoscopy)
Patient factors
  Preference
  Physiology (eg, pulmonary reserve)
  Pathology (eg, ischemic heart disease)
  Pharmacology (eg, recreational opioid use)
Resource factors
  Anesthetic expertise with technique
  Infrastructure (acute pain service)

control with systemic opioids is generally poor, many other strategies are now used in place of (or in addition to) systemic opioids. In our unit, more than 95% of patients undergoing esophagectomies or open lung resections receive thoracic epidural analgesia. We usually treat the remaining patients with a combination of systemic opioids, paravertebral blocks, and nonopioid analgesic drugs.

Systemic Opioids

Accurate titration of systemic opioids postthoracotomy is required if a balance between beneficial effects (analgesia sufficient to preserve FRC by prevent splinting and enabling passive expiration) and detrimental effects (sedation, hypoventilation, cough inhibition, and reduced sighing) is to be achieved. Achieving this balance is complicated by the many-fold variation between patients in postoperative opioid requirement (26) and the exponential decrease in opioid requirements that occurs after surgery (26, 27). In addition, a small group of patients may experience minimal postsurgical pain (28). In comparison to intramuscular opioids, the widely used in PCA (patient-controlled analgesia) systems provide superior analgesia and improves patient satisfaction. There is, however, no evidence to suggest that they improve outcome (12). When used in isolation, the pain control achieved in the early postthoracotomy period with systemic opioids is generally poor. Systemic opioids are best given as part of a multimodal strategy that includes nonopioid analgesic drugs and nerve blocks.

Nonopioid Analgesic Drugs

Nonsteroidal Anti-Inflammatory Drugs

Pain perception is dependent, in part, on prostaglandins. Nonsteroidal anti-inflammatory drugs (NSAIDs) block the synthesis of prostaglandins by inhibiting the enzyme cyclo-oxygenase. The NSAIDs also have centrally mediated (29) and peripheral nonprostaglandin (30) analgesic effects. The side effects of NSAIDs are potentially serious. Gastrointestinal bleeding as a result of impaired gastric mucus production is well known (31). Creatinine clearance decreases transiently during the postoperative period in normal patients receiving NSAIDs for analgesia (32). There is an increased risk of developing NSAID-induced renal failure in elderly patients undergoing major surgery (33, 34), patients with pre-existing renal failure, hypovolemic patients, and patients with congestive heart failure. Two different isoenzymes of the cyclo-oxygenase enzyme exist: COX-1 and COX-2 (35). The COX-1 isoenzyme has physiological functions, whereas the COX-2 isoenzyme is induced during inflammation.

Selective COX-2 inhibition should produce less impairment of the homeostatic functions of prostaglandins. The NSAIDs vary in their selectivity for inhibiting the cyclo-oxygenase isoenzymes. The COX-2-selective inhibitors (Celecoxib, etodolac, meloxicam, and rofecoxib) have a lower risk of serious upper gastrointestinal side effects and cause less platelet inhibition than nonselective NSAIDs. Future developments of COX-2 inhibitors that are more selective may further increase the safety profile of NSAIDs.

For more than 20 years, NSAIDs have been used to control post-thoracotomy pain (36). They have been shown to significantly improve pain control in patients receiving systemic opioids after thoracotomy (37, 38), but they have not been shown to significantly reduce pain scores in patients receiving thoracic epidural analgesia after thoracotomy (39). The NSAIDs may be effective in controlling the ipsilateral shoulder pain after thoracotomy in patients receiving thoracic epidural analgesia (21), although research in this area has been limited.

Paracetamol (Acetaminophen)

Paracetamol is a basic analgesic that is frequently used to supplement postthoracotomy analgesia (40). Because the effects of paracetamol and NSAIDs are additive (41, 42), these drugs can be combined to provide additional postthoracotomy analgesia. Used alone, paracetamol is considered to be safe for patients at risk of renal failure (43). When administered rectally, the dosage should exceed the oral dose by 50%, and its slower onset should be considered (43). The place in the treatment of postthoracotomy pain of the recently developed precursor of paracetamol, proparacetamol, which can be administered intravenously, is still being established.

Paravertebral Blocks

Paravertebral blocks were introduced into clinical practice in 1906 (44). After some initial popularity, thoracic paravertebral blocks were largely abandoned (45); however, they were reintroduced in 1979 (46). Since then, substantial experience has been gained in the use of thoracic paravertebral block, and its safety has been established. For patients undergoing thoracotomy, thoracic paravertebral block are probably best established by a catheter placed surgically into the paravertebral space, deep to the endothoracic fascia (47) and brought out of the chest by a separate intercostal puncture. An earlier surgical technique was to create a subpleural paravertebral pocket by reflecting the parietal pleura from the wound margin (48). For patients undergoing video-assisted surgery, video assistance for surgical placement of the catheter (49) may be appropriate, but an alternative is the percutaneous placement of a paravertebral catheter.

A number of different techniques for the percutaneous placement of paravertebral catheters have been described. We insert a Tuohy needle 2.5 cm lateral to the rostral edge of the appropriate spinous process. The needle is the advanced perpendicular to the skin until contact is made with the underlying transverse process. If contact with bone is not made at the expected depth, the needle is withdrawn and then readvanced slowly, while fanning it in the sagittal plane, until contact with bone is made. At this point, the needle is walked off the rostral edge of the transverse process and advanced slowly for approximately 1 cm until a loss of resistance (less complete than that in the epidural space) is encountered. This is frequently preceded by a subtle click as the costotransverse ligament is penetrated. After aspiration to confirm that the needle is extravascular, approximately 20 mL of 0.25% bupivacaine is administered to open up the paravertebral space and to facilitate threading of a catheter into the paravertebral space. Consideration may be given to adding a small quantity of dye to the local anaesthetic that is administered so that correct placement of the block can be confirmed visually at thoracoscopy.

The reported effectiveness of thoracic paravertebral block varies, but when used appropriately, thoracic paravertebral block can provide analgesia similar (50) or, in one study (51), superior to a local anaesthetic-only thoracic epidural. Patients receiving thoracic paravertebral block rarely report ipsilateral shoulder pain, possibly because shoulder pain is masked by significant incisional pain. Because the analgesia produced by paravertebral block alone is rarely good, analgesia is usually supplemented with systemic opioids and NSAIDs.

Thoracic paravertebral blocks are technically simple to perform, but they have a failure rate of approximately 10% (52). Complications include inadvertent pleural puncture, pulmonary hemorrhage, hypotension, nerve injury, inadvertent dural puncture, and central nervous system local anaesthetic toxicity. The latter is of concern, because mean plasma concentrations have been shown to exceed the threshold for central nervous system toxicity 48 hours after commencing a 0.1 mL kg^{-1} h^{-1} (usual rate) infusion of 0.5% bupivacaine (53). In a separate study (51), 7% of patients receiving paravertebral 0.5% bupivacaine at this rate developed temporary confusion attributed to bupivacaine accumulation. Because lower concentrations of bupivacaine are less effective, the addition of adrenaline to the bupivacaine or use of the newer, less toxic ropivacaine should be considered. Thoracic paravertebral blocks are, however, safe, and as of this writing, no fatality directly related to their use has been reported (54).

The relatively short duration of local anesthetic agents necessitates the use of an infusion or repeated blocks to provide ongoing postthoracotomy analgesia with the associated risks of local anesthetic toxicity and catheter dislodgement. Efforts to develop ultralong-acting local anesthetics may mean that it will someday be possible to place ultralong-acting local anesthetics in the paravertebral space. Efforts to develop ultralong-acting local anesthetics have recently focussed on new drug-delivery systems.

Biodegradable bupivacaine containing polylactic-coglycolic acid polymer microcapsules have been developed and shown to produce prolonged local anesthesia (55). The addition of glucocorticoid within the microcapsule further prolongs this local anaesthesia (56). In sheep, bupivacaine-dexamethasone microcapsules produced a prolonged block without development of the granulomatous reactions that occurred around the bupivacaine-only microspheres (57). In humans, the use of bupivacaine-dexamethasone microcapsules has been shown to produce an intercostal nerve block with a duration of as long as 4 days (58).

Bupivacaine has been incorporated into liposomes (59). Liposomal bupivacaine has been shown to have a prolonged action in animals (60), and it has been used to provide postoperative epidural analgesia in humans (61).

Intrapleural Blocks

The terminology used to describe the deposition of local anesthetic between the parietal and visceral pleura is confusing. Some authors have called this block interpleural (62), and others have suggested the term pleural block (63). The issue is further confused by use of the term interpleural block to describe both intrapleural and paravertebral blocks (64). Although a large number of studies have shown intrapleural blocks to be effective after cholecystectomy (64), the efficacy of intrapleural blocks after thoracotomy is, at best, variable. Some advantage was in seen early studies (65, 66), but most (mainly later) studies showed little or no benefit (67–70). The pleura are normally closely applied to each other, and the wide spread of local anesthetic within this potential space probably accounts for the effectiveness of intrapleural blocks after cholecystectomy. After thoracotomy, the pleural space contains blood and air, and dependent pooling of local anesthetic is promoted and the spread of local anesthetics limited. Dilution of local anaesthetic with blood (65) and loss of local anesthetic into the chest drains (70, 71) further reduce the efficacy of this technique. We now rarely use this technique to provide postthoracotomy analgesia in adults.

Epidural Analgesia

Postthoracotomy thoracic epidural analgesia was introduced into clinical practice during the 1970s (72). It was not until the 1990s, however, that thoracic epidural analgesia became the mainstay of postthoracotomy analgesia in most high-volume units, including our own (40). Widespread use of the thoracic epidural for routine postthoracotomy analgesia occurred because it provides effective and reliable postthoracotomy analgesia, reduces the postthoracotomy complication rate, and is believed to improve outcome. Thoracic epidurals are best placed at the dermatomal level of the surgical incision. In some reported studies, 10% to 15% of epidural catheters could not be inserted or failed to provide postoperative analgesia (73). These technical failures are of significance to individual patients and also limit the potential benefits of thoracic epidural analgesia. In the future, increased familiarity with insertion and accurate confirmation of thoracic epidural placement may reduce these technical failures. Unsuccessful catheter placement rates of 1% and failed epidural rates of less than 1% have already been reported (74), and it is anticipated that these rates will become the norm.

When unsupplemented epidural local anaesthetics are used to provide postthoracotomy analgesia, high concentrations provide effective analgesia, but the incidence of side effects is high (75). Lower concentrations are less effective. Unlike epidural local anaesthetics, epidural opioids have not been shown to reduce the incidence of postoperative pulmonary complications (12). The synergistic antinociceptive interactions of epidural local anesthetics and opioids (76) enable the amount of each drug administered to be minimized, thereby decreasing the incidence and severity of the associated side effects. Mixtures of local anesthetics and opioids are therefore widely used to provide postthoracotomy analgesia (40, 77). Although probably no epidural mixture is optimal for all patients, a mixture of 4 μg mL^{-1} of fentanyl in 0.125% bupivacaine is close (78), and this or similar mixtures are widely used. In our unit, we routinely use 5 μg mL^{-1} of fentanyl in 0.1% bupivacaine and administer a 0.1 mL kg^{-1} bolus before surgery. We then infuse the epidural mixture at 0.1 mL kg^{-1} h^{-1}, adjusting the infusion rate if appropriate.

Epinephrine improves the analgesic effect of epidural opioids and local anesthetics. Epinephrine-mediated epidural vasoconstriction is thought to be the major cause of this effect, but an α_2-adrenergic action of epinephrine in the substantia gelatinosa may contribute to the analgesia (79). Concerns about the vasoconstrictive effects on vessels to the central nervous system have limited the use of epidural epinephrine. There is, however, considerable clinical experience with epidural clonidine, another α_2-adrenergic agonist. When combined with epidural opioids, clonidine reduces opioid requirements and opioid-related side effects

(80). The addition of clonidine did not significantly improve analgesia in a study using an optimization model to find the best epidural combination of fentanyl, bupivacaine, and clonidine to administer after laparotomy (78). Although epidural clonidine is not widely used to provide postthoracotomy analgesia in the United Kingdom (77), the addition of clonidine to the epidural mixture should be considered for some patients who are particularly sensitive to epidural opioids.

Urinary Retention

Urinary retention is a complication of epidural opioid use (81). This is thought to result from inhibition of the sacral parasympathetic outflow and of the pontine micturition center (82). Epidural morphine decreases detrusor muscle function in human volunteers, and this decrease is antagonized by naloxone (83). Naloxone can reverse bladder dysfunction without reversing analgesia in patients receiving epidural morphine analgesia after uterine surgery (84). Concerns about late respiratory depression have limited the use of epidural hydrophilic opioids after thoracotomy, and bupivacaine-fentanyl mixtures are widely used (77). Young men in particular experience considerable discomfort because of urgency if they awaken with a functioning thoracic epidural and urinary catheter after thoracotomy. When given to postthoracotomy patients receiving a bupivacaine-fentanyl thoracic epidural analgesia, low-dose naloxone reverses the analgesic effects of the epidural fentanyl without reducing the need for urinary catheterization (85). Naloxone should not be used to treat nonlife-threatening complications in patients receiving bupivacaine-fentanyl thoracic epidural analgesia.

Gastric Emptying

Patients receiving thoracic epidural analgesia after thoracotomy for lung resection are usually comfortable. Normal diet and oral medication can be resumed a few hours postoperatively. Gastric emptying, the rate-limiting step for the absorption of most orally administered drugs, is variably affected by anesthesia and surgery (86–89). Gastric emptying has been shown to be normal in patients receiving bupivacaine epidural analgesia after cholecystectomy (89). The stomach receives its innervation through branches of the vagus nerve and T6–10 sympathetic nerves (90). Epidural opioids cause gastric hypomobility, whereas sympathetic blockade by epidural local anesthetic may, in contrast, hasten gastric emptying. Gastric emptying is delayed for more than 48 hours postthoracotomy in patients receiving 10 µg mL^{-1} of fentanyl in 0.1% bupivacaine via a thoracic epidural for analgesia (91). It is not known if this delay would be reduced by using a lower concentration of epidural fentanyl. The delayed gastric emptying after thoracotomy is of significance, because it may lead to reflux or regurgitation, with possible aspiration. In addition, the desired effect of orally administered drugs may not be achieved.

Awake Vs Asleep Insertion of Thoracic Epidurals

For many years, controversy has existed regarding whether thoracic epidurals are best inserted with the patient awake or asleep (92–94). In Britain during the mid-1990s, most thoracic epidurals were inserted with the patient anesthetized (77). Although no study has shown that awake insertion reduces the incidence of iatrogenic spinal injury, the incidence of awake insertion of thoracic epidurals is increasing (95).

A number of factors have contributed to this change in practice. It was once argued that cord injury during awake insertion might not be recognized. It is now accepted, however, that needle injury to the cord is associated with pain (96–98). Medicolegal positions have also changed, and now in Germany, for example, guidelines require all thoracic epidurals to be inserted in awake patients. Greater use of thoracic epidurals has improved confidence in their insertion. For those patients unable to receive a thoracic epidural while awake, treatment with a combination of thoracic paravertebral block, systemic opioids, and NSAIDs is now seen as providing an acceptable alternative (54). This has reduced the perceived need to insert thoracic epidurals into anesthetized patients. Unrecognized malplacement of a thoracic epidural is becoming less acceptable as the advantages of thoracic epidural analgesia are increasingly recognized. Awake insertion followed by testing and, if necessary, replacement before the induction of anesthesia can greatly reduce—if not eliminate—this problem.

POSTTHORACOTOMY ANALGESIA AND OUTCOME

Although effective analgesia reduces postthoracotomy morbidity and mortality, not all equianalgesic techniques are equivalent in this respect. Evidence is accumulating that thoracic epidurals containing local anesthetics are superior to other techniques in reducing postthoracotomy morbidity and mortality.

Chronic Postthoracotomy Pain

Chronic postthoracotomy pain is a continuous dysesthetic pain, occurring in 50% to 80% of patients after thoracotomy (99, 100). Most patients experience mild pain, but 3% to 5% experience severe pain (100). The etiology is thought to be intercostal nerve damage during thoracotomy. Cryoanalgesia, the direct application of a cryoprobe to intercostal nerves during thoracotomy, is associated with the development of chronic postthoracotomy pain (93, 101). A correlation between acute postthoracotomy pain and the development of chronic postthoracotomy pain has been noted (15, 100), and evidence suggests that preoperative initiation of epidural analgesia can reduce the incidence of chronic postthoracotomy pain (17, 102).

Respiratory Complications

Good evidence indicates that thoracic epidural analgesia reduces the incidence of respiratory complications after thoracic surgery. Epidural analgesia has been shown, in a randomized study, to reduce respiratory failure after major abdominal surgery (73). A recent meta-analysis showed that neuraxial blocks reduce the incidence of pneumonia after a range of operations and that this reduction was greatest for patients receiving thoracic epidural analgesia (11). An earlier meta-analysis showed that epidurals containing local anesthetics, but not solely opioid epidurals, reduced the incidence of pulmonary complications after a variety of surgeries (12). For patients undergoing pneumonectomy, it has been shown that thoracic epidural analgesia is associated with a significant reduction in respiratory complications (13). There are a number of possible mechanisms whereby thoracic epidural analgesia may reduce respiratory complications after thoracotomy. These include better preservation of FRC; improved mucociliary clearance; reduction of inhibitory effects on the diaphragm; less pain, nausea, and sedation; and better co-ordination with physiotherapy.

Improved Postoperative Diaphragmatic Dysfunction

Prolonged diaphragmatic dysfunction occurs after thoracic (103) and upper abdominal (104) surgery. It has been postulated that this dysfunction is secondary to reflex inhibition of the phrenic nerve from stimulation of afferent nerves in the viscera, diaphragm, and chest wall (105). Diaphragmatic function is not improved by epidural opioid analgesia (104), and pain is not considered to be a major mediator (106). The contractility of the diaphragm is not impaired (105, 107). Thoracic epidural local anesthetics can improve diaphragmatic function after upper abdominal surgery (108) and after thoracotomy in animals (106). Thoracic epidural local anesthetics have not been shown to improve the impaired diaphragmatic segmental shortening after thoracotomy in humans, although other ventilatory parameters did improve. However, because epidural local anaesthetics can alter other respiratory muscle functions, an improvement in diaphragmatic function may have been masked (103).

Functional Residual Capacity

A number of factors, including pain, contribute to the fall in FRC that occurs after thoracotomy. The analgesic effects of a thoracic epidural analgesia may moderate this decrease in FRC by enabling passive expiration. In addition, thoracic epidural analgesia may directly affect FRC after thoracotomy, because an increase in FRC occurs in healthy patients receiving thoracic epidural analgesia (109).

Cardiovascular Complications

Postoperative myocardial infarction contributes significantly to total postthoracotomy morbidity and mortality. Thoracic epidural analgesia can block the T1–5 sympathetic nerve fibers to the heart and have been used to treat refractory angina (110, 111). Thoracic epidural analgesia can improve hemodynamic stability, reduce postoperative hypercoagulability (112), and dilate constricted coronary arteries of patients undergoing thoracic surgery. If not accompanied by excessive hypotension, these changes have the potential to reduce myocardial ischemia. A recent meta-analysis of patients undergoing various surgeries has confirmed this potential as well as shown that epidural analgesia reduces the rate of postoperative myocardial infarctions by 40% and that thoracic epidural analgesia is superior to lumber epidural analgesia in this respect (113).

Supraventricular arrhythmias, usually atrial fibrillation, occur in 20% to 30% of patients after thoracotomy (114, 115) and are associated with increased mortality (116, 117). Some evidence suggests that decreasing the sympathetic tone by using thoracic epidural local anesthetics reduces the incidence of supraventricular arrhythmias (118).

Mortality

The recent reduction in postthoracotomy mortality has, in part, resulted from improvements in postthoracotomy analgesia. The debate as to whether thoracic epidural analgesia specifically reduces mortality is ongoing. There are good theoretical reasons to believe that thoracic epidural analgesia may reduce postthoracotomy mortality. Epidural analgesia can reduce postoperative pulmonary complications (11–13), decrease perioperative myocardial infarctions (113), and reduce the incidence of thromboembolic events (119, 120). These potential advantages, however, must be balanced against the rare—and potentially fatal—risks associated with thoracic epidural use. In addition, hypotension induced by epidural analgesia or vasoconstrictors used to treat the hypotension may adversely affect outcome (121). A meta-analysis reviewing 30 years of randomized, controlled studies showed that neuraxial blocks reduce mortality after surgery (11). Retrospective analysis has shown thoracic epidural analgesia to be associated with a lower mortality rate after thoracoabdominal esophagectomy (122). In contrast, a large, prospective, randomized study of patients undergoing major abdominal surgery did not show epidural analgesia to be associated with reduced mortality (73).

In high-risk thoracic patients, there would be considerable difficulties in undertaking a prospective, randomized study to determine the influence of thoracic epidural analgesia on mortality. There may never be such a study.

CONCLUSIONS

Pain control is central to the care of patients undergoing thoracic surgery. Recent advances in postoperative analgesia have resulted in most patients experiencing less postthoracotomy pain. In itself, this represents a significant advance, but there is now convincing evidence that thoracic epidural analgesia can reduce postthoracotomy morbidity, particularly respiratory complications. The influence of thoracic epidurals on mortality after thoracotomy is less clear, although evidence suggests that they may reduce mortality in high-risk patients undergoing esophagectomy or lung resections. It is anticipated that in the future, additional data regarding the risk:benefit ratio for thoracic epidural analgesia will aid in the difficult decision whether to use epidural insertion for high-risk patients who are also at increased risk of epidural-related complications.

It is now possible to enable patient to experience minimal pain after thoracotomy. Postthoracotomy analgesia should minimize mortality, patient suffering, and other morbidity. It is unlikely, however, that a single technique will optimally fullfil all these objectives for all patients.

In the future, the development of clinically useable, ultralong-acting local anesthetics might enable significant further advances to be made in the provision of postthoracotomy analgesia.

References

1. Ferlay J, Black RJ, Pisani P, et al.: Cancer in the European Union: IARC Cancer-Base. Lyon, France, International Agency for Cancer Research, 1996.
2. Cohen S, Parkman HP: Heartburn—a serious symptom. N Engl J Med 1999; 340:878–9.
3. Landis SH, Murray T, Bolden S, Wingo PA: Cancer statistics: 1999. CA Cancer J Clin 1999; 49:8–31.
4. Massard G, Moog R, Wihlm JM, Kessler R, Dabbagh A, Lesage A, Roeslin N, Morand G: Bronchogenic cancer in the elderly: operative risk and long-term prognosis. Thorac Cardiovasc Surg 1996; 44:40–5.
5. Lewis RJ, Caccavale RJ, Sisler GE, Bocage JP, Mackenzie JW: One hundred video-assisted thoracic surgical simultaneously stapled lobectomies without rib spreading. Ann Thorac Surg 1997; 63:1415–21.
6. Walker WS: Video-assisted thoracic surgery (VATS) lobectomy: the Edinburgh experience. Semin Thorac Cardiovasc Surg 1998; 10:291–9.
7. BTS Guidelines: Guidelines on the selection of patients with lung cancer for surgery. Thorax 2001; 56:89–108.
8. Conacher ID: Pain relief after thoracotomy. Br J Anaesth 1990; 65:806–12.
9. Rigg JR: Does regional block improve outcome after surgery? Anaesth Intensive Care 1991; 19:404–11.
10. Liu S, Carpenter RL, Neal JM: Epidural anesthesia and analgesia. Their role in postoperative outcome. Anesthesiology 1995; 82: 1474–506.
11. Rodgers A, Walker N, Schug S, McKee A, Kehlet H, van Zundert A, Sage D, Futter M, Saville G, Clark T, MacMahon S: Reduction of postoperative mortality and morbidity with epidural or spinal anaesthesia: results from overview of randomized trials. BMJ 2000; 321:1493–97.
12. Ballantyne JC, Carr DB, deFerranti S, Suarez T, Lau J, Chalmers TC, Angelillo IF, Mosteller F: The comparative effects of postoperative analgesic therapies on pulmonary outcome: cumulative meta-analyses of randomized, controlled trials. Anesth Analg 1998; 86:598–612.
13. Licker M, Spiliopoulos A, Frey JG, Robert J, Hohn L, de Perrot M, Tschopp J: Risk factors for early mortality and major complications following pneumonectomy for non-small cell carcinoma of the lung. Chest 2002; 121:1890–7.
14. Tsui SL, Law S, Fok M, Lo JR, Ho E, Yang J, Wong J: Postoperative

analgesia reduces mortality and morbidity after esophagectomy. Am J Surg 1997; 173:472–8.

15. Katz J, Jackson M, Karanagh, et al.: Acute pain after thoracic surgery predicts long term postthoracotomy pain. Clin J Pain 1996; 12:50–5.

16. d'Amours RH, Riegler FX, Little AG: Pathogenesis and management of persistent postthoracotomy pain. Chest Surg Clin N Am 1998; 8:703–22.

17. Senturk M, Ozcan PE, Talu GK, Kiyan E, Camci E, Ozyalcin S, Dilege S, Pembeci K: The effects of three different analgesia techniques on long-term postthoracotomy pain. Anesth Analg 2002; 94:11–5.

18. Benumof JL: Anesthesia for Thoracic Surgery. 2nd ed. Philadelphia, WB Saunders, 1995.

19. Mark JBD, Brodsky JB: Ipsilateral shoulder pain following thoracic operations. Anesthesiology 1993; 79:192.

20. Burgess FW, Anderson DM, Colonna D, Sborov MJ, Cavanaugh DG: Ipsilateral shoulder pain following thoracic surgery. Anesthesiology 1993; 78:365–8.

21. Scawn ND, Pennefather SH, Soorae A, Wang JY, Russell GN: Ipsilateral shoulder pain after thoracotomy with epidural analgesia: the influence of phrenic nerve infiltration with lidocaine. Anesth Analg 2001; 93:260–4.

22. Macintosh RR, Mushin WW: Anaesthetics research in wartime. Medical Times 1945; 253–5.

23. Kirchner A, Birklein F, Stefan H, Handwerker HO: Left vagus nerve stimulation suppresses experimentally induced pain. Neurology 2000; 55:1167–71.

24. Tan N, Agnew NM, Scawn ND, Pennefather SH, Chester M, Russell GN: Suprascapular nerve block for ipsilateral shoulder pain after thoracotomy with thoracic epidural analgesia: a double-blind comparison of 0.5% bupivacaine and 0.9% saline. Anesth Analg 2002; 94:199–202.

25. Eghert LD, Battit GE: Reduction of postoperative pain by encouragement and instruction of patients. N Engl J Med 1964; 270:825–7.

26. Bullingham RE: Optimum management of postoperative pain. Drugs 1985; 29:376–86.

27. Bullingham RES. Postoperative pain. Postgrad Med J 1984; 60: 847–51.

28. Loan WB, Morrison JD: The incidence and severity of postoperative pain. Br J Anaesth 1967; 39:695–8.

29. Bjørkman R, Hedner T, Hallman KM, Henning M, Hedner J: Localization of the central antinociceptive effects of diclofenac in the rat. Brain Res 1992; 590:66–73.

30. Rømsing J, Møiniche S, Østergaard D, Dahl JB: Local infiltration with NSAIDs for postoperative analgesia: evidence for a peripheral analgesic action. Acta Anaesthesiol Scand 2000; 44:672–83.
31. Hawkey CJ: Nonsteroidal anti-inflammatory drugs and peptic ulcers. BMJ 1990; 300:278–84.
32. Lee A, Cooper MC, Craig JC, Knight JF, Keneally JP: The effecs of nonsteroidal anti-inflammatory drugs (NSAIDs) on postoperative renal function: a meta-analysis. Anaesth Intensive Care 1999; 27: 574–80.
33. Appadurai IR, Power I: NSAIDS in the postoperative period. Use with caution in elderly people. BMJ 1993; 307:257.
34. Gibson P, Weadington D, Winney RJ: NSAIDs in the postoperative period. Clinical experience confirms risk. BMJ 1993; 307:257–8.
35. Goppelt-Struebe M: Regulation of prostaglandin endoperoxide synthase (cyclo-oxygenase) isoenzyme expression. Prostaglandins Leukot Essent Fatty Acids 1995; 52:213–22.
36. Keenan DJ, Cave K, Langdon L, Lea RE: Comparative trial of rectal indomethacin and cryoanalgesia for control of early postthoracotomy pain. BMJ 1983; 287:1335–7.
37. Pavy T, Medley C, Murphy DF: Effect of indomethacin on pain relief after thoracotomy. Br J Anaesth 1990; 65:624–7.
38. Rhodes M, Conacher I, Morritt G, Hilton C: Nonsteroidal anti-inflammatory drugs for postthoracotomy pain. A prospective controlled trial after lateral thoracotomy. J Thorac Cardiovasc Surg 1992; 103:17–20.
39. Bigler D, Moller J, Kamp-Jensen M, Berthelsen P, Hjortso NC, Kehlet H: Effect of piroxicam in addition to continuous thoracic epidural bupivacaine and morphine on postoperative pain and lung function after thoracotomy. Acta Anaesthesiol Scand 1992; 36:647–50.
40. Cook TM, Riley RH: Analgesia following thoracotomy: a survey of Australian practice. Anaesth Intensive Care 1997; 25:520–4.
41. Montgomery JE, Sutherland CJ, Kestin IG, Sneyd JR: Morphine consumption in patients receiving rectal paracetamol and diclofenac alone and in combination. Br J Anaesth 1996; 77:445–7.
42. Seymor RA, Kelly PJ, Hawkesford JE: The efficacy of ketoprofen and paracetamol (acetaminophen) in postoperative pain after third molar surgery. Br J Clin Pharmacol 1996; 41:581–5.
43. Dahl V, Ræder JC. Nonopioid postoperative analgesia. Acta Anaesthesiol Scand 2000; 44:1191–203.
44. Sellheim H. Verh Dtch Ges Gynak 1906; 176.
45. Atkinson RS, Rushman GB: A Synopsis of Anaesthesia. 8th ed. Bristol, UK, Wright, 1977.
46. Eason MJ, Wyatt R: Paravertebral thoracic block—a reappraisal. Anaesthesia 1979; 34:638–42.

47. Karmakar MJ, Chung DC: Variability of a thoracic paravertebral block. Are we ignoring the endothoracic fascia? Reg Anesth Pain Med 2000; 25:325–7.
48. Sabanathan S, Smith PJ, Pradhan GN, Hashimi H, Eng JB, Mearns AJ: Continuous intercostal nerve block for pain relief after thoracotomy. Ann Thorac Surg 1988; 46:425–6.
49. Soni AK, Conacher I, Waller DA, Hilton CJ: Video-assisted thoracoscopic placement of paravertebral catheters. BJA 1994; 72:462–4.
50. Matthews PJ, Govenden V: Comparison of continuous paravertebral and extradural infusions of bupivacaine for pain relief after thoracotomy. Br J Anaesth 1989; 62:204–5.
51. Richardson J, Sabanathan S, Jones J, Shah RD, Cheema S, Mearns AJ: A prospective, randomized comparison of preoperative and continuous balanced epidural or paravertebral bupivacaine on postthoracotomy pain, pulmonary function and stress responses. Br J Anaesth 1999; 83:387–92.
52. Lonnqvist PA, MacKenzie J, Soni AK, Conacher ID: Paravertebral blockade. Failure rate and complications. Anaesthesia 1995; 50: 813–5.
53. Berrisford RG, Sabanathan S, Mearns AJ, Clarke BJ, Hamdi A: Plasma concentrations of bupivacaine and its enantiomers during continuous extrapleural intercostal nerve block. BJA 1993; 70:201–4.
54. Karmakar MK: Thoracic paravertebral block. Anesthesiology 2001; 95:771–80.
55. Curley J, Castillo J, Hotz J, et al.: Prolonged regional nerve blockade. Injectable biodegradable bupivacaine/polyester microspheres. Anesthesiology 1996; 84:1401–10.
56. Castillo J, Curley J, Hotz J, et al.: Glucocorticoids prolong rat sciatic nerve blockade in vivo from bupivacaine microspheres. Anesthesiology 1996; 85:1157–66.
57. Drager C, Benziger D, Gao F, Berde CB: Proloned intercostal nerve blockade in sheep using controlled-release of bupivacaine and dexamethasone from polymer microspheres. Anesthesiology 1998; 89:969–79.
58. Kopacz DJ, Lacouture PG, Wu D, Nandy P, Swanton R, Landau C: The dose response and effects of dexamethasone on bupivacaine microcapsules for intercostal blockade (T9 to T11) in healthy volunteers. Anesth Analg 2003; 96:576–82.
59. Grant GJ, Vermeulen K, Langerman L, Zakowski M, Turndorf H: Prolonged analgesia with liposomal bupivacaine in a mouse model. Reg Anesth 1994; 19:264–9.
60. Grant GJ, Lax J, Susser L, Zakowski M, Weissman TE, Turndorf H:

Wound infiltration with liposomal bupivacaine prolongs analgesia in rats. Acta Anaesthesiol Scand 1997; 41:204–7.

61. Boogaerts JG, Lafont ND, Declercq AG, Luo HC, Gravet ET, Bianchi JA, Legros FJ: Epidural administration of liposome-associated bupivacaine for the management of postsurgical pain: a first study. J Clin Anesth 1994; 6:315–20.
62. Covino BG: Interpleural regional analgesia. Anesth Analg 1988; 67:427–9.
63. Baumgarten RK: Intrapleural, interpleural, or pleural block? Simpler may be better. Reg Anesth 1992; 17:116.
64. Murphy DF: Interpleural analgesia. Br J Anaesth 1993; 71:426–34.
65. Kambam JR, Hammon J, Parris WC, Lupinetti FM: Intrapleural analgesia for postthoracotomy pain and blood levels of bupivacaine following intrapleural injection. Can J Anaesth 1989; 36:106–9.
66. Symreng T, Gomez MN, Rossi N: Intrapleural bupivacaine v saline after thoracotomy—effects on pain and lung functions—a double-blind study. J Cardiothorac Anesth 1989; 3:144–9.
67. Schneider RF, Villamena PC, Harvey J, Surick BG, Surick IW, Beattie EJ: Lack of efficacy of intrapleural bupivacaine for postoperative analgesia following thoracotomy. Chest 1993; 103:414–6.
68. Miguel R, Hubbell D: Pain management and spirometry following thoracotomy: a prospective, randomized study of four techniques. J Cardiothorac Vasc Anesth 1993; 7:529–34.
69. Raffin L, Fletcher D, Sperandio M, Antoniotti C, Mazoit X, Bisson A, Fischler M: Interpleural infusion of 2% lidocaine with 1:200,000 epinephrine for postthoracotomy analgesia. Anesth Analg 1994; 79:328–34.
70. Rosenberg PH, Scheinin BM, Lepantalo MJ, Lindfors O: Continuous intrapleural infusion of bupivacaine for analgesia after thoracotomy. Anesthesiology 1987; 67:811–3.
71. Broome IJ, Sherry KM, Reilly CS: A combined chest drain and intrapleural catheter for postthoracotomy pain relief. Anaesthesia 1993; 48:724–6.
72. Griffith DPG, Diamond AW, Cameron JD: Postoperative epidural analgesia following thoracic surgery: a feasibility study. Br J Anaesth 1975; 47:48–55.
73. Rigg JR, Jamrozik K, Myles PS, SIlbert BS, Peyton PJ, Parsons RW, Collins KS: MASTER Anaethesia Trial Study Group. Epidural anaesthesia and analgesia and outcome of major surgery: a randomized trial. Lancet 2002; 359:1276–82.
74. Giebler RM, Scherer RU, Peters J: Incidence of neurologic complications related to thoracic epidural catheterization. Anesthesiology 1997; 86:55–63.

75. Conacher ID, Paes ML, Jacobson L, Phillips PD, Heaviside DW: Epidural analgesia following thoracic surgery. Anaesthesia 1983; 38:546–51.

76. Kaneko M, Saito Y, Kirihara Y, Collins JG, Kosaka Y: Synergistic antinociceptive interaction after epidural coadministration of morphine and lidocaine in rats. Anesthesiology 1994; 80:137–50.

77. Romer HC, Russell GN: A survey of the practice of thoracic epidural analgesia in the United Kingdom. Anaesthesia 1998; 53: 1016–22.

78. Curatolo M, Schnider TW, Petersen-Felix S, Weiss S, Signer C, Scaramozzino P, Zbinden AM: A direct search procedure to optimize combinations of epidural bupivacaine, fentanyl, and clonidine for postoperative analgesia. Anesthesiology 2000; 92:325–37.

79. Niemi G, Breivik H: Epinephrine markedly improves thoracic epidural analgesia produced by a small-dose infusion of ropivacaine, fentanyl, and epinephrine after major thoracic or abdominal surgery: a randomized, double-blinded cross-over study with and without epinephrine. Anest Analg 2002; 94:1598–605.

80. Eisenach JC, De Kock M, Klimscha W: α_2-Adrenergic agonists for regional anesthesia. A clinical review of clonidine (1984–1995). Anesthesiology 1996; 85:655–74.

81. Bromage PR, Camporesi EM, Durant PA, Nielsen CH: Nonrespiratory side effects of epidural morphine. Anesth Analg 1982; 61: 490–5.

82. Yaksh TL: Spinal opiate analgesia: characteristics and principles of action. Pain 1981; 11:293–346.

83. Rawal N, Mollefors K, Axelsson K, Lingardh G, Widman B: An experimental study of urodynamic effects of epidural morphine and of naloxone reversal. Anesth Analg 1983; 62:641–7.

84. Husted S, Djurhus JC, Husegaard HC, Jepsen J, Mortensen J: Effect of postoperative extradural morphine on lower urinary tract function. Acta Anaesthesiol Scand 1985; 29:183–5.

85. Wang J, Pennefather S, Russell G: Low-dose naloxone in the treatment of urinary retention during extradural fentanyl causes excessive reversal of analgesia. Br J Anaesth 1998; 80:565–6.

86. Goldhill DR, Whelpton R, Winyard JA, Wilkinson KA: Gastric emptying in patients the day after cardiac surgery. Anaesthesia 1995; 50:122–5.

87. Petring OU, Dawson PJ, Blake DW, Jones DJ, Bjorksten AR, Libreri FC, Leadbeater M: Normal postoperative gastric emptying after orthopaedic surgery with spinal anesthesia and im ketorolac as the first postoperative analgesic. Br J Anaesth 1995; 74:257–60.

88. Au J, Hawkins T, Venables C, Morritt G, Scott CD, Gascoigne AD,

Corris PA, Hilton CJ, Dark JH: Upper gastrointestinal dysmotility in heart-lung transplant recipients. Ann Thorac Surg 1993; 55:94–7.

89. Thorn SE, Wattwil M, Naslund I: Postoperative epidural morphine, but not epidural bupivacaine, delays gastric emptying on the first day after cholecystectomy. Reg Anesth 1992; 17:91–4.
90. Bonica JJ: Autonomic innervation of the viscera in relation to nerve block. Anesthesiology 1968; 29:793–813.
91. Guha A, Scawn NDA, Rogers SA, Pennefather SH, Russell GN: Gastric emptying in post thoracotomy patients receiving a thoracic fentanyl-bupivacaine epidural infusion. Eur J Anaesth 2002; 19: 652–7.
92. Bromage PR: The control of postthoracotomy pain. Anaesthesia 1989; 44:445–6.
93. Gough JD, Williams AB, Vaughan RS, Khalil JF, Butchart EG: The control of postthoracotomy pain. A comparative evaluation of thoracic epidural fentanyl infusions and cryoanalgesia. Anaesthesia 1988; 43:780–3.
94. Fischer HBJ: Regional anaesthesia—before or after general anaesthesia? Anaesthesia 1998; 53:727–9.
95. Minzter BH, Johnson RF, Grimm BJ: The practice of thoracic epidural analgesia: a survey of academic medical centers in the United States. Anesth Analg 2002; 95:472–5.
96. Reynolds F: Damage to the conus medullaris following spinal anaesthesia. Anaesthesia 2001; 56:238–47.
97. Absalom AR, Martinelli G, Scott NB: Spinal cord injury caused by direct damage by local anaesthetic infiltration needle. Br J Anaesth 2001; 87:512–5.
98. Horlocker TT, McGregor DG, Matsushige DK, Schroeder DR, Besse JA: A retrospective review of 4,767 consecutive spinal anesthetics: central nervous system complications. Perioperative Outcomes Group. Anesth Analg 1997; 84:578–84.
99. Dajczman E, Gordon A, Kreisman H, Wolkove N: Long-term postthoracotomy pain. Chest 1991; 99:270–4.
100. Perttunen K, Tasmuth T, Kalso E: Chronic pain after thoracic surgery: a follow-up study. Acta Anaesthesiol Scand 1999; 43:563–7.
101. Muller LC, Salzer GM, Ransmayr G, Neiss A: Intraoperative cryoanalgesia for postthoracotomy pain relief. Ann Thorac Surg 1989; 48:15–9.
102. Obata H, Saito S, Fujita N, Fuse Y, Ishizaki K, Goto F: Epidural block with mepivacaine before surgery reduces long-term postthoracotomy pain. Can J Anaesth 1999; 46:1127–32.
103. Fratacci MD, Kimball WR, Wain JC, Kacmarek RM, Polaner DM,

Zapol WM: Diaphragmatic shortening after thoracic surgery in humans. Effects of mechanical ventilation and thoracic epidural anesthesia. Anesthesiology 1993; 79:654–65.

104. Simonneau G, Vivien A, Sartene R, Kunstlinger F, Samii K, Noviant Y, Duroux P: Diaphragm dysfunction induced by upper abdominal surgery. Role of postoperative pain. Am Rev Respir Dis 1983; 128:899–903.

105. Dureuil B, Viires N, Cantineau JP, Aubier M, Desmonts JM: Diaphragmatic contractility after upper abdominal surgery. J Appl Physiol 1986; 61:1775–80.

106. Polaner DM, Kimball WR, Fratacci MD, Wain JC, Zapol WM: Thoracic epidural anesthesia increases diaphragmatic shortening after thoracotomy in the awake lamb. Anesthesiology 1993; 79:808–16.

107. Torres A, Kimball WR, Qvist J, Stanek K, Kacmarek RM, Whyte RI, Montalescot G, Zapol WM: Sonomirometric regional diaphragmatic shortening in awake sheep after thoracic surgery. J Appl Physiol 1989; 67:2357–68.

108. Manikian B, Cantineau JP, Bertrand M, Kieffer E, Sartene R, Viars P: Improvement of diaphragmatic function by a thoracic extradural block after upper abdominal surgery. Anesthesiology 1988; 68:379–86.

109. Warner DO, Warner MA, Ritman EL: Human chest wall function during epidural anesthesia. Anesthesiology 1996; 85:761–73.

110. Richter A, Cederholm I, Jonasson L, Mucchiano C, Uchto M, Janerot-Sjoberg B: Effect of thoracic epidural analgesia on refractory angina pectoris: long-term home self-treatment. J Cardiothorac Vasc Anesth 2002; 16:679–84.

111. Gramling-Babb P, Miller MJ, Reeves ST, Roy RC, Zile MR: Treatment of medically and surgically refractory angina pectoris with high thoracic epidural analgesia: initial clinical experience. Am Heart J 1997; 133:648–55.

112. Tuman KJ, McCarthy RJ, March RJ, DeLaria GA, Patel RV, Ivankovich AD: Effects of epidural anesthesia and analgesia on coagulation and outcome after major vascular surgery. Anesth Analg 1991; 73:696–704.

113. Beattie WS, Badner NH, Choi P: Epidural analgesia reduces postoperative myocardial infarction: a meta-analysis. Anesth Analg 2001; 93:853–8.

114. Oka T, Ozawa Y: Correlation between intraoperative hemodynamic variability and postoperative arrhythmias in patients with pulmonary surgery. Masui 1999; 48:118–123.

115. Ritchie AJ, Bowe P, Gibbons JR: Prophylactic digitalization for thoracotomy: a reassessment. Ann Thorac Surg 1990; 50:86–8.

116. Krowka MJ, Pairolero PC, Trastek VF, et al.: Cardiac dysrhythmia

following pneumonectomy: clinical correlates and prognostic significance. Chest 1987; 91:490–5.

117. Von Knorring J, Lepantalo M, Lindgren L, Lindfors O: Cardiac arrhythmias and myocardial ischemia after thoracotomy for lung cancer. Ann Thorac Surg 1992; 53:642–7.

118. Oka T, Ozawa Y, Ohkubo Y: Thoracic epidural bupivacaine attenuates supraventricular tachyarrhythmias after pulmonary resection. Anesth Analg 2001; 93:253–9.

119. Modig J, Borg T, Karlstrom G, Maripuu E, Sahlstedt B: Thromboembolism after total hip replacement: role of epidural and general anesthesia. Anesth Analg 1983; 62:174–80.

120. Sharrock NE, Cazan MG, Hargett MJ, Williams-Russo P, Wilson PD Jr: Changes in mortality after total hip and knee arthroplasty over a 10-year period. Anesth Analg 1995; 80:242–8.

121. Golledge J, Goldstraw P: Renal impairment after thoracotomy: incidence, risk factors, and significance. Ann Thorac Surg 1994; 58: 524–8.

122. Watson A, Allen PR: Influence of thoracic epidural analgesia on outcome after resection for esophageal cancer. Surgery 1994; 115: 429–32.

John M. Alvarez, FRACS

9 | Postpneumonectomy Pulmonary Edema

Much has been written; little has been learnt.

Dr. P.A. Fuentes

INTRODUCTION

The syndrome of postpneumonectomy pulmonary edema (PPPE) refers to the development of an acute lung injury (ALI) characterized by relentless, severe, and often fatal pulmonary edema of unknown cause. It is therefore a diagnosis of exclusion (1). Numerous names have been attached to this syndrome: noncardiogenic pulmonary edema, postperfusion pulmonary edema, postoperative acute lung injury (ALI), and post-lung resection pulmonary edema (2). Recently, in an endeavor to achieve consensus, Williams et al. (2) proposed accepting the guidelines of the American-European consensus committee, categorizing this syndrome within the spectrum of ALI-acute respiratory distress syndrome (ARDS) (Table 9.1). The limited evidence from autopsy findings in these patients reveals that the histological changes identified in PPPE are identical to those in ARDS. Hence, I will use these terms (ie, PPPE/ARDS) synonymously.

Controversy has surrounded this syndrome since Zeldin and Peters postulated that a cause-and-effect relationship existed because of overzealous intraoperative administration of intravenous crystalloid fluids by anesthetists (3). Two decades later, the absence of a precise

Progress in Thoracic Anesthesia, edited by Peter Slinger,
Lippincott Williams & Wilkins, Baltimore © 2004.

TABLE 9.1 Recommended Criteria for the Diagnosis of Acute Lung Injury and Acute Respiratory Distress Syndrome

Diagnosis	Timing	Oxygenation[a]	Chest radiography (frontal)	PCWP[b]
ALI	Acute	$PaO_2/FIO_2 < 300$ mm Hg	Bilateral infiltrates	<18 mm Hg
ARDS	Acute	$PaO_2/FIO_2 < 200$ mm Hg	Bilateral infiltrates	<18 mm Hg

ALI = acute lung injury; ARDS = acute respiratory distress syndrome; PaO_2/FIO_2 = arterial partial pressure of oxygen/fraction of inspired oxygen; PCWP = pulmonary capillary wedge pressure.
[a]Regardless of positive end-expiratory pressure.
[b]When measured or no clinical evidence of left atrial hypertension.

definition, the absolute requirement for prompt exclusion of potential causes, and a not fully elucidated multifactorial pathogenesis has translated into continued misdiagnosis and, thus, underreporting. However, PPPE is not rare. It is universally fatal if unrecognized, and it has been responsible for the majority of all mortality postpneumonectomy in centers with an awareness of this syndrome. In the 20 years since Zeldin and Peters brought our attention to this syndrome, advances have been achieved that limit the incidence of PPPE and that significantly improve the survival in patients who develop PPPE. Some findings, however, challenge the entrenched dogma of how patients undergoing pneumonectomy are treated (during surgery, during anesthesia, and in the intensive care unit [ICU]); thus, further controversy has added inertia to the goal of achieving consensual guidelines to better manage and assess results in dealing with PPPE. This monograph will endeavor to address the clinical perspective of PPPE and to propose working solutions.

THE PROBLEM OF PPPE: IS IT REAL?

The first report by Peters of PPPE in 1982 was subsequently associated with a dire prediction of "a new complication—an iatrogenic one . . . by failure to understand the effects of pneumonectomy on lung fluid exchange. There is now a worldwide epidemic of postpneumonectomy pulmonary edema" (4) (p. 876). Because pneumonectomies had been successfully performed for the previous 32 years, either "the problem" (ie, PPPE) was present and unrecognized or a new phenomenon had arrived. However, via the efforts of Gibbon and Gibbon (5) as well as Macklin and Macklin (6), physicians had been aware that pulmonary edema could be produced in animals having lung resections by either excessive administration of plasma or hyperinflation of the lungs.

Ginsberg et al. (7), in a landmark mortality analysis of 2220 lung resections (569 pneumonectomies) in North America, make no mention of PPPE. Hirschler-Schulte et al. (8) from Holland also make no mention of PPPE, despite assessing the need for mechanical ventilation for acute respiratory failure among 365 lung resections (115 pneumonectomies). Hence, in 1982, I suggest that PPPE was unrecognized by a majority of physicians, despite strong animal data that it was a real entity; however, the occurrence of PPPE was not of epidemic proportions.

In 2003, how much has changed? Despite semantic issues, PPPE is recognized as a distinct clinical entity by a growing number of anesthetists, intensivists, and surgeons. The reported incidence of PPPE ranges from 2.5% to 14% (Table 9.2) as reported by numerous authors, albeit retrospectively, from around the world. Furthermore, two groups have recently described a premanifest syndrome of pulmonary edema occurring in 12.2% and 15% of pneumonectomies (9, 10).

Nevertheless, a persistent and glaring disparity exists regarding the reported incidence of PPPE in many large surgical series addressing outcomes following major lung resection (Table 9.3). Hence, Harpole et al. (11), assessing prognostic models of mortality following lung resection, make no mention of PPPE. This was a prospective study involving 123 U.S. Veterans Affairs centers from 1991 to 1995, with 3,516 lung resections (569 pneumonectomies). Wada et al. (12), analyzing mortality data for 1994 from all 312 centers of the Japanese Association for Chest Surgery (7,099 resections and 586 pneumonectomies), also make no mention of PPPE. From Europe, recent series analyzing outcomes following lung resection (2,856 patients and 673 pneumonectomies) either make no or scarce mention of PPPE (13–18). In many of these series, unquantified respiratory failure requiring mechanical ventilation occurred at a rate of 5% to 8%, with an associated high mortality rate (<26%) (17). Ostensibly, therefore, one may conclude that PPPE remains unrecognized in many centers.

RELATIONSHIP OF PPPE TO MORTALITY FOLLOWING PNEUMONECTOMY

Alvarez et al. (19) reported that PPPE accounted for 75% of all in-hospital deaths following 180 lung resections (28 pneumonectomies) and for all deaths following pneumonectomy. Kutlu et al. (10) reported that ALI/ARDS accounted for 72.5% of the total mortality among 1,139 patients having lung resection (198 pneumonectomies) from 1991 to 1997. Ruffini et al. (20), reporting a series of 1,221 patients (188 pneumonectomies) from 1993 to 1999, stated that ALI/ARDS was the main cause of death, accounting for 41% of their total in-hospital mortality. Martin et

TABLE 9.2 Reported Incidence of Postpneumonectomy Pulmonary Edema

Series	Year	Incidence (%)	PPPE/ Pneumonectomies (n/n)	Right (%)	Left (%)	Mortality (%)
Verheijen-Breemhaar et al. (37)	1988	4	11/243	7.1	2.3	27
Turnage and Lunn (23)	1993	2.6	21/806	Ratio: 16	5	100
Waller et al. (24)	1993	4.4	9/205	5.1	4.0	55
Parquin et al. (39)[a]	1996	3.4	5/146	—	—	40
Van der Werff et al. (9)	1997	2.5	5/197	—	—	100
Alvarez et al. (19, 68)	1998/2003					
Era 1:1993–1996		14	4/28	18	11	60
Era 2:1996–2000		0	0/29	0	0	0
Mathisen et al. (28)[b]	1998		7/?			
Era 1:1986–1993		4.4		Ratio: 5	2	86
Era 2:1993–1997		7.5[c]	8/83	Ratio: 3	5	25
Deslauriers et al. (27)	1998	4.5	13/291	6.3	2.8	85
Kutlu et al. (10)[b]	2000	5.1	10/198	6.6	5.5[c]	80[c]
Ruffini et al. (20)[d]	2001	3.8	7/188	4.5	3.0	59

PPPE = Postpneumonectomy pulmonary edema

[a]Twenty-two patients had mild pulmonary edema; 5 patients had severe PPPE.

[b]Use definition of acute respiratory distress syndrome.

[c]Frequency for right/left is for combined acute lung injury/acute respiratory distress syndrome.

[d]Incidence and frequency is for combined acute lung injury/acute respiratory distress syndrome.

TABLE 9.3   Mortality Associated with Pneumonectomy and
Incidence of Postpneumonectomy Pulmonary Edema

Series	Year	Number	Mortality (%)	PPPE (%)
Ginsberg et al. (7)	1983	569	6.2	0
Keagy et al. (93)	1983	90	12.2	0
Hirschler-Schulte et al. (8)	1985	115	6–10	0
Krowka et al. (94)	1987	236	11	0
Wahi et al. (95)	1989	197	7	0
Patel et al. (13)	1992	197	8.6	0
Romano and Mark (96)	1992	1592	11.6	0
Wada et al. (12)	1994	586	3.2	0
Harpole et al. (11)	1995	567	11.5	0
Swartz et al. (40)	1997	92	10.9	0
Mizushima et al. (80)	1997	27 (>70 years)	22	0
		95 (<70 years)	3.2	
Licker et al. (14)	1999	151	7.9	0
Stephan et al. (15)	2000	87	7	0
Myrdal et al. (17)	2001	157	5.7	0
Alexiou et al. (18)	2001	206	6.8	0
Martin et al. (21)	2001	97	11.3	0
Joo et al. (44)	2001	105	10.5	0

PPPE = postpneumonectomy pulmonary edema.

al. (21) reported a 23.9% operative mortality rate among patients having a right pneumonectomy following neoadjuvant therapy. Postpneumonectomy ARDS was responsible for all six in-hospital deaths and for a further one of seven deaths (21–95 days) postsurgery; ARDS thus accounted for 64% of all deaths (21). To quote Slinger, "as other early causes of post lung resection mortality have decreased . . . the importance of PPPE is now becoming more evident" (p. 49) (22).

Why are there such disparities in the incidence and the impact of PPPE among these series? I concur with the view of Kutlu et al.: "This high incidence may be partially due to heightened awareness of the problem at our institution . . . the mortality . . . is unacceptably high, representing a major challenge to the thoracic surgeon and intensivist for the next decade" (10). I would include in this challenge the anesthetist as well.

CLINICAL PRESENTATION AND DIAGNOSIS

The clinical syndrome of PPPE requires the exclusion of factors known to produce ARDS. For a correct diagnosis to be made, two factors are required: a high index of suspicion and the prompt exclusion of other possible causes (19). In addition to establishing either the ALI or ARDS status of the patient, the criteria proposed by Turnage and Lunn (23) are clinically useful:

1. The presence of respiratory distress at clinical examination.
2. The presence of pulmonary infiltrates on chest radiography and documented progression of extravascular lung water (EVLW).
3. No indication of cardiac failure at the time of diagnosis by hemodynamic measurements.
4. No evidence of pneumonia by culture of airway secretions.
5. No evidence of sepsis by blood cultures
6. No clinically evident episodes of aspiration.

This syndrome does not follow a uniform course, possibly reflecting a multifactorial cause that, once triggered and reaching a critical level, follows an inexorable and fatal pathway. The onset of PPPE is variable (24). We noted that the first clinical sign was oliguria (<20 mL/h); this sign manifested at a mean of 11 hours (range, 6–25 hours) following surgery (19). The oliguria was associated with low central venous pressure (CVP) in all five cases. Others have not documented oliguria as a presenting feature (3, 25). However, to my knowledge, ours is the sole report documenting a precise temporal sequence of clinical events with PPPE. Furthermore, our patients were unequivocally "dry": No net fluid overload was observed, and these patients had normal preoperative renal function (19). This may explain why Zeldin et al. (3) noted polyuria in their series (four patients), because all patients had unphysiologically high net 24-hour perioperative fluid balances (2.8 ± 1.4 L). The five patients with PPPE reported by Mathru et al. (26) had a mean 24-hour urine output (UO) of 47 mL/h (range, 35–75 mL/h), and Deslauriers et al. (27) reported 11 patients with PPPE and a mean 48-hour UO of 56 mL/h. However, neither Zeldin et al. (3), Mathru et al. (26), nor Deslauriers et al. (27) correlated the changes in hourly UO to the onset of symptoms or changes on chest radiography. To my knowledge, these four reports are the sole commentary on UO and PPPE.

We hypothesized that our patients were hypovolemic secondary to sequestration of intravascular fluid in the "leaking" lung, thus producing oliguria. However, it is equally tenable that if the renal function is normal, excessive intravascular expansion will induce polyuria regardless of the pathophysiology occurring in the lungs until the intravascular volume becomes depleted.

Concurrent with the development of oliguria was the appearance of infiltrates on the chest radiograph. We unequivocally demonstrated that the chest radiographic changes preceded the development of dyspnea by a mean of 23 hours (range, 13–30 hours) (19). Although this is generally agreed on (22, 27), Kutlu et al. (10) reports that "radiological changes lag behind the clinical deterioration." Apropos, Deslauriers et al. (27)

comment that "[r]adiologically, the first signs of impending PPPE can be very subtle and are often missed even by experienced surgeons."

Hence, the onset of PPPE based on the occurrence of dyspnea has ranged from 12 hours to 13 days following surgery. However, the retrospective nature of all these reports suggests caution. The series of Kutlu et al. (10) was based on patients admitted to the ICU; hence, the mean time to ARDS was 5.2 ± 1.7 days. Waller et al. (24), however, noted that PPPE became manifest in the operating theatre (ie, immediately) in 18% (2/11 cases). This immediate onset of PPPE is supported by the series of van der Werff et al. (9), who in a retrospective review of chest radiographs found that 40% (2/5 cases) and 33% (8/24 cases) had PPPE and premanifest PPPE, respectively, within 24 hours following surgery. That up to one in five cases may occur immediately following surgery supports a multifactorial pathogenesis, but it also clearly implicates what occurs in the operating theater.

Dyspnea is associated with tachycardia, tachypnea, lung rales, and hypoxemia. Fever (>38°C) and leukocytosis have been reported in as many as 60% of cases. A telling feature is that despite oxygen therapy and diuretic use, including renal-dose dopamine (ie, 2–4 µg/kg/min), the hypoxemia is refractory and progressive; clinical deterioration occurs at a variable yet rapid rate (1, 19, 23, 27). We observed a need for endotracheal intubation in all cases at a mean of 29 hours (range, 6–69 hours) following dyspnea (19). All our patients had been transferred to the ICU for a mean of 6.4 hours before being intubated. The role of corticosteroids is uncertain, and to my knowledge, only three reports have described their use (19, 27, 28). We reported their use, noting that it may have delayed the time of intubation and the avoidance of hemodynamic collapse associated with intubation but that it did not prevent the need for mechanical ventilation (19). However, of our survivors, all received steroids. Mathisen et al. (28) administered steroids to five patients, three of whom died, in their series of 10 cases. Deslauriers et al. (27) also advocated a 48-hour course of high-dose steroids. However, although theoretically appealing, the available evidence is, as Deslauriers et al. note, anecdotal.

Differential Diagnosis

The exclusion of other pathologies is critical, because these may become inextricably superimposed on PPPE (1, 19, 23, 27). Turnage and Lunn (23), with the largest autopsy series, reported superimposed bacterial pneumonia in all 21 cases and pulmonary emboli in 18%. We noted that 60% of our series also developed positive blood and sputum cultures (19).

The causes that must be excluded are cardiogenic pulmonary edema, pulmonary emboli, intrapulmonary sepsis, aspiration pneumonia, bronchopleural fistula, extrapulmonary systemic sepsis, and drugs and blood transfusions. The judicious use of bronchoscopy, echocardiography, pulmonary arterial catheterization, computed tomographic (CT) angiography, serum biochemical markers, and microbiological sampling together with careful examination and observation of the patient will, in the vast majority of cases, confirm or refute the diagnosis of PPPE (19, 27).

Cardiogenic Pulmonary Edema

Possible causes include supraventricular arrhythmia, myocardial infarction, valvular heart disease, cardiomyopathy, and iatrogenic fluid overload. A careful history, electrocardiography, biochemical assays (ie, serum troponin), and echocardiography will elucidate this cause. Use of a Swan-Ganz catheter will confirm or deny raised left ventricular filling pressures. The caveat, known since 1986, is that in some of these patients, the occlusion of a pulmonary artery branch by the balloon catheter may adversely impact left ventricular filling such that the pulmonary capillary wedge pressure (PCWP) reading is artificially low. However, this is identified by a concurrent reduction in the mean systemic arterial pressure of 6 to 10 mm Hg (29). Reports of PPPE dealing with such hemodynamic measurements are few, and fewer still record whether this phenomenon actually occurred (19, 27, 30). The favorable response of cardiogenic pulmonary edema to traditional therapy, and the obverse encountered with PPPE, is an important hallmark strongly suggesting that a raised pulmonary hydrostatic pressure is not the sole operating pathogenetic factor (1, 22, 27, 28).

Pulmonary Emboli

Although the patient history is unhelpful, patients with pulmonary emboli rarely develop progressive and severe infiltrates (31, 32). Anticoagulation is advocated until the diagnosis of pulmonary embolism is eliminated, usually by ventilation-perfusion scanning or CT angiography.

Intrapulmonary Sepsis

Bacterial pneumonia is often lobar in distribution. Thus, sputum sampling, especially by early bronchoscopy, is mandatory.

Aspiration Pneumonia

Although clinical history (eg, obtundancy, previous gastrointestinal disease, advanced age, recurrent nerve palsy), radiographic findings (ie, infiltrates in the most dependant lung segments), and bronchoscopy (ie, foreign debris) may be definitive, concerns about the role of microaspiration in association with epidural anesthesia in triggering PPPE have recently been raised (27).

Bronchopleural Fistula

Apart from the clinical and radiographic features, early bronchoscopy should be definitive.

Extrapulmonary Systemic Sepsis

Blood cultures, CT scanning, and a careful history and physical examination should exclude iatrogenic sources (ie, infected vascular catheters) and other uncommon pathology (eg, severe pancreatitis).

Drugs and Blood Transfusions

Transfusion associated ARDS is well-described. Drugs (ie, amiodarone) have also been implicated in inducing ARDS.

Pathophysiology

By definition, the pathophysiology is not wholly understood. However, in the nearly 50 years since the Gibbons' original research (5), much has been learned, forgotten, and rediscovered. A detailed treatise on each component is beyond the scope of this monograph and is readily available elsewhere (1, 22, 27, 33, 34). However, from the clinical perspective, several points are worth noting regarding six factors

Volume Overload

No single factor has caused greater controversy between anesthetists and surgeons in this field than the recommendation by Zeldin et al. (3) that "the most important thing that we can do in terms of recognizing this problem is to watch our anesthetists as they start loading the patient up with fluid." This view from 1984 remains prevalent today. As Slinger (22) stated, "fluid overload is vital . . . our anaesthetic colleagues believe you can oxygenate the patient with Ringer's lactate . . . the patients . . . only remaining lung gets flooded by the overadministration of this dangerous fluid."

It is noteworthy that the landmark article by Zeldin et al. (3) was based on 10 patients studied retrospectively from seven centers; fluid data were available only on four patients, three of whom had a pulmonary catheter inserted and only one of whom had a measured cardiac output. From the clinical data, however, it is perturbing to note that despite an estimated blood loss of 550 mL, total iv fluid input over the first 24 hours was 4.9 ± 1.1 L, even in their six controls for a similar blood loss (579 mL); the total iv fluid load over 24 hours was 3.5 ± 0.9 L (3). The net fluid intake over the first 24 hours was 2.8 L and 2.0 L for patients with PPPE and controls, respectively. No comment was made regarding who (surgeon or anesthetist) ordered the fluid load over this period or whether it was excessive even in their controls (3). Slinger (1, 22) correctly identifies inherent flaws in the conclusions of Zeldin et al. Namely, intraoperative zealous iv fluid administration should cause problems well before the reported onset of PPPE 2 to 3 days later, and none of the measured PCWPs were above normal. I would add if it was solely a hydrostatic problem, it should have responded to conventional therapy; however, it did not.

The animal experiments reported by Zeldin et al. (3) appear to be the cornerstone supporting the "zealot anesthetic overload theory." In these experiments, 13 dogs were subjected to either a 100 mL/kg immediate iv Ringer's lactate load pre-right pneumonectomy (group A) or a 50 mL/kg bolus on induction followed by a further 50 mL/kg during surgery (group B). In addition, crystalloid replacement of blood loss occurred in both groups, and crystalloid was administered over the ensuing 48 hours to keep the PCWP to at least 5 mm Hg and to maintain a positive fluid balance of 100 mL/kg^3. These were compared to control dogs administered fluid as in group A but without a thoracotomy. The diagnosis of PPPE was based on a ratio of left lung weight to right lung weight of greater than 1. Although no control dog developed PPE, 46% (6/13) of the pneumonectomied group, 37.5% of group A dogs, and 20% group B dogs developed PPPE. Zeldin et al. accepted that "this disease has variable penetrance," yet no data were provided regarding when the dogs first manifested pulmonary edema. This is important, because Zeldin et al.'s human data imply a delay to onset of PPPE. However, the dog data are silent regarding when the pulmonary edema became clinically evident, yet it was blatant at autopsy. Also, no detailed data are provided regarding total iv load given per animal or daily changes in PCWP, especially regarding when the boluses of fluid were given (except for three dogs in which the PCWP was noted to rise from 14 to 20 ± 2 mm Hg), or if plasma oncotic pressure was affected. It is noteworthy that despite these massive fluid challenges, the majority (54%) of a normal dog's lung subjected to pneumonectomy resists edema formation, as should be expected (33).

Guyton and Lindsey (35), in a landmark paper involving dogs that preceded the report by Zeldin et al. (3) by 24 years, evidenced the near-linear relationship of EVLW to left atrial pressure (LAP) either once the LAP exceeded 23 mm Hg (colloid oncotic pressure normal) or once the LAP exceeded 10 mm Hg (colloid oncotic pressure decreased). We should not be surprised that giving 7 L (ie, 70-kg patient at 100 mL/kg) acutely to the type of patients who require pneumonectomy could lead to pulmonary edema.

Lee et al. (36) compared the effects of artificially raising LAP in a measured, stepwise fashion from 10 to 25 mm Hg by inflating a Foley catheter in the left atrium acutely for 30 minutes in pneumonectomied versus control dogs (36). Their conclusion, based on measured EVLW, was that the pneumonectomied dogs were no more susceptible to increases in EVLW caused by a hemodynamic challenge than the controls up to an LAP of 25 mm Hg. However, "all dogs had definite pulmonary edema evidenced by copious frothy sputum" (36).

Even in the often-quoted paper of Gibbon and Gibbon (5), the acute administration of 15 mL/kg plasma over 30 minutes in cats (~25–30% of the blood volume) immediately following removal of 70% of their lung mass is unsurprising in causing pulmonary edema and increasing feline mortality from 20% to 73%.

Despite a cause-and-effect relationship being further supported by Verheijen-Bremhaar et al. (37) (11 cases) and Margolis (38) (three cases), Turnage and Lunn (23) were the first to unequivocally disprove this hypothesis. Further convincing support was subsequently provided by Waller et al. (24), Kutlu et al. (10), and Deslauriers et al. (27). We demonstrated that PPPE will occur despite patients being intentionally either euvolemic or hypovolemic (19). So, too, Mathison et al. (28), from a quaternary teaching institution, having been aware of the problem of PPPE from the work of Peters, categorically states that "none of the patients had excessive fluid administration (intraoperatively or in the first 48 hours)," because "our anesthesiologists pay strict attention to intraoperative fluid balance because of our concern over the role of excessive fluid administration and ARDS." Yet, despite these surgeons stopping their anesthetists from "boldly loading their patients" with "dangerous solutions," the incidence of PPPE at the Massachusetts General hospital was 4.4% from 1986 to 1993 and 7.5% from 1993 to 1997 (25). As Slinger (1, 22) emphasized, there is more to PPPE than just withholding iv fluids.

One cannot, however, discount the suspicion that excessive iv fluids are administered both intraoperatively but also postoperatively (21). Verheijen-Bremhaar et al. (37) and Margolis (38) reported net 24-hour fluid balances of approximately 2 to 2.5 L (PPPE)/1 L (non-PPPE) and of 86 mL/kg (ie, 70-kg patient = 6 L) [PPPE]/47 mL/kg (ie, 70-kg patient = 3.3 L) [non-PPPE].

Are contemporary patients getting too much iv fluid intraoperatively?

Patel et al. (13) reported that 12% of postpneumonectomy patients received 24-hour iv fluid infusions of more than 3 L and that the mean iv volume load was 2.6 L (range, 1.5–5.0 L) despite a mean operative blood loss of 1.1 L (range, 0.3–5 L). Patients receiving more than 3 L of iv fluid had a mortality rate of 22%($p < 0.05$). Parquin et al. (39) reported that an intraoperative iv load of more than 2 L was an independent predictor of PPPE on multivariate analysis. Swartz et al. (40) identified excess fluid administration in the first 12 hours postoperatively as an independent predictor for death after pneumonectomy. Moller et al. (41) reported that 12.4% of patients undergoing pneumonectomy received more than 4 L during anesthesia! Regression analysis demonstrated that this was associated with a higher risk than blood loss of more than 1 L and was the strongest risk factor for postoperative complications and in-hospital mortality. Moller, an anesthetist, strongly suggests that trials comparing fluid restriction and vasopressor use versus current anesthetic practices must be instituted. I disagree . . . but yes, many patients are getting unnecessary iv loads.

Why the large iv load if patients are not bleeding?

Use of an iv fluid load during anesthesia, especially at induction and in the absence of significant blood loss during surgery, is ostensibly for defense of the systemic blood pressure. However, by definition, if the blood pressure drops during induction, it is related either to cardiac output or to reduced vasomotor tone. If the rate is sinus, the electrocardiogram is normal, and given the rarity that surgeons would continue a pneumonectomy in the face of an evolving myocardial infarction or the scarcity of details (if any) regarding the use of inotropes either intra- or postpneumonectomy, then the cause of the loss of blood pressure is a reduced peripheral vascular resistance secondary to anesthesia. It is illogical to bolster the preload with crystalloid when the cause is best served by a vasopressor, the antidote for a reduced systemic vascular resistance. Brodsky and Fitzmaurice (42) advocate that "in most situations small amounts of a vasopressor . . . rather than intravenous fluid, should be used to improve cardiac performance during thoracotomy." I agree, but not because you are treating cardiac dysfunction rather than reduced afterload.

Given what is known about PPPE and the effects of acute elevation in LAP in animals, it is untenable to persist with a practice of acute volume loading affecting 10% or more of these patients. Based on the animal data, I concur with Slinger (22) that "there may be an individual critical pulmonary capillary pressure for patients at which edema will rapidly develop." Particularly because use of a Swan-Ganz catheter or intraoperative trans oesophageal echocardiography (TOE) is not standard practice during pneumonectomy, the response of the left and right ventricle is unmeasured and, thus, unnoticed. Yet, 18% to 33% (or more) of patients undergoing a pneumonectomy have a history of ischemic heart disease (14, 18). It is worth remembering that in unselected series, pneumonectomy carries a mortality rate that has remained unchanged for the last decade or longer (~10%) (21, 43, 44). Hence, I suggest that no such trials as Moller desires are warranted and that the anesthetist should treat the primary cause (systemic vasodilatation) by a vasopressor, not by a variable (ie, intraoperative crystalloid volume load) that remains implicated in the pathogenesis of a devastating complication—PPPE.

Increased Permeability of the Alveolar Epithelial-Capillary Endothelial Barrier

The poor response to diuretics and the development of PPPE despite the absence of excessive intra- or postoperative volume loading could not be explained by volume overload alone. Mathru et al. (26), in five patients with PPPE, demonstrated that the ratio of the protein content of edema fluid to serum was greater than 0.6. This was the first clear evidence that a pulmonary membrane leak pathology existed. All of these patients had raised mean pulmonary artery pressure, normal to high cardiac output, and normal left (bar one) and right ventricular filling pressures. Based on the animal data from Staub (45) Mathru et al. (26) postulated that the increased protein leak was secondary to the mechanical disruption of the endothelial junctions from the increased flow velocity of blood following pneumonectomy. Mathru et al. further elaborated that at least two causative factors were at play: one being hydrostatic from fluid overload and the other being injury to the alveolar capillary membrane. However, all of these patients recovered with presumably conventional treatment, suggesting that the lung injury may have been ALI rather than ARDS/PPPE. West and Mathieu-Costello (46) demonstrated in rabbits that increases in capillary pressure above 40 mm Hg could produce destruction of all components of the alveolar epithelial-endothelial membrane.

Waller et al. (47), having previously demonstrated that their postpneumonectomy patients had noncardiogenic PPPE, measured pulmonary capillary permeability by means of radioisotopic tracer differential accumulation between the remaining lung and the heart in 21 men undergoing pneumonectomies and lobectomies. All pneumonectomies demonstrated increased tracer accumulation (ie, a leaky lung). One of their 10 pneumonectomies, serendipitously, developed PPPE. This membrane leak was observed solely in the pneumonectomy group and was maximal in the first 5 hours following surgery. Two factors appeared to be linked to increased protein leak following pneumonectomy: preoperative expression of neutrophil activation (ie, via changes in serum elastase) and increased pulmonary vascular resistance (PVR; >100 dynes · sec/cm^5) following pneumonectomy. Waller et al. suggested that two forces may be at play—activated neutrophils and intraoperative hemodynamic forces—thus suggesting that pulmonary vasodilators had a theoretically positive benefit. Finally, van der Werff et al. (9) implicated a potential immunological reaction adversely affecting the lung membrane from the administration of Fresh Frozen Plasma (FFP).

Mediastinal Lymphatic Damage

Based on Nohl-Oser's seminal description of metastatic deposits in resected lungs (48), the right lung is drained in the main (94%) via the right paratracheal lymph chain; however, the left has a significant component (56%) that is drained contralaterally. Hence, following a right pneumonectomy with mediastinal dissection, the left lung may have impaired lymphatic drainage with a higher incidence of PPPE. This is questionable, however, because despite what was previously thought, the incidence of PPPE may actually be equal regarding the site of surgery (9, 10, 20, 27, 39). Furthermore, the lymphatic drainage reserve of the lung is enormous. Zarins et al. (49) demonstrated in baboons that despite reductions in plasma oncotic pressure of 76% with a constant pulmonary hydrostatic pressure, resulting in a 7-fold increased lymph flow, no pulmonary edema occurred. Little et al. (50) noted no difference in the increase in EVLW between pneumonectomied dogs with or without mediastinal nodal dissection acutely challenged with a crystalloid load to an LAP of 23 mm Hg. Furthermore, Broaddus et al. (51) has presented evidence that lung lymph flow may not be a transvascular filtration steady-state process; instead, it can leak into the pleura (23–29% of all lymph flow) to further compensate for increased demands following permeability-induced pulmonary edema. However, gross pleural effusions are not reported with PPPE. Thus, lymphatic disruption may play a role, albeit an unlikely one, in triggering PPPE.

One-Lung Anesthesia and Volume Trauma

Intraoperative considerations

Conventional treatment of ventilated patients undergoing pneumonectomy uses tidal volumes of 10 to 12 mL/kg, respiratory rates of 10 to 12 breaths/min, inspiratory:expiratory ratios of 1 to 1.5:2, and accepts peak inspiratory pressures of less than 30 cm H_2O and end-tidal CO_2 of less than 30 mm Hg (22, 42, 52, 53). With one-lung ventilation (OLV), these parameters remain essentially unchanged (21, 42). Anesthetic practice, however, is not uniform. The fraction of inspired oxygen used by anesthetists in patients with OLV ranges from 0.3 to 1.0; so, too, some anesthetists reduce tidal volumes by 1 to 2 mL/kg with OLV (42, 53–55). The single dependent lung is thus variably subjected to hyperoxia and hyperinflation capable of damaging the alveolar-endothelial barrier (2, 56–58).

Hyperoxia

Shimizu et al. (55) recorded arterial partial pressure of oxygen (PaO_2) levels of 338 to 364 mm Hg and 139.7 to 179 mm Hg at the start and 30 minutes, after OLV, respectively. Moutafis et al. (59) recorded PaO_2 levels of 305 and 178 mm Hg at 10 and 30 minutes of OLV, respectively. Indeed, Moutafis et al. advocate the use of nitric oxide (NO) and almitrine to prevent episodes of arterial desaturation; with these two drugs, the corresponding PaO_2 values at 20 and 30 minutes of OLV were 354 and 325 mm Hg respectively. These policies aim to minimize the incidence of hypoxemia (arterial oxygen saturation [SaO_2], <90%) associated with OLV.

How frequently does arterial desaturation actually occur? Moutafis et al. reported an incidence of 45% in 20 patients requiring Video Assisted Thoracoscopy (VAT) surgery. However, Fradj et al. (53) stated that only "a relatively small percentage of patients experienced hypoxemia." Schwarzkopf et al. (52) recorded an incidence of 1.3% (2/151 patients) during thoracotomy.

The oxidative stress effects of OLV with the generation of cytotoxic reactive oxygen species (ROS) has been implicated in the etiology of PPPE (57). In rats subjected to OLV with and without pneumonectomy, hydroxyl radical damage with increased albumin permeability of the lung, impaired oxygenation, and raised pulmonary pressures occurred; these changes were absent in controls (58). Interestingly, pretreatment with an ROS scavenger (superoxide dismutase) and an NO synthetase inhibitor (NNL-arginine methyl ester) attenuated and abolished these changes, respectively. Williams et al. (60), using plasma surrogate markers (thiols and protein carbonyls) of ROS, also demonstrated that oxidative damage occurs with all lung resections in humans. Lases et al. (57), using surrogate parameters of oxidative stress (urine malondialdehyde [MDH] and expired H_2O_2), also revealed that oxidative stress occurs after lung resection. One patient developed PPPE and displayed significantly elevated levels of H_2O_2 and MDH. Carvalho et al. (61) suggest, however, that the human lung is more resistant to hyperoxic damage than previously expected.

Hyperinflation

Subjecting one abnormal lung (ie, that vast majority of patients undergoing pneumonectomies) in a decubitus position to twice its physiological tidal volume potentially exposes this lung to added injury. In ventilated dogs, increases in alveolar pressures greater than 10 cm H_2O resulted in significant increases in EVLW and pulmonary edema (62, 63). Grosfeld et al. (64) induced severe interstitial emphysema causing "air block syndrome" in cats by raising intratracheal pressure greater than 40 cm H_2O. Major et al. (65) demonstrated a linear relationship between the severity of interstitial perivascular emphysema from induced overinflation and rises in PVR. West and Mathieu-Costello (46) demonstrated that overinflation produces "stress failure" of the alveolar-capillary membrane with severe pulmonary edema. In rabbits, Bregeon et al. (66) provided evidence that tidal volumes of 10 mL/kg produced a proinflammatory cytokine upregulation in alveolar macrophages associated with increased alveolar macrophage numbers, cytokine production, and significant increases in EVLW.

In humans, Larson et al. (56) revealed that the FRC immediately following left pneumonectomy was increased by 30%. Slinger (21) comments that the lung is maximally compliant at its normal Functional Residual Capacity (FRC). The combination of 10 mL/kg tidal volumes and the development of auto-positive end-expiratory pressure with OLV, with a raised FRC, results in end-inspiratory lung volumes at high risk for volotrauma (67). So, too, at these levels of FRC, the PVR and pulmonary pressures will increase, potentially compounding the Starling effect on an already-abnormal lung receiving the entire cardiac output. Van der Werff et al. (9) found higher intraoperative ventilation pressures (>40 cm H_2O) significantly associated with the development of PPPE (relative risk, 3.0; 95% confidence interval, 1.2–7.3.). Critically, the incidence of premanifest PPPE was 34.3% with raised ventilation pressures versus 13% without; 17% of the premanifest group developed PPPE, with a 100% mortality. This is the first report clinically linking intraoperative hyperinflation with causation in PPPE (9). Slinger (22) thus advocates limiting peak airway and plateau pressures to 35 and 25 cm H_2O, respectively (67).

Fuentes (43), on the basis of a 22% significant reduction in mortality reported by the Acute Respiratory Distress Syndrome Network Trial using 6 mL/kg tidal volumes and concerns of volotrauma with OLV, has started a clinical trial of "protective" low tidal volumes (5–7 mL/kg), the results of which are eagerly awaited. Given that as much as 20% of cases of PPPE occur in the operating theatre (24), that biochemical evidence of lung injury (ROS) is either common or universal following lung resection (2), and that extensive animal data link pulmonary overinflation to alveolar-capillary damage, it is apparent that contemporary anesthetic practices of ventilation for thoracic surgery (ie, OLV) are far from per-fect. At the very least, trials of reduced tidal volumes, permissive hyper-capnia, or alternative means of ventilatory modes (ie, high-frequency in-termittent positive-pressure ventilation with jet ventilation) must be performed. Fundamentally, OLV is for the benefit of the surgeon, and pneumonectomy may be possible to perform safely without OLV, as has been my experience with sheep (unpublished data).

Postoperative hyperinflation

Air egress from the empty hemithorax can occur at a variable rate via the thoracotomy (ie, with sneezing or coughing). Consequently, the reduc-tion in intrathoracic pressure in the empty hemithorax can induce medi-astinal shift, with hyperinflation of the remaining lung. If this hyperin-flation is severe enough, given the plethora of factors occurring following pneumonectomy, then alveolar-capillary membrane damage leading to PPPE may occur (68). The induced hyperinflation in the remaining lung can be substantial, acute, and unrecognized. The surgical management of the drainage of the empty hemithorax is variable. Three options exist: no intercostal tube (ICT) drainage, clamped ICT drainage with intermittent release to an underwater seal (UWS), or a balanced ICT-UWS drainage, as described by Laforet and Boyd (69) roughly 40 years ago (Figure 9.1). Only the latter allows for automatic correction of changes in intrathoracic pressure in the empty hemithorax, thus preventing mediastinal shift.

Neonatal correction of diaphragmatic hernia (CDH) can be associ-ated with a syndrome nearly identical to PPPE both in clinical presen-tation and in outcome. The hypoplastic lung on the side of the corrected

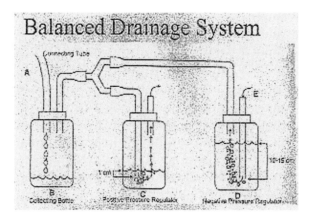

FIGURE 9.1 Postpneumonectomy balance drainage system.

hernia fails to fully expand, causing hyperinflation of the contralateral lung and severe pulmonary hypertension. Often, a "honeymoon period" of adequate gas exchange occurs, followed by progressive respiratory distress, ARDS, and death (70, 71). The development of extensive and severe pulmonary interstitial emphysema (PIE) and alveolar disruption induces progressive centripetal air dissection, with the consequent effects of producing collapse of peripheral and central blood vessels (ie, air-block syndrome) (6, 64).

Ramenofsky (70) analyzed the effect of the empty pleural space following pneumonectomy on the remaining lung. Newborn beagle puppies subjected to a left pneumonectomy were divided into two groups: In group 1, the ICT was drained to UWS at -2 cm H_2O, and in group 2, the ICT was attached to a pressure manometer and air-filled syringe, with the mediastinal shift being prevented by air injection. By 4 and 24 hours following surgery, 50% and 100% of group 1 animals, respectively, had died from histologically confirmed ARDS, compared to 36.3% in group 2. Critically, all group 2 deaths were technical (ie, non-ARDS). Impressively, in group 1, the intrapleural pressures exceeded -10 cm H_2O by 4 hours following surgery. Raffensperger et al. (72) similarly conducted left pneumonectomies on beagle puppies and demonstrated that the removal of air in the empty hemithorax produced immediate hypoxemia, hypercapnia, and increased alveolar-arterial CO_2 gradients. The removal of such air caused mediastinal shift and overdistension of the remaining lung, with histologically confirmed PIE and disrupted alveoli. Raffensperger et al. thus advocated that the mediastinum should be stabilized in the midline following repair of CDH. De Luca et al. (73), in fetal lambs with surgically created CDH followed by delayed (>30 days) repair, noted that PIE developed in all lambs and that ICT drainage promoted barotrauma from hyperinflation of the remaining lung.

Deslauriers et al. (27), reviewing their incidence of PPPE among 291 pneumonectomies from 1988 to 1993, identified the type of postoperative pleural drainage system to be a very significant risk factor for developing PPPE ($p = 0.009$). Multivariate analysis was not included regarding the two other variables associated with PPPE: extent of resection (simple or extended, $p = 0.04$) and length of surgery ($p = 0.005$). Nevertheless, no patient (0/77) with a balanced drainage system developed PPPE, compared to 6.5% (13/199) without (PPPE: no ICT drainage, 2.6% [2/78]; ICT-UWS, 9.1% [11/121]).

We also were concerned about the possibility of unrecognized hyperinflation of the remaining lung secondary to a vacuum effect from reduced intrathoracic pressure in the operated hemithorax (68). We therefore changed from an ICT-UWS drainage clamped with an intermittent-release system (era 1, 1993–1996), in which no injection of air was performed, because it appeared not to be required clinically and also based on serial postoperative chest radiography. Our incidence of PPPE from 1993 to 1996 was 14.3% (4/28 pneumonectomies). Following use of the balanced drainage system (era 2, 1996–2000), we reported no cases (0%) in 29 pneumonectomies ($p = 0.001$). Importantly, no cases of postpneumonectomy space infection occurred in our series, nor was this reported by Laforet and Boyd (69) or by Deslauriers et al. (27). This is the theoretical Achilles' heel associated with allowing the ingress of outside air.

Right Ventricular Dysfunction

Reed et al. (74), in 15 lung resections (two pneumonectomies) in patients without a history of cardiac disease and with preoperative echocardiography available in 33%, demonstrated increases in right ventricular end-diastolic volume (RVEDV; >20mL) and reductions in right ventricular ejection fraction (RVEF; >0.9) from baseline by day 2 postsurgery. Furthermore, Reed et al. (75) demonstrated that these changes were independent of intrinsic right ventricular myocardial contractility. Importantly, Reed et al. (74) demonstrated that conventional indices of right ventricular performance do not accurately reflect actual right ventricular performance. Hence, the CVP remained unaltered despite significant changes to RVEDV and RVEF.

The effects of pneumonectomy differ markedly between rest and exercise. Van Mieghen and Demedts (76) demonstrated a less than 30% rise of PVR and mean pulmonary arterial pressure (MPAP) from baseline with exercise that was also associated with reduced arterial saturation. Lindgrem et al. (77) incidentally documented significant increases in right ventricular pressures in controls (54%) compared to verapamil-treated patients (13%) on withdrawal of oxygen in patients following thoracotomy. Slinger (1) thus cogently states that premature withdrawal of oxygen therapy could exacerbate the right ventricular dysfunction that occurs following lung resection and "points to the potential benefits of monitoring oxygenation and right heart function post thoracotomy." Amar et al. (78) noted that pneumonectomy patients had higher MPAP manifest from day 2 postsurgery and that right ventricular enlargement occurred in both lobectomy and pneumonectomy patients and heralded a poor prognosis if respiratory failure ensued.

Right ventricular dysfunction can interfere with lymphatic clearance from the lung and, by adversely affecting left ventricular performance, cause higher PCWP, thus having a net Starling effect on pulmonary capillaries favoring edema formation. Ostensibly, although right ventricular dysfunction may likely contribute adversely to the course of PPPE, the etiological importance remains undefined.

Occult Microaspiration

Deslauriers et al. (27) have implicated the possible role of microaspiration secondary to a reduced state of airway protection/consciousness from the effect of effective analgesia. In a retrospective review of 1,045 consecutive patients undergoing lung resections, significant respiratory complications occurred in 14.8% (79). However, respiratory insufficiency "occurred much more often between 1980–90 than 1990–2000." Aubree et al. (79) suggest that this may be due to the effect of excessive postoperative analgesia (particularly epidural analgesia).

The undeniable, overwhelming weight of evidence both in animal and human data, I suggest, clearly demands that we, at the very least, reassess conventional surgical and anaesthetic axioms of intra- and postoperative management of pneumonectomy cases.

WHO IS AT RISK OF DEVELOPING PPPE?

Examining the data from series containing in excess of 50 patients subjected to pneumonectomy and/or reporting more than three cases of PPPE reveals conflicting results. There are several reasons. Not all series address each variable; Ruffini et al. (20) make no analysis of perioperative fluid load. Kutlu et al. (10) and Ruffini et al. (20) do not separate ALI from ARDS, and interestingly, only Kutlu et al. (10) include nonlung cancer surgery. Critically important, no series has been conducted in a prospective fashion. However, unequivocal agreement exists that this syndrome occurs more often after pneumonectomy than after lobectomy (by a factor of 5- to 10-fold). From the available data, 14 variables have been associated with the syndrome of PPPE (Table 9.4.).

Recently, Caras (30) suggested, albeit based on only two patients, that advanced emphysema measured by quantitative CT scan emphysema scores may predict patients at risk for PPPE, because a poor relationship exists between spirometric assessment and actual histopathology.

MANAGEMENT STRATEGIES FOR PNEUMONECTOMY AND PPPE

Contemporary standard pneumonectomy continues to carry a significant risk of death, with a very broad range of reported mortality rates (2.1–22%) (20, 80). However, right-sided pneumonectomies unquestionably have a higher risk, with an average mortality rate of 10%; the range is also broad (10–24%), depending on factors such as age and use of neoadjuvant therapy (21, 40, 44). As Fuentes (43) stated, this risk is

TABLE 9.4   Variables Associated with Development of
Postpneumonectomy Pulmonary Edema

Variable	Yes[a]	No[a]
Preoperative		
Age > 60 years	10	19, 27
Male sex	10	19, 20, 27, 39
Neoajuvant chemo/radiotherapy	39	20
Cancer surgery	10	—
Remaining lung perfusion < 55%	39	—
Intraoperative		
Right pneumonectomy	3, 19, 23, 37	9, 10, 20, 24, 27, 28, 39
Extended/completion pneumonectomy	10, 27	20
Return thoracotomy	37	9
Administration of FFP	9	—
Duration of surgery > 143 minutes	27	9
Reduction in preoperative serum elastase	47	—
Anaesthetic		
Intraoperative iv fluid load > 2 L	39	—
Maximum inspiratory pressure > 40cm H$_2$O	9	—
Postoperative		
Excess net 24-hour fluid balance > 1.8 L	3, 37, 38	9, 20, 19, 23, 24, 27
Nonbalanced drainage of the empty hemithorax	27, 68	—

FFP = Fresh Frozen Plasma.
[a]References cited.

"one of the highest that may be encountered by patients having non-emergent surgery." Based on this reality, plus the added reality of PPPE and the data just reviewed, the following recommendations for prophylaxis and treatment are suggested.

Prophylaxis

Anesthetic Considerations

1. Avoid exacerbating hypotension from fasting-related hypovolemia (ie, preload) and associated perianesthetic hypotension (ie, systemic afterload) by iv replacement at 1 mL/kg/h from commencement of the fasting state.
2. Use vasopressors (eg, metaraminol, ephedrine) instead of rapid volume replacement for nonhemorrhagic hypotension (3).
3. Avoid intraoperative volume loads greater than 2 L. Aim to replace solely ongoing physiological and surgical losses. The chest has no third space (1, 22).

4. Use the lowest tidal volume consistent with an SaO_2 of greater than 90%, a peak airway pressure of less than 35 cm H_2O, and plateau end-inspiratory pressure of less than 25 cm H_2O.
5. Minimize the risk of excessive analgesia following surgery. (No epidurals?)

Surgical Considerations

1. Expeditious, precise, and hemostatic surgery (ie, avoid FFP) must be "de rigeur."
2. Total positive fluid balance for the first 48 hours should be physiological to minimal (<20 mL/kg/day).
3. Use a balanced drainage system.
4. Continue oxygen therapy for at least 3 days, aiming to keep the SaO_2 greater than 91%.
5. Avoid the decubitus position to the operated side.
6. Preoperative neoadjuvant therapy must be used solely as part of a clinical trial.

Additional Considerations

For logical decisions regarding volume replacement and hemodynamics to be achieved intra- and postoperatively, baseline preoperative echocardiography with particular quantification of right ventricular dimensions and function should be standard. This may identify patients who may be at increased risk of ventricular dysfunction (right or left), thus facilitating appropriate and early use of inotropes. Given that 18% to 33% (18, 33) of patients have a history of coronary artery disease, at the very least continuous CVP monitoring should be established before surgery, with a low threshold for Swan-Ganz catheterization and serial echocardiography following surgery.

A "one shoe fits all" mentality regarding pneumonectomy has not produced excellent outcomes; hence, tailoring therapies to patients may do so. Therefore, preoperative optimization of renal function in patients, and in particular those with chronic renal impairment (serum creatinine, >130mmol/L), using renal-dose dopamine and prophylactic saline-mannitol has been successful in cardiac surgery and merits consideration (81). Our aim is to maintain the lowest ventricular filling pressure (based on CVP/PCWP) consistent with adequate tissue perfusion based on a systolic blood pressure of greater than 100 mm Hg, a UO of greater than 0.5 mL/kg/h, warm peripheries, and if available, CI of greater than 2.0 L/min/m^2 both intra- and postoperatively (19).

Treatment

Based on the relentless, severe nature of this syndrome, we have outlined an aggressive approach once PPPE is suspected (68). A high index of suspicion cannot be overstated, particularly as a premanifest syndrome (ALI?), at least on a plausible theoretical basis of a continuum of disease progression, may allow therapies to abort progression to the severe and irreversible stage of PPPE/ARDS. Arguably, the focus thus relies, in patients who are kept "dry," on detecting the development of oliguria secondary to fluid sequestration in the chest. The irreconcilable initial sign is the radiographic onset of at times subtle pulmonary infiltrates on chest radiography. If a balanced drainage system is not used, reliance on daily chest radiography for evidence of mediastinal shift with correction by air injection is folly given Ramenofsky's evidence (70). Remembering that the first sign in as many as 20% of patients may be increased ventilatory pressures and arterial desaturation in the operating theatre, detubation and initiation of therapy may be required intraoperatively.

Immediate exclusion of pulmonary embolism by CT angiography with pre-emptive anticoagulation based on the patient history is essential. Immediate bronchoscopy allows assessment of the bronchial stump, bronchial toilet, and accessing secretions for microbiological culture.

Empiric antibiotic therapy is advisable until the results of microbiological assays (eg, urine, blood) are available. Transfer to the ICU is essential, and use of a Swan-Ganz catheter, together with serial echocardiography, will assist with guiding early and appropriate inotropic therapy. On theoretical grounds, high-dose corticosteroids for 48 to 72 hours appears to be justified; similarly, colloids should be avoided. Oxygen therapy is guided by oximetry aiming to keep the SaO_2 at greater than 90%, and an enforced diuresis with loop diuretics should be added to the prophylactic renoprotective regimen as required.

The key decision is whether to intubate the patient early and electively (19, 28). We, like others, advocated elective intubation on demonstration of progression of radiographic changes consistent with a diagnosis of PPPE. However, recent data have made the role of CPAP controversial for two reasons. First, despite a sole report by Nabers et al. (82) of successful CPAP management of PPPE for 6 days with survival, we, like most others, have not advocated CPAP use. We found that CPAP provided variable, temporary relief, but all patients required intubation, at times in an emergent fashion (19, 27). However, Auriant et al. (83) recently reported that in a randomized trial of 48 patients admitted to the ICU for ARDS following lung resection, those treated by immediate CPAP had, compared to medical therapy, significantly improved survival (12.5% vs 37%) and need for intubation and mechanical ventilation

(21% vs 50%). Second, the early use of NO on diagnosis of ARDS to treat PPPE has recently produced the best survival outcomes to date (28).

Use of pulmonary-specific vasodilators, such as prostacyclin and NO, to treat PPPE has cogent appeal on theoretical grounds, but translation into consistent, demonstrable clinical improvement has been elusive (84, 85). Hence, despite NO being introduced and widely used in clinical practice since 1993, a recent large, prospective, observational study analyzing outcomes in treating ARDS revealed that although mortality was significantly reduced (from 66% to 34%), this resulted from by better ICU organizational changes (ie, better treatment of sepsis and changed ventilatory strategies); specifically, the effect of widespread use of other therapeutic interventions (ie, including NO) could not be "meaningfully assessed" (84).

Use of pulmonary vasodilators, such as prostacyclin and NO, to treat PPPE had been reported with inconsistent success (22, 86, 87). However, Mathisen et al. (28) reported a 65% reduction in mortality subsequent to the introduction of NO use for PPPE. In 10 consecutive patients (1993–1997) with PPPE and meeting accepted criteria for ARDS compared to a historical control group (1986–1993) of seven consecutive patients with PPPE, the use of NO reduced the mortality rate from 86% to 30%. Nitric oxide was introduced immediately on diagnosis of ARDS, which implies, given their stated policy of early intubation, that it commenced on endotracheal intubation. The concentration of NO varied from 5 to 20 ppm. The median number of days that NO was required was 6.5 (range, 3–39 days). None of the three deaths were ARDS-related. Clearly, the impact of NO use was striking (25).

There were, however, confounding variables in the Mathisen et al. (28) study. Half the patients received simultaneous high-dose iv corticosteroids for 48 hours, with apparent (but not statistically significant) improvement in gas-exchange parameters, but the historical controls did not receive corticosteroids. Furthermore, although this is a unit with a stated "high index of awareness for PPPE" and a stated prompt, aggressive policy of early intervention (eg, bronchoscopy, antibiotics), intubation, and enforced diuresis, no mention is made of other potentially confounding variables (eg, changes to intraoperative anaesthetic ventilatory parameters, postoperative management of the empty hemothorax, perioperative net fluid status). Nevertheless, no better results have been achieved, and adhering to the guidelines for the use of NO proposed by Mathisen et al. appears to be prudent.

The impact of previously mentioned strategies would be sabotaged if the process of mechanical ventilation enhanced further alveolar-endothelial damage. As Abel et al. (84) have demonstrated, better ventilation strategies (ie, smaller tidal volumes) have contributed to improved survival. Extensive animal data have demonstrated that the deleterious effects, termed barotrauma, are in the main caused by hyperinflation, or "volotrauma" (21, 88). Conventional tidal volumes used during mechanical ventilation range from 10 to 15 mL/kg, compared to physiological values of 6 to 8 mL/kg. The clear priority is normocapnia, normoxemia, and a normal pH—at the potential expense of added lung damage. In patients with PPPE, the lung damage is severe, so a priority of ventilatory management may be contributing to the poor outcomes. Although uncontrolled studies suggested better outcomes in ARDS with lower tidal volumes, four randomized trials revealed no benefit (89). Weaknesses with these four trials, however, were addressed by the Acute Respiratory Distress Syndrome Network Study (89), which investigated the effect of traditional treatment (tidal volume, 12 mL/kg; end-inspiratory airway pressure, <50 cm H_2O) versus "lung friendly" treatment (tidal volume, 6 mL/kg; end-inspiratory airway pressure, <30 cm H_2O) (89). The trial was terminated prematurely, however, because the lung-friendly group demonstrated a 22% reduced mortality rate (31% vs 39.8%, $p = .005$). Guidelines on specific gas-exchange/acid-base status management neutralized pretrial theoretical concerns (89). It would be hoped that adoption of this strategy may further improve outcomes in patients with PPPE.

Use of extracorporeal support in patients with PPPE has also been anecdotally described with variable success (90). Use of Extra Corporeal Membrane Oxygenation (ECMO) for ARDS is controversial in adults and beyond the scope of this monograph. Suffice it to say that the vision of Deslauriers and Awad (91) of a future means of performing "lung dialysis" by the arrival of technologically friendly, reliable, and inexpensive equipment is both challenging and interesting. This remains a personal decision between the physician and the patient/family. If it is to be considered, it should be finite in duration and cognizant of the Tumor Node Metastasis (TNM) status of the patient, associated comorbidities, and reality-based data regarding long-term survival expectations for that specific patient.

PPPE: FACTS AND WEAKNESSES

The uncommon, but not rare, incidence of PPPE as well as the associated problems of nomenclature, recognition, and diagnosis have translated into a body of literature accurately described as "sparse" (10). Only 19 reports could be identified in the English-language literature specifically dealing with this syndrome, and 42% (8/19) included fewer than five patients with PPPE (30, 31, 38, 39, 47, 86, 87, 80). This literary corpus dealt with 172 cases of PPPE/ARDS and 48 cases of ALI/pre-manifest PPPE. Hence, despite near 20 years having passed since Zeldin's (3) seminal description, the total English-speaking worldwide number of reported PPPE cases is approximately equal to the annual expected rate of PPPE in the United Kingdom (165 cases/year) (2).

Furthermore, all these reports are retrospective and nonuniform in both documentation and analysis of potentially important variables dealing with causation and prognosis. It is therefore clear that a concerted effort should be undertaken to achieve consensus regarding definition, diagnosis, and treatment. This would necessitate multicenter collaboration as an absolute prerequisite.

The British Thoracic Society guidelines regarding selection of patients with lung cancer for surgery state that the mortality rate for pneumonectomy should not be in excess of 8% (92). Fuentes (43), however believes—and I concur—regarding pneumonectomy that "it is however obvious that there is almost one out of ten who will die after such an operation, whatever the surgical group, the institution or the country may be." Clearly, it is apparent that Fuentes and others pragmatically believe that the true mortality rate without selection bias is actually 10%, with a broad range (44) (Table 9.3). Because the reality for right pneumonectomy is an operative mortality rate in excess of 8% and because the leading cause of death is PPPE, decisions regarding how we assess and treat these patients (anesthetically, surgically, and in the ICU) should be made in an environment of collaborative, prospective data accumulation and rational scientific analysis of therapeutic interventions. That is the challenge to which physicians treating these patients must rise, because unquestionably, there certainly is far more to this puzzle (PPPE) than simply withholding fluids.

References

1. Slinger PD: Perioperative fluid management for thoracic surgery: the puzzle of postpneumonectomy pulmonary edema. J Cardiothorac Vasc Anesth 1995; 9:442–51.
2. Williams EA, Evans TW, Goldstraw P: Acute lung injury following lung resection: is one lung anaesthesia to blame? Thorax 1996; 51:114–6.
3. Zeldin RA, Normandin D, Landtwing D, Peters RM: Postpneumonectomy pulmonary edema. J Thorac Cardiovasc Surg 1984; 87:359–65.
4. Peters RM. Pulmonary resection and gas exchange. J Thorac Cardiovasc Surg. 1984; 88(5 pt 2):872–9.
5. Gibbon JH, Gibbon MH: Experimental pulmonary edema following lobectomy and plasma infusion. J Thorac Surg 1942; 12:694–704.
6. Macklin MT, Macklin CC: Malignant interstitial emphysema of the lungs and mediastinum as an important occult complication in

many respiratory diseases and other conditions: an interpretation of the clinical literature in the light of laboratory experiment. Medicine 1944; 23:281–358.

7. Ginsberg RJ, Hill LD, Eagan RT, Thomas P, Mountain CF, Deslauriers J, Fry WA, Butz RO, Goldberg M, Waters PF, et al.: Modern thirty-day operative mortality for surgical resections in lung cancer. J Thorac Cardiovasc Surg 1983; 86:654–8.

8. Hirschler-Schulte CJ, Hylkema BS, Meyer RW: Mechanical ventilation for acute postoperative respiratory failure after surgery for bronchial carcinoma. Thorax 1985; 40:387–90.

9. Van der Werff YD, van der Houwen HK, Heijmans PJ, Duurkens VA, Leusink HA, van Heesewijk HP, de Boer A: Postpneumonectomy pulmonary edema. A retrospective analysis of incidence and possible risk factors. Chest 1997; 111:1278–84.

10. Kutlu CA, Williams EA, Evans TW, Pastorino U, Goldstraw P: Acute lung injury and acute respiratory distress syndrome after pulmonary resection. Ann Thorac Surg 2000; 69:376–80.

11. Harpole DH, Liptay MJ, DeCamp MM Jr, Mentzer SJ, Swanson SJ, Sugarbaker DJ: Prospective analysis of pneumonectomy: risk factors for major morbidity and cardiac dysrhythmias. Ann Thorac Surg 1996; 61:977–82.

12. Wada H, Nakamura T, Nakamoto K, Maeda M, Watanabe Y: Thirty-day operative mortality for thoracotomy in lung cancer. J Thorac Cardiovasc Surg 1998; 115:70–3.

13. Patel RL, Townsend ER, Fountain SW: Elective pneumonectomy: factors associated with morbidity and operative mortality. Ann Thorac Surg. 1992; 54:84–8.

14. Licker M, Spiliopoulos A, Frey JG, Robert J, Hohn L, de Perrot M, Tschopp JM: Risk factors for early mortality and major complications following pneumonectomy for non-small cell carcinoma of the lung. Chest 2002; 121:1890–7.

15. Stephan F, Boucheseiche S, Hollande J, Flahault A, Cheffi A, Bazelly B, Bonnet F: Pulmonary complications following lung resection: a comprehensive analysis of incidence and possible risk factors. Chest 2000; 118:1263–70.

16. Bernard A, Ferrand L, Hagry O, Benoit L, Cheynel N, Favre JP: Identification of prognostic factors determining risk groups for lung resection. Ann Thorac Surg 2000; 70:1161–7.

17. Myrdal G, Gustafsson G, Lambe M, Horte LG, Stahle E: Outcome after lung cancer surgery. Factors predicting early mortality and major morbidity. Eur J Cardiothorac Surg 2001; 20:694–9.

18. Alexiou C, Beggs D, Rogers ML, Beggs L, Asopa S, Salama FD: Pneumonectomy for non-small cell lung cancer: predictors of operative mortality and survival. Eur J Cardiothorac Surg 2001; 20:476–80.

19. Alvarez JM., Bairstow BM, Tang C, Newman MAJ: Post-lung resection pulmonary edema: a case for aggressive management. J Cardiothorac Vasc Anesth 1998; 12:199–205.
20. Ruffini E, Parola A, Papalia E, Filosso PL, Mancuso M, Oliaro A, Actis-Dato G, Maggi G: Frequency and mortality of acute lung injury and acute respiratory distress syndrome after pulmonary resection for bronchogenic carcinoma. Eur J Cardiothorac Surg 2001; 20:30–6.
21. Martin J, Ginsberg RJ, Abolhoda A, Bains MS, Downey RJ, Korst RJ, Weigel TL, Kris MG, Venkatraman ES, Rusch VW: Morbidity and mortality after neoadjuvant therapy for lung cancer: the risks of right pneumonectomy. Ann Thorac Surg 2001;72:1149–54.
22. Slinger P: Postpneumonectomy pulmonary edema: is anaesthesia to blame? Curr Opin Anaesthesiol 1999; 12:49–54.
23. Turnage WS, Lunn JJ: Postpneumonectomy pulmonary edema. A retrospective analysis of associated variables. Chest 1993; 103:1646–50.
24. Waller DA, Gebitekin C, Saunders NR, Walker DR: Noncardiogenic pulmonary edema complicating lung resection. Ann Thorac Surg 1993; 55:140–3.
25. Alvarez JM. Nitric oxide for ARDS. Ann Thorac Surg 1999; 68:2387.
26. Mathru M, Blakeman B, Dries DJ, Kleinman B, Kumar P: Permeability pulmonary edema following lung resection. Chest 1990; 98:1216–8.
27. Deslauriers J, Aucoin A, Gregoire J: Postpneumonectomy pulmonary edema. Chest Surg Clin N Am 1998; 8:611–31.
28. Mathisen DJ, Kuo EY, Hahn C, Moncure AC, Wain JC, Grillo HC, Hurford WE, Wright CD: Inhaled nitric oxide for adult respiratory distress syndrome after pulmonary resection. Ann Thorac Surg 1998; 66:1894–902.
29. Wittnich C, Trudel J, Zidulka A, Chiu RC: Misleading "pulmonary wedge pressure" after pneumonectomy: its importance in postoperative fluid therapy. Ann Thorac Surg 1986; 42:192–6.
30. Caras WE. Postpneumonectomy pulmonary edema: can it be predicted preoperatively? Chest 1998; 114:928–31.
31. Shapira OM, Shahian DM: Postpneumonectomy pulmonary edema. Ann Thorac Surg 1993; 56:190–5.
32. Satur CM, Robertson RH, Da Costa PE, Saunders NR, Walker DR: Multiple pulmonary microemboli complicating pneumonectomy. Ann Thorac Surg 1991; 52:122–6.
33. Staub NC: Pulmonary edema: physiological approaches to management. Chest 1978:74:559–64.
34. Jordan S, Mitchell JA, Quinlan GJ, Goldstraw P, Evans TW: The

pathogenesis of lung injury following pulmonary resection. Eur Respir J 2000; 15:790–9.

35. Guyton AC, Lindsey AW: Effect of elevated left atrial pressure and decreased plasma protein concentration on the development of pulmonary edema. Circ Res 1959; 7:649–57.
36. Lee E, Little AG, Wen-Hu H, Skinner DB: Effect of pneumonectomy on extravascular lung water in dogs. J Surg Res 1985; 38:568–73.
37. Verheijen-Breemhaar L, Bogaard JM, van den Berg B, Hilvering C: Postpneumonectomy pulmonary oedema. Thorax 1988; 43:323–6.
38. Margolis M: Postpneumonectomy pulmonary oedema. Thorax 1990; 45:239.
39. Parquin F, Marchal M, Mehiri S, Herve P, Lescot B: Postpneumonectomy pulmonary edema: analysis and risk factors. Eur J Cardiothorac Surg 1996; 10:929–32.
40. Swartz DE, Lachapelle K, Sampalis J, Mulder DS, Chiu RC, Wilson J: Perioperative mortality after pneumonectomy: analysis of risk factors and review of the literature. Can J Surg 1997; 40:437–44.
41. Moller AM, Pedersen T, Svendsen PE, Engquist A: Perioperative risk factors in elective pneumonectomy: the impact of excess fluid balance. Eur J Anaesthesiol 2002; 19:57–62.
42. Brodsky JB, Fitzmaurice B: Modern anesthetic techniques for thoracic operations. World J Surg 2001; 25:162–6.
43. Fuentes PA: Pneumonectomy: historical perspective and prospective insight. Eur J Cardiothorac Surg 2003; 23:439–45.
44. Joo JB, DeBord JR, Montgomery CE, Munns JR, Marshall JS, Paulsen JK, Anderson RC, Meyer LE, Estes NC: Perioperative factors as predictors of operative mortality and morbidity in pneumonectomy. Am Surg 2001; 67:318–21.
45. Staub NC: New concepts about the pathophysiology of pulmonary edema. J Thorac Imaging 1988; 3:8–14.
46. West JB, Mathieu-Costello O: Stress failure of pulmonary capillaries: role in lung and heart disease. Lancet 1992; 340:762–7.
47. Waller DA, Keavey P, Woodfine L, Dark JH: Pulmonary endothelial permeability changes after major lung resection. Ann Thorac Surg 1996; 61:1435–40.
48. Nohl-Oser HC: An investigation of the anatomy of the lymphatic drainage of the lungs. Ann R Coll Surg Engl 1972; 51:157–76.
49. Zarins CK, Rice CL, Peters RM, Virgilio RW: Lymph and pulmonary response to isobaric reduction in plasma oncotic pressure in baboons. Circ Res 1978; 43:925–30.
50. Little AG, Langmuir VK, Singer AH, Skinner DB: Hemodynamic pulmonary edema in dog lungs after contralateral pneumonectomy and mediastinal lymphatic interruption. Lung 1984; 162:139–45.
51. Broaddus VC, Wiener-Kronish JP, Staub NC: Clearance of lung

edema into the pleural space of volume-loaded anesthetized sheep. J Appl Physiol 1990; 68:2623–30.

52. Schwarzkopf K, Klein U, Schreiber T, Preussetaler NP, Bloos F, Helfritsch H, Sauer F, Karzai W: Oxygenation during one-lung ventilation: the effects of inhaled nitric oxide and increasing levels of inspired fraction of oxygen. Anesth Analg 2001; 92:842–7.

53. Fradj K, Samain E, Delefosse D, Farah E, Marty J: Placebo-controlled study of inhaled nitric oxide to treat hypoxaemia during one-lung ventilation. Br J Anaesth 1999; 82:208–12.

54. Wilson WC, Kapelanski DP, Benumof JL, Newhart JW II, Johnson FW, Channick RN: Inhaled nitric oxide (40 ppm) during one-lung ventilation, in the lateral decubitus position, does not decrease pulmonary vascular resistance or improve oxygenation in normal patients. J Cardiothorac Vasc Anesth 1997; 11:172–6.

55. Shimizu T, Abe K, Kinouchi K, Yoshiya I: Arterial oxygenation during one lung ventilation. Can J Anaesth 1997; 44:1162–6.

56. Larsson A, Malmkvist G, Werner O: Variations in lung volume and compliance during pulmonary surgery. Br J Anaesth 1987; 59:585–91.

57. Lases EC, Duurkens VA, Gerritsen WB, Haas FJ: Oxidative stress after lung resection therapy: a pilot study. Chest 2000; 117:999–1003.

58. Williams EA, Quinlan GJ, Anning PB, Goldstraw P, Evans TW: Lung injury following pulmonary resection in the isolated, blood-perfused rat lung. Eur Respir J 1999; 14:745–50.

59. Moutafis M, Liu N, Dalibon N, Kuhlman G, Ducros L, Castelain MH, Fischler M: The effects of inhaled nitric oxide and its combination with intravenous almitrine on PaO_2 during one-lung ventilation in patients undergoing thoracoscopic procedures. Anesth Analg 1997; 85:1130–5.

60. Williams EA, Quinlan GJ, Goldstraw P, Gothard JW, Evans TW: Postoperative lung injury and oxidative damage in patients undergoing pulmonary resection. Eur Respir J 1998; 11:1028–34.

61. Carvalho CR, de Paulo Pinto Schettino G, Maranhao B, Bethlem EP: Hyperoxia and lung disease. Curr Opin Pulm Med 1998; 4:300–4.

62. Albert RK, Lakshminarayan S, Kirk W, Butler J. Lung inflation can cause pulmonary edema in zone I of in situ dog lungs. J Appl Physiol 1980; 49:815–9.

63. Pang LM, Rodriguez-Martinez F, Stalcup SA, Mellins RB: Effect of hyperinflation and atelectasis on fluid accumulation in the puppy lung. J Appl Physiol 1978; 45:284–8.

64. Grosfeld JL, Boger D, Clatworthy HW: Hemodynamic and manometric observations in experimental air-block syndrome. J Pediatr Surg 1971; 6:339–344.

65. Major D, Cloutier R, Fournier L: Lung overexpansion, perivascular emphysema and pulmonary hypertension: preliminary results. Ital J Pediatr Surg Sci 1992; 6:7–10.
66. Bregeon F, Roch A, Delpierre S, Ghigo E, Autillo-Touati A, Kajikawa O, Martin TR, Pugin J, Portugal H, Auffray JP, Jammes Y: Conventional mechanical ventilation of healthy lungs induced pro-inflammatory cytokine gene transcription. Respir Physiol Neurobiol 2002: 132:191–203.
67. Dreyfuss D, Saumon G: Role of tidal volume, FRC and end inspiratory volume in the development of pulmonary edema following mechanical ventilation. Am Rev Respir Dis 1993; 148:1194–203.
68. Alvarez JM, Panda RK, Newman MAJ: Postpneumonectomy pulmonary edema: is the answer balanced pleural drainage? J Cardiothorac Vasc Anaesth 2003; 17:388–95.
69. Laforet EG, Boyd TF: Balanced drainage of the postpneumonectomy space. Surg Gynaecol Obstet 1964; 18:1051–64.
70. Ramenofsky ML. The effects of intrapleural pressure on respiratory insufficiency. J Pediatr Surg 1979; 14:750–56.
71. Srouji MN, Buck B, Downes JJ: Congenital diaphragmatic hernia: deleterious effects of pulmonary interstitial emphysema and tension extrapulmonary air. J Pediatr Surg 1981; 16:45–54.
72. Raffensperger JG, Luck SR, Inwood RJ: The effect of overdistension of the lung on pulmonary function in beagle puppies. J Pediatr Surg 1979; 14:757–60.
73. De Luca U, Cloutier JM, Laberge L, Fournier L, Prendt H, Major D, Edgell D, Roy PE, Roberge S, Guttman FM: Pulmonary barotrauma in congenital diaphragmatic hernia: experimental study in lambs. J Pediatr Surg 1987; 22:311–6.
74. Reed CE, Dorman BH, Spinale FG: Assessment of right ventricular contractile performance after pulmonary resection. Ann Thorac Surg 1993; 56:426–31.
75. Reed CE, Spinale FG, Crawford FA Jr: Effect of pulmonary resection on right ventricular function. Ann Thorac Surg 1992; 53:578–82.
76. Van Mieghem, Demedts M: Cardiopulmonary function after lobectomy or pneumonectomy for neoplasm. Respir Med 1989; 93:199–206.
77. Lindrem L, Lepantalo M, Van Knorring J, et al.: Effect of verapamil on right ventricular pressure and atrial tachyarrhythmia after thoracotomy. Br J Anaesth 1991; 66:205–11.
78. Amar D, Burt ME, Roistacher N, Reinsel RA, Ginsberg RJ, Wilson RS: Value of perioperative Doppler echocardiography in patients undergoing major lung resection. Ann Thorac Surg 1996; 61:516–20.

79. Aubree N, Gregoire G, Jacques LF, Piraux M, Guojin L, Lacasse Y, Deslauriers J: Respiratory complications after pneumonectomy. An analysis of incidence, risks factors and outcome. Presented at the 83rd AATS meeting, Boston, USA 2003.

80. Mizushima Y, Noto H, Sugiyama S, Kusajima Y, Yamashita R, Kashii T, Kobayashi M: Survival and prognosis after pneumonectomy for lung cancer in the elderly. Ann Thorac Surg 1997; 64:193–8.

81. Alvarez JM, Chatwin C, Fahrer C: The prevention of anuric renal failure post cardiac surgery in at risk patients by the prophylactic use of iv mannitol and normal saline. Heart Lung Circ 2000; 9:74–7.

82. Nabers J, Hoogsteden HC, Hilvering C: Postpneumonectomy pulmonary edema treated with a continuous positive airway pressure face mask. Crit Care Med 1989; 17:102–3.

83. Auriant I, Jallot A, Herve P, Cerrina J, Le Roy Ladurie F, Fournier JL, Lescot B, Parquin F: Noninvasive ventilation reduces mortality in acute respiratory failure following lung resection. Am J Respir Crit Care Med 2001; 164:1231–5.

84. Abel SJC, Finney SJ, Brett SJ, Keogh BF, Morgan CJ, Evans TW: Reduced mortality in association with the acute respiratory distress syndrome. Thorax 1998; 53:292–4.

85. Van Heerden PV, Webb SAR, Hee G, Corkeron M, Thompson WR: Inhaled aerosolised prostacyclin as a selective pulmonary vasodilator for the treatment of severe hypoxaemia. Anaesth Intensive Care 1996; 24:87–90.

86. Chiche JD, Canivet JL, Damas P, Joris J, Lamy M: Inhaled nitric oxide for hemodynamic support after postpneumonectomy ARDS. Intensive Care Med 1995; 21:675–8.

87. Rabkin DG, Sladen RN, DeMango A, Steinglass KM, Goldstein DJ: Nitric oxide for the treatment of postpneumonectomy pulmonary edema. Ann Thorac Surg. 2001; 72:272–4.

88. Hickling KG, Wright T, Laubscher K, Town IG, Tie A, Graham P, Monteath J, A'Court G: Extreme hypoventilation reduces ventilator-induced lung injury during ventilation with low positive end-expiratory pressure in saline-lavaged rabbits. Crit Care Med 1998; 26:1690–7.

89. The Acute Respiratory Distress Syndrome Network: Ventilation with lower tidal volumes as compared with traditional tidal volumes for acute lung injury and the acute respiratory distress syndrome. N Engl J Med 2000, 342:1301–8.

90. Verhelst H, Vranken J, Muysoms F, Rondelez L, Schroe H, De Jongh R: The use of extracorporeal membrane oxygenation in postpneumonectomy pulmonary oedema. Acta Chir Belg 1998; 98:269–72.

91. Deslauriers J, Awad JA: Is extracorporeal CO_2 removal an option in the treatment of adult respiratory distress syndrome? Ann Thorac 1997; 64:1581–2.
92. British Thoracic Society, Society of Cardiothoracic Surgeons of Great Britain, and Ireland Working Party: Guidelines on the selection of patients with lung cancer for surgery. Thorax 2001; 56:89–108.
93. Keagy BA, Schorlemmer GR, Murray GF, et al.: Correlation of preoperative pulmonary function testing with clinical course in patients after pneumonectomy. Ann Thorac Surg 1983; 36:253–57.
94. Krowka MJ, Pairolero P, Trastek VF, Spencer Payne W, Bernatz PE: Cardiac dysrhythmia following pneumonectomy. Chest 1987; 91:490–5.
95. Wahi R, McMurtrey MJ, DeCaro LF, et al.: Determinants of perioperative morbidity and mortality after pneumonectomy. Ann Thorac Surg 1989; 48:33–7.
96. Romano PS, Mark DH: Patient and hospital characteristics related to in hospital mortality and morbidity after lung cancer resection. Chest 1992; 101:1332–7.

Paul M. Heerdt, MD, PhD
Jaideep Malhotra, MD

The Right Ventricular Response to Lung Resection

10

INTRODUCTION

Although cardiac complications account for a large percentage of the perioperative morbidity associated with thoracic surgery (1–5), but extensive clinical experience has demonstrated that hemodynamically significant complications generally do not occur until after a 48- to 72-hour window of relative stability (6). These observations suggest that the cardiopulmonary response to lung resection evolves over time, with an initial, acute "reactive phase" that is different than the "adaptive phase" that becomes apparent during a period of cellular and structural adaptation within the heart, which in turn may be different than the steady-state "compensated phase" that is achieved after stabilization of delayed processes both intrinsic and extrinsic to the heart. Specific clinical study of the mechanisms by which lung resection influences performance of the heart, however, have been impeded by the fact that complete assessment of the individual factors dictating cardiac function often require invasive techniques that are not easily applied in patients. Furthermore, the complexities of dissociating primary sequelae from secondary events (ie, induced ischemia) and the common overlay of parenchymal lung disease only serve to heighten physiological complexity of thoracic surgical patients.

Progress in Thoracic Anesthesia, edited by Peter Slinger,
Lippincott Williams & Wilkins, Baltimore © 2004.

LUNG RESECTION AND ACUTE CHANGES IN CARDIAC FUNCTION

Intraoperative Considerations

During the course of any intrathoracic procedure, a variety of imposed physiological stresses can acutely influence—both individually and collectively—cardiovascular function and initiate secondary processes that are maintained postoperatively.

Entrance to the Chest Cavity

Simply opening the thorax stimulates primary (eg, reflex) and secondary (eg, elaboration of inflammatory mediators, pain, and autonomic activity) processes that can affect cardiovascular performance regardless of the magnitude of lung resected. Appreciation of this situation has helped to foster the notion that minimally invasive lung resection may provide multiple levels of patient benefit, including improved postoperative cardiac performance. Although the data are limited and the studies not well controlled, investigation has begun to suggest enhanced right ventricular (RV) mechanical function in high-risk elderly patients (3) following video-assisted thoracoscopy as compared to open thoracotomy.

Single-lung ventilation

During most thoracic surgical procedures, one lung is selectively collapsed to facilitate surgical exposure. Because of the acute changes in distending airway pressure coupled with vascular reactive processes such as hypoxic vasoconstriction and the mechanical consequences of physical atelectasis, cardiac-loading conditions can change during single-lung ventilation. As shown in Figure 10.1, single-lung ventilation in healthy subjects elicits a modest, progressive rise in pulmonary arterial (PA) pressure but relatively little change in systemic arterial pressure. Although of minimal global significance in normal patients, the imposition of single-lung ventilation in those with parenchymal lung disease and baseline pulmonary hypertension can produce more pronounced hemodynamic effects. In addition to the direct effects of lung collapse during single-lung ventilation, secondary physical and metabolic consequences may occur following re-expansion (7, 8).

Lung manipulation and vascular ligation

Implicit even in limited lung resection is the fact that lung tissue must be grasped and retracted to facilitate access to the lesion as well as to

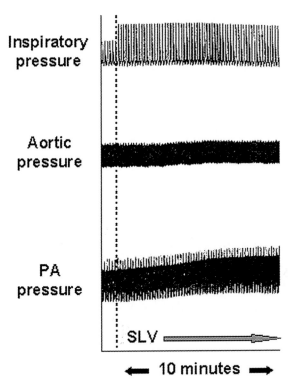

Inspiratory pressure

Aortic pressure

PA pressure

SLV

← 10 minutes →

FIGURE 10.1   Representative tracings of inspiratory pressure along with aortic and pulmonary arterial (PA) pressures during the first 10 minutes of single-lung ventilation (SLV) in a normal subject.

vascular and bronchial structures. In contrast to the reversible effects of single-lung ventilation, ligation of major branches of the pulmonary artery produces both acute and sustained hemodynamic effects that influence both the resistive and elastic components of RV afterload (discussed later).

Lymphatic disruption and pulmonary capillary dysfunction

After thoracotomy and lung resection, approximately 5% of patients will manifest radiographic and/or functional evidence of pulmonary edema, a phenomenon generally categorized as "postpneumonectomy pulmonary edema" regardless of whether or not an entire lung was removed (9, 10). Although this response was initially attributed to over-hydration (9), more recent data have implicated a primary capillary injury secondary to processes such as baro- or volutrauma or reperfusion injury after single-lung ventilation (7, 8). Whatever the mechanism, three important features are evident. First, the response is rarely acute, with the vast majority of cases evolving over several days postopera- tively. Second, there is a spectrum of severity, ranging from largely asymptomatic, diffuse pulmonary infiltrates to an acute lung injury syndrome (normal left heart-filling pressures but a ratio of arterial par- tial pressure of oxygen (PaO_2) to fraction of inspired oxygen (FIO_2) of <300) or fulminant adult respiratory distress syndrome (normal left heart-filling pressures but PaO_2:FIO_2 ratio of <200). Finally, and most importantly, is the reported mortality rate—often caused, at least in part, by heart failure—of 33% for acute lung injury and up 100% for acute respiratory distress syndrome (8–12).

Postoperative Hemodynamic Response to Lung Resection

Despite extensive clinical experience with lung resection, the subse- quent direct effect on performance of the heart remains remarkably con- fused. In general, changes in cardiac pump function and postoperative arrhythmogenesis independent of exacerbation of pre-existing disease have been attributed to an acute increase in RV afterload secondary to PA ligation (Figure 10.2). This simple paradigm is attractive, but ques- tions posed by both clinical and experimental observations complicate its universal application.

Is the RV Inherently Dysfunctional after Lung Resection?

Although the anatomic disruption imposed by lung resection remains fixed, resting mean PA pressure and vascular resistance (PVR) tend to normalize postoperatively (13, 14), with the magnitude of change de- pending on the extent of resection (eg, lobectomy vs pneumonectomy). However, despite relative normalization of PA pressure, RV ejection fraction continues to fall during the first few postoperative days, sug- gesting that evolving reactive and/or adaptive processes influence this index of RV performance (4, 13, 14). Other studies indicate that resting RV ejection fraction may then remain depressed indefinitely despite the normal propensity for the heart to hypertrophy as a compensation for increased load (15).

From a functional standpoint, resting hemodynamics alone do not provide a clear picture; thus, multiple studies have focused on the post- operative response to exercise. Results of these investigations, however, must be interpreted in the context of the amount of lung resected and the stress of the exercise challenge. For example, Okada et al. (14) ex-

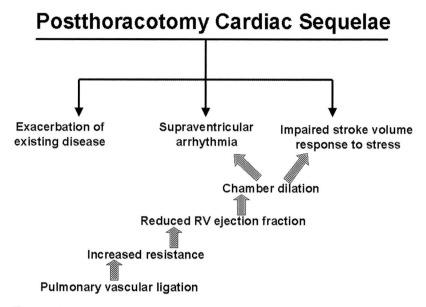

FIGURE 10.2 Conventional paradigm for the genesis of changes in cardiac function following lung resection. RV = right ventricular.

amined hemodynamic variables, including thermodilution RV ejection fraction at rest and during submaximal exercise (sufficient to produce an ~25% increase in heart rate), before and 3 weeks after lobectomy or pneumonectomy. With data from all patients combined, no significant pre- versus postoperative differences in heart rate, mean arterial pressure, pulmonary capillary wedge pressure, mean PA pressure, central venous pressure, RV volumes, or cardiac index were found under resting conditions. There was, however, a modest reduction in both stroke volume index (48 ± 8 vs 41 ± 8) and RV ejection fraction (43 ± 3 vs 37 ± 6). As shown in Figure 10.3, during submaximal exercise both mean PA pressure and PVR rose to a much greater relative degree after lung resection. However, despite these changes, no marked difference was seen in the RV ejection fraction response, whereas stroke volume and cardiac output actually increased to a greater relative degree.

Although Okada et al. conclude that after lung resection the RV is compensated at rest but becomes dysfunctional during exercise (ie, the ejection fraction falls), the results of the study demonstrate that the capacity to increase both stroke volume and cardiac output was preserved—if not enhanced—during submaximal exercise. In contrast, another study examining more strenuous exercise in pneumonectomy patients up to 10 years after resection indicates that stroke volume eventually becomes fixed at some maximal value (ie, cannot rise with in-

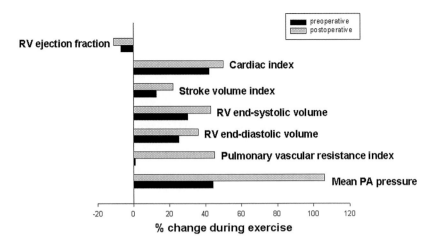

FIGURE 10.3 Comparison of the hemodynamic response to submaximal exercise before and after lung resection. PA = pulmonary arterial; RV = right ventricular. [Data from Okata et al. (4).]

creasing workload) despite more than sufficient time for compensatory hypertrophy of the heart (16). This study also highlights two very important points. First, it clearly demonstrates that despite fixed ventilatory deficits and a ceiling on stroke volume and cardiac output, exercise training after pneumonectomy improves maximal oxygen uptake (VO_2max) by enhancing peripheral oxygen extraction. Second, it reinforces the prospect that changes in cardiac performance after pneumonectomy (and, possibly, lesser resections) are not exclusively the result of altered RV afterload but may involve changes in left ventricular function as well.

Is the Left Ventricle Influenced by Lung Resection?

In general, studies using PA catheterization or echocardiography have indicated preservation of LV mechanical performance both at rest and during exercise after lung resection. However, one investigation using nuclear stethoscope technology indicated reductions in LV ejection fraction and ejection rate that could not be explained by altered RV function (17). Similar conclusions were reached in an animal study that assessed the hemodynamic response to exercise in dogs after pneumonectomy (18). That study did not elucidate a specific mechanism, but it did raise the prospect of reorientation of the heart within the cardiac fossa producing mechanical impairment of LV filling and/or ejection. A similar conclusion has been reached in a clinical investigation based on the observation that pleuromediastinal adhesion and organized hemofibrothorax in combination with overexpansion of the remaining lung may reduce compliance of the cardiac fossa and restrict the Starling mechanism on both sides of the heart (16).

Have Adequate Methods Been Applied for Clinical Assessment of RV-Pulmonary Vascular Coupling?

In an effort to more closely characterize the relationship between post-thoracotomy changes in RV afterload (characterized as PVR) and pump function in patients having lesser resections, Reed et al. (13) examined the influence of the relatively selective pulmonary vasodilator prostaglandin (PG) E_1 on thermodilution-derived RV ejection fraction before and 48 hours after lobectomy. Despite a modest decline in calculated PVR during PGE_1 under both conditions, these investigators were unable to demonstrate any augmentation of RV ejection fraction regardless of whether or not lung had been removed.

The finding that RV ejection fraction was reduced after lung resection independent of changes in PVR suggested that other factors such as depressed contractility contributed to the response. Accordingly, Reed et al. attempted to characterize postoperative changes in RV contractility in conjunction with simultaneous alteration in afterload. To the authors' credit, they carefully considered that although contractility is relatively simple to quantify in isolated muscle systems or intact hearts beating isovolumically, load-independent quantification in the ejecting heart is much more complex. Accordingly, Reed et al. used an adaptation of the preload recruitable stroke work (PRSW) concept (essentially a linearized Frank-Starling plot) to determine changes in contractility. Using rapid infusion of colloid to increase preload, these investigators plotted RV stroke work over a range of end-diastolic volumes, and they found that whereas the starting point of the curve was different for lung resection patients (ie, higher baseline end-diastolic volume), the slope of the relationship was the same. The sample size was quite small, but this study concluded that neither changes in RV afterload nor contractility contribute to decreased RV ejection fraction after lung resection.

Although seemingly straightforward, the conclusions of this study as well as those of others need to be carefully interpreted within the context of several technical considerations. The first relates to the basic concept of ventricular afterload. Commonly summarized as vascular resistance (calculated as mean pressure/mean flow), the pressure and flow generated by the heart are not steady and continuous but are intermittent and pulsatile. Ejection, therefore, is opposed not only by steady-state resistive forces but also by elastic (large vessels are distended with each beat and recoil during diastole to maintain pressure and flow) and reflective (pressure and flow waves reflected backward) forces. Accordingly, expression of RV afterload in terms of simple resistance is incomplete. Functional significance of this concept can be found in the fact that when the impact of increased PA pressure secondary to a primary change in resistance (eg, vasoconstriction of small pulmonary vessels) is compared to a similar pressure response produced by a primary change in compliance (eg, ligation of a large pulmonary artery), a different functional alteration in RV hydraulic work is evident (19). To incorporate all components, proximal PA pressure and flow characteristics can be mathematically resolved into individual frequency components (because each waveform actually represents summation and cancellation of forward and backward waves of multiple frequencies) and used to calculate input impedance (Z_{in}). This "frequency domain" analysis of pressure and flow throughout the entire cardiac cycle allows for creation of an impedance spectrum in which the pressure-flow amplitude and phase ratios over a range of frequencies are plotted (20). Analysis of this spectrum then allows characterization of the different components of afterload. Unfortunately, precise generation of impedance spectra requires complex and invasive instrumentation; thus, the impact of lung resection on these measurements in humans have not been widely reported. However, in laboratory animals undergoing thoracotomy, our laboratory and others have used PA pressure and flow data obtained with intravascular micromanometers and extravascular probes, respectively, to generate impedance spectra. These data indicate that whereas major lung resection acutely produces only a modest increase in PVR (small vessel load), it results in an approximately 50% rise in "characteristic impedance," which is the pulsatile, elastic load imparted by large vessels (21). Other investigators have reported maintenance of increased characteristic impedance years after left pneumonectomy in dogs (22), suggesting that facilitatory adaptation within the pulmonary circulation does not occur. Thus, clinical studies appropriately conclude that reduced RV ejection fraction following lung resection is independent of a change in PVR, but when the definition of afterload is expanded to include changes in large vessel elasticity, alterations in RV ejection fraction are indeed linked to altered afterload.

Both clinical and experimental studies also support the prospect that more than just an acute increase in RV afterload influences cardiac performance after lung resection. Although mean PA pressure and PVR have been reported to be 20% to 27% lower in normal subjects than in pneumonectomy patients both at rest and during submaximal exercise (23), the highest PA pressure achieved in the pneumonectomy patients never exceeded that measured in normal subjects at maximal exercise (24). Furthermore, clinical studies have demonstrated the capacity of the heart to continually increase cardiac output up to a mean PA pressure of nearly 60 mm Hg in normal subjects exercising under hypoxic conditions (25). As shown in Figure 10.4*A,* conventional application of the PRSW concept involves plotting the area of individual ventricular pressure-volume loops (stroke work for that cardiac cycle) during acute changes in venous return (eg, over seconds) as a function of end-diastolic volume (preload). Within this framework, chamber work for any given preload can be defined; with impaired contractility, less work is performed per cycle for the same preload. In that the study by Reed et al. (13) used a rather unorthodox application of the preload recruitable stroke work principal thermodilution measurements of RV volume during colloid infusion over minutes) that cannot exclude the influence of homeostatic reflexes, the suggestion of a dissociation between RV ejection fraction and both afterload (expressed as PVR) and contractility following limited lung resection cannot be definitively supported.

Recent work from our laboratory has focused on using direct measurements of RV pressure and volume to characterize chamber performance before, during, and after lung resection (26). As shown in Figure 10.5, plotting data from the same animal shows that RV pressure and volume are relatively dynamic in the perioperative period. Importantly, immediately after removal of the left upper lobe and resumption of double-lung ventilation, the heart is initially hyperdynamic, with increased heart rate and stroke volume that occur in conjunction with normalization of ejection fraction. In contrast, 3 hours after lobectomy, RV pressure and volume have both begun to increase at end-systole (minimum volume achieved) and end-diastole (maximum volume achieved),

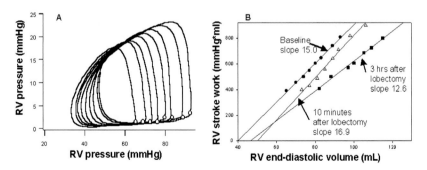

FIGURE 10.4   (A) Right ventricular (RV) pressure-volume loops during transient occlusion of the inferior vena cava. The area of each loop represents stroke work with preload for that cardiac cycle (maximal end-diastolic volume) designated as an open circle. (B) RV stroke work (area of individual loops) plotted as a function of end-diastolic volume (preload) during transient occlusion of the inferior vena cava under various conditions. The slope of this relationship is designated as preload recruitable stroke work and represents a relatively load-independent index of contractility.

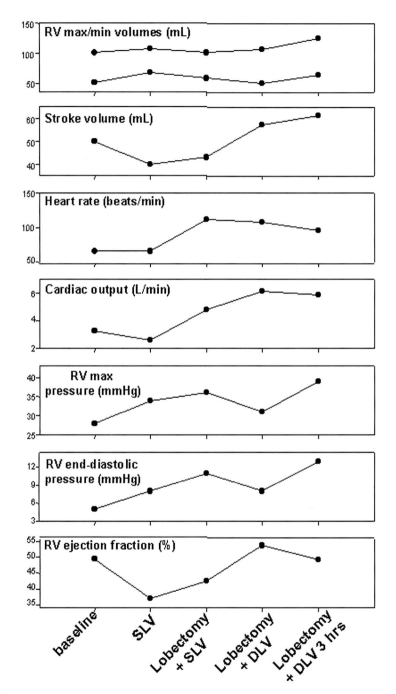

FIGURE 10.5 Hemodynamic variables before, during, and after left upper lobectomy in a domestic swine. DLV = double-lung ventilation; RV = right ventricular; SLV = single-lung ventilation.

which is indicative of chamber dilation. Nonetheless, although ejection fraction has begun to trend downward, stroke volume is maintained because of the fall in heart rate. Plotting RV pressure-volume data obtained during acute inferior venal caval occlusion at different time points (Figure 10.4*B*) demonstrates that RV PRSW was slightly increased immediately after lung removal but modestly depressed 3 hours postoperatively.

Table 10.1 compares RV pressure, volume, ejection fraction, and PRSW data obtained in swine 72 hours after left pneumonectomy to those obtained in nonoperated controls. Consistent with the trend beginning to emerge 3 hours after lobectomy, animals that had undergone pneumonectomy exhibit significantly higher RV volumes in conjunction with a decline in PRSW and ejection fraction. Importantly, however, these data demonstrate that nonstressed (ie, measured while anesthetized) cardiac output is relatively maintained despite a reduction in heart rate and evidence of depressed RV contractility and ejection fraction.

What Is the Global Significance of Altered RV Ejection Fraction after Lung Resection?

Multiple studies conducted at rest have indicated RV dilation and significant reduction in RV ejection fraction but preserved stroke volume after major lung resection in the absence of concomitant parenchymal lung compromise, suggesting adequate Frank-Staring compensation (14, 27). Indeed, one study demonstrated that a low perioperative RV ejection fraction, even in the presence of poor respirometric pulmonary function tests, is not generally predictive of perioperative morbidity (15). However, when the RV is acutely challenged by postoperative pulmonary

TABLE 10.1   Hemodynamic Response to Pneumonectomy

	Control (n = 4)	Pneumonectomy (n = 7)
Maximum RV pressure (mm Hg)	27 ± 2	31 ± 2
RV end-diastolic pressure (mm Hg)	5 ± 2	7 ± 1
RV end-systolic volume (mL)	89 ± 6	113 ± 14
RV end-diastolic volume (mL)	44 ± 5	66 ± 9
Preload recruitable stroke work (mm Hg · mL/mL)	16 ± 0.8	11.2 ± 1.2
Heart rate (beats/min)	84 ± 8	68 ± 5
Cardiac output (L/min)	3.6 ± 0.3	3.1 ± 0.2
RV ejection fraction (%)	49 ± 2	41 ± 4

Data are presented as mean ± SEM.
RV = right ventricular.

embolism, pneumonia, acute lung injury, or frank adult respiratory distress syndrome, it will fail (12). In the context of long-term outcome (ie, =6 months), exercise limitation has been conventionally regarded as a cardiac phenomenon, with dyspnea being a manifestation of a fixed, maximal RV stoke volume. This concept is supported by increased long-term morbidity in patients with an RV ejection fraction of less than 35% after pulmonary vascular ligation (15). However, recent data demonstrating that in many postpneumonectomy patients exercise limitation is actually respiratory and not cardiac (discussed later) challenges application of the fixed stroke volume paradigm to all patients (28).

Assessment of RV pump function in the thoracic surgical population is often technically complex, and the interpretation is subjective. For example, in two relatively large studies using transthoracic echocardiography to assess RV function after pneumonectomy (27, 29), both sets of investigators concluded that RV dilation occurred during the early postoperative period, but only one (29) interpreted this response as being indicative of significant RV dysfunction. Importantly, the two studies used different approaches to analyzing data. Because of technical limitations with visualizing the RV proper (particularly in patients with obstructive lung disease), the study that was negative for RV dysfunction (27) focused on regional wall motion, the velocity of any tricuspid regurgitation jet, and estimated peak RV pressure. In contrast, the positive study (29) used a subtraction technique based on a hemiellipsoid model and the area-length method to calculate ejection fraction. Other investigations have used label imaging or fast response thermodilution to directly measure RV ejection fraction. Thermodilution measurements in particular have been widely used in the perioperative setting and have the advantage of also supplying right heart pressures, because the technique requires placement of a pulmonary artery catheter. Unfortunately, accuracy and, thus, clinical utility of these measurements may be diminished by tricuspid regurgitation (30), a condition that is common in elderly patients and exacerbated by acute increases in RV afterload.

Does Altered RV Systolic and Diastolic Function Facilitate Supraventricular Arrhythmias?

Although pericardial restraint does not influence RV function under normal conditions, with the increased volumes that accompany increased afterload the pericardium does become limiting, and diastolic compliance falls (31). Consistent with this observation, echocardiographic assessment of biventricular diastolic function has indicated a much greater impact on the RV than the left ventricle (LV) after lung resection (32). Accordingly, the cardiac response to leg raising or loss of atrial contraction will be expected to be more pronounced after lung resection. Functional significance of altered right heart pressure-volume relationships is heightened by the fact that supraventricular arrhythmias are the most common complication of thoracotomy, occurring in approximately 20% of patients (33). Within this subset of patients, 64% exhibit atrial fibrillation (AF), 23% supraventricular tachycardias, and 13% atrial flutter (34). In general, the primary risk factors of supraventricular arrhythmias are age greater than 70 years, extent of resection, and pre-existing cardiac disease (33, 35, 36). As with the progressive postoperative decline in RV ejection fraction, supraventricular arrhythmias generally do not develop for 48 to 72 hours, suggesting a reactive, inflammatory, or autonomic component that acts to initiate the arrhythmia (the arrhythmogenic stimulus), which is then facilitated or perpetuated by cellular or structural changes (the arrhythmogenic substrate) within the myocardium.

Multiple lines of investigation suggest that atrial arrhythmogenesis in general can be linked to alterations in myocyte ion transients dictated by stretch-sensitive ion channels (37–39). Thus, a common perception is that distension of the right atrium secondary to impaired RV ejection is a primary stimulus for postpneumonectomy AF. However, some clinical studies have failed to find any association between RV distension, atrial size, and arrhythmia after pneumonectomy (40). Analogous to ventricular tachycardia, AF is thought to result from re-entrant mechanisms, with the atria requiring areas of abnormal dispersion of refractoriness to initiate and maintain the re-entrant circuit (33). Accordingly, conditions that alter the atrial effective refractory period (ERP) tend to be proarrhythmic. To date, the specific stimuli for initiating AF after lung resection are unknown, although factors such as sympathovagal imbalance, myocarditis, and pericarditis have been implicated along with myocyte stretch (33, 39). Alternatively, specific anatomic substrates, particularly atrial fibrosis, have been consistently implicated in the perpetuation of arrhythmia once initiated. Aging alone induces fibrosis and other degenerative changes in atrial anatomy that are accompanied by potentially proarrhythmic physiological alterations, such as shorter ERP, longer sinoatrial and atrioventricular nodal conduction times, atrial stiffening, and splitting of the atrial excitation waveform by the pectinated trabeculae (41, 42).

PROLONGED COMPENSATION

End Points for Quantifying Functional Adaptation to Lung Resection

In many ways, the alterations in cardiopulmonary function elicited by lung resection parallel those produced by progression of intrinsic parenchymal pulmonary disease. Ultimately, the efficacy of functional adaptation/compensation to each process can be characterized in terms of oxygen uptake and peripheral extraction. Important, however, is an appreciation that adaptation to alterations in oxygen transport is a co-ordinated, whole-body phenomenon involving multiple steps. Within this framework, the disturbance of one step elicits adaptive changes in other steps to establish a new functional equilibrium (43).

Fundamentally, oxygen transport is a sequential process of venti-lation matched with blood flow, diffusion through lung and capillaries, chemical interaction with hemoglobin and myoglobin, and ultimately, mitochondrial oxidative phosphorylation. In most subjects (eg, those who are not physically trained), VO_2max is limited by maximal cardiac output and peripheral oxygen extraction, not by pulmonary diffusing capacity or maximal ventilation. Accordingly, augmenting maximal cardiac output and enhancing oxygen extraction with regular exercise markedly increases VO_2max, whereas increasing maximal ventilation or diffusing capacity has minimal effect (43). In the perioperative period as well as during the subsequent postoperative convalescence, secondary processes such as physical deconditioning and anemia can augment the primary deficit created by lung removal and/or disruption of ventila-tion by chest wall dysfunction. After recovery and assumption of a steady-state compensated phase, physical limitation will be influenced by the extent of resection and magnitude of deconditioning, both within the context of pre-existing disease. Ultimately, however, whether phys-ical limitation after lung resection—often presenting not only as dysp-nea but also as leg fatigue—is cardiac or pulmonary in origin remains somewhat controversial.

Two obvious considerations in the assessment of how lung resec-tion alters exercise capacity are the extent of resection and the time frame during which data are acquired. Miyoshi et al. (44) measured VO_2max in a group of 16 patients (13 lobectomies, three pneumonec-tomies) before surgery and at 9 ± 2 and 26 ± 12 days postoperatively. In comparison to preoperative values, they found, on average, a 27% de-cline in VO_2max at the first time point but only an 18% reduction at the later one. Analysis of their data suggested that the early drop was both respiratory and circulatory in origin, with subsequent short-term im-provement resulting from the augmented respiratory performance pro-vided by recovery from the surgical insult and normalization of chest wall mechanics. In contrast, Nezu et al. (45) examined the initial loss and subsequent recovery of exercise capacity (characterized as VO_2max) 3 and 6 months after lobectomy or pneumonectomy. Their data show that the initial decline in VO_2max was approximately twice as great in the pneumonectomy group. In addition, 6 months after resection, a modest improvement was seen in the lobectomy group, but no change was seen in patients having pneumonectomy. A subsequent report of pulmonary function up to 4 years after lung resection (46) showed no major changes in comparison to data acquired after the first 4 to 6 months, with the exception of modest improvements in airway resistance and diffusing capacity. However, 80% of the patients exhibiting physical limitation 4 to 6 months postoperatively demonstrated long-term improvement in daily activity. Although the results of multiple studies (47–49) are consistent with a close relationship between extent of resection and functional loss of exercise capacity, some investigators have failed to find a direct correlation (45, 50), thus raising the issue of other factors. In that maximal cardiac output may be limited along with ventilatory capacity and pulmonary diffusing capacity (16, 50–52), many authors believe that a postresection decline in VO_2max is primarily a circulatory phenomenon (16, 46, 53, 54). However, other studies, including one that compared thoracotomy alone to limited resection and pneumonectomy, implicate a primary reduction in ventilatory reserve (28, 49).

Cardiopulmonary Structural Adaptation

Under most circumstances, the distortion of myocytes that accompanies increased pressure and volume within any heart chamber triggers a sequence of events, many of which are calcium-regulated (55), that eventually lead to adaptive hypertrophy of individual cells. The major hypertrophic stimulus probably is physical stretch of the myocardium, but this process also involves autonomic neurotransmitters and intracardiac paracrine/autocrine mediators. These individual factors coalesce to produce a cascade of immediate and, ultimately, prolonged molecular and cellular events that are mediated, in part, by altered expression of a variety of genes within both myocytes and noncontractile elements of the myocardium (56). The clinical observation that most hemodynamically significant cardiac sequelae after lung resection occur after 48 to 72 hours raises the question of whether or not an evolving response to both the trauma of surgery and increased right heart volumes play a part. Similarly, the acute increase in blood flow and, possibly, inspiratory volume to the remaining lung are most likely sufficient to initiate a variety of secondary responses within the pulmonary parenchyma.

Cardiac Hypertrophy

Although the myocardial response to increased pressure or volume is generally linked to progressive alterations in myocyte size over weeks to months, multiple genes encoding for transcription factors and other proteins can be rapidly (minutes to hours) influenced by acute changes in cardiac pressure and volume (56, 57). Remarkably, despite both experimental and clinical data demonstrating acute dilation of the right heart after lung resection, limited data are available specifically relating to either the time course or the magnitude of secondary molecular and structural myocardial remodeling. Studies in rats after right pneumonectomy (58) have indicated three stages of RV reaction:

1. Acute disturbances and initiation of secondary responses (0–10 days).
2. Steady hypertrophy of the RV (10–90 days).
3. A stage of decompensation (>90 days).

Histological analysis of myocardium over this time frame revealed a progressive loss of cardiomyocytes and their nuclei. Other data from rats indicate up to a 72% increase in RV mass after right pneumonectomy (59). Experimental studies in small dogs have also demonstrated hypertrophy (increases in both length and width of myocytes) of the right atrium and RV (60) that correlate both with the extent of lung resected and with the postoperative period of observation and that is nonuniform within the heart, perhaps contributing to eventual decompensation. In contrast, significant RV hypertrophy is not evident up to 70 days postresection after left pneumonectomy in sheep (61).

How these experimental data relate to humans is unclear, particularly in light of the supervening influences of age and pre-existing disease. Multiple lines of investigation indicate that when major lung resection is performed at a very young age, cardiopulmonary adaptation in general is more extensive and efficient (62–64). For example, Murray et al. (62) studied the cardiovascular response to hypoxia in dogs 5 years after pneumonectomy performed at 6 to 10 weeks or 1 year of age. They found that although both groups exhibited similar increases in PVR and pulmonary characteristic impedance while breathing a low FIO_2, the RV response was clearly more hyperdynamic in animals undergoing pneumonectomy as puppies, a response attributed to an enhanced performance of the RV as a pump that was independent of afterload. Also evident within that study was that although the animals operated on as adults failed to show as robust an RV response to hypoxia as those operated on as puppies, they did not mount a less dynamic response than the nonoperated control animals, and they exhibited no sign of RV pump failure despite a greater than 60% rise in mean PA pressure.

At the opposite end of the age spectrum, senescence alters characteristics of myocardial systolic function and dampens the cardiac response to increased pressure-volume load. As a probable adaptation to generalized age-induced arterial stiffening, myocardial excitation-contraction coupling is lengthened, thus allowing individual cells to experience a prolongation of both the calcium transient and the force-bearing capacity (65, 66). This response, in turn, enhances ventricular ejection into a stiff circulation. Age-related alterations in excitation-contraction coupling have largely been attributed to downregulation of the gene encoding for the sarcoplasmic endoreticular calcium adenosine triphosphatase subtype 2a, which is responsible for calcium uptake into the sarcoplasmic reticulum from the cytosol (65). Aging also dampens the chronotropic and inotropic responses to sympathetic stimulation because of a decline in the ability of myocardial β-receptors to augment calcium influx via the L-type calcium channel (65, 66). Accordingly, the elderly heart maintains stroke volume during stress more by dilation ("in situ adaptation") than marked increases in contractility. This may have particular importance in the post-lung resection RV, because aging alone produces chamber dilation in humans (67). In the LV, aging has been reported to diminish the hypertrophic response to exercise (68), to both pressure and volume overload (69,70), and possibly, to thyroid hormone stimulation (71). However, fundamental differences between the LV and RV in regard to embryology, structure, load, and growth with maturation complicate direct extension of data derived from one chamber to the other. For example, in both animals and humans, normal senescence produces an increase in the mass of the LV but not of the RV (65). Furthermore, the aging process produces greater cellular hypertrophy, fibrosis, myosin heavy-chain isoform shift, and prolongation of contraction duration in the LV than in the RV. To date, and to our knowledge, no reports have appeared describing how myocardial hypertrophic remodeling secondary to increased RV pressure-volume load after lung resection is influenced by senescence. However, data clearly indicate age-related diminution of both cellular and biochemical indices of RV hypertrophy after PA banding (72).

Not uncommonly, patients requiring lung resection suffer from underlying pulmonary parenchymal disease that has already elicited cardiac adaptation to chronic changes in cardiac loading. In particular, chronic obstructive pulmonary disease (COPD) can alter RV afterload by reducing the area of the pulmonary vascular bed, by initiating regional hypoventilation with secondary hypoxic vasoconstriction, or simply by compressing the vasculature by hyperinflation (73). Alternatively, preload of both ventricles can be altered by lung hyperinflation and septal shift secondary to RV dilation. Compounding hemodynamic alterations is the possibility that the increased work of breathing associated with chronic lung disease, particularly restrictive disease, can lead to a "circulatory steal" phenomenon, whereby blood is diverted to the diaphragm and away from other skeletal muscle during exercise (73). In most patients with COPD, resting PA pressures tend to be normal, and in those with elevated PA pressures, the increase is usually characterized as being mild to moderate (73, 74). During exercise, however, PA pressures may rise rapidly, even in patients with normal pressures at rest, because of a combination of dynamic hyperinflation, regional hypoxic vasoconstriction, and structural changes in the pulmonary vascular bed. Although the maximal PA pressures attained do not usually exceed those observed in normal subjects during strenuous exercise, they occur at much lower work rates and cardiac output, which is consistent with a prominent shift in the PA pressure-flow relationship. Accordingly, a level of pre-existing (and, perhaps, even subclinical) COPD may contribute to the disparity between experimental and clinical observations regarding PA pressure-flow relationships after lung resection. Not surprisingly, RV ejection fraction has been reported to be reduced in patients with COPD and not to increase with exercise (75). Nonetheless, patients with COPD tend to exhibit a normal increase in cardiac output relative to VO_2max, probably resulting more from an augmented heart rate response than from increased stroke volume (76). To our knowledge, no data are available describing how underlying lung disease specifically influences cardiac adaptation to lung resection. However, in a study of 20 patients with modest, pre-existing COPD and low-normal RV ejection fraction who underwent lung resection, Lewis et al. (15) could not demonstrate any correlation between perioperative PA pressure or PVR and RV ejection fraction nor any value of RV ejection fraction in predicting short-term morbidity. However, these investigators did demonstrate that if RV ejection fraction declined to less than 35% or the RV ejection fraction:PVR ratio rose to greater than 5 after ligation of the PA supply to the resected area, this response was predictive for long term (>6 months) morbidity. While not conclusive, this study suggests that although these patients had sufficient cardiac reserve to tolerate the acute insult of lung resection, a diminished capacity for long-term adaptation influenced the eventual outcome.

Compensatory Lung Growth

It has long been known that after removal of lung tissue, the remaining lung expands. Functionality of this expanded lung, however, is not necessarily proportional to the increase in size. As with cardiac compensation, the magnitude of pulmonary adaptation appears to depend on the extent of lung resected, age, and underlying disease. Furthermore, experimental data are influenced by species variation, with mice and rats in particular exhibiting a marked compensatory growth of remaining lung. In larger animals and humans, adaptation to altered gas exchange has been characterized as occurring at three different levels (77):

1. Recruitment of diffusing capacity reserves in remaining lung.

2. Enlargement of remaining alveolar airspaces and thinning of the alveolar tissue barrier.
3. Compensatory lung growth.

In immature animals, pneumonectomy stimulates alveolar regeneration of sufficient magnitude to return lung volume, diffusing capacity, and extravascular septal tissue volume to normal (77, 78). Aspects of lung mechanical function remain abnormal, however, and regeneration of extra-alveolar airways and blood vessels is limited. Similar responses appear to occur in humans (79). In mature animals, compensatory growth appears to occur only after removal of the left lung (80). This finding suggests a threshold of resection below which the existing lung can adapt via physiological recruitment and structural remodeling. Nonetheless, unlike immature animals, mature ones maintain long-term cardiopulmonary deficits regardless of which lung was removed (77).

A variety of stimuli have been proposed to account for adaptive changes in the lung. Recent data examining the impact of mediastinal shift on remaining lung after pneumonectomy have concluded that although mechanical strain is a major stimulus for regenerative lung growth (81), other signals account for a significant amount of the compensatory response (82, 83). Also implicated has been the increased blood flow to remaining lung, because augmentation of shear forces within vessels elicits a variety of responses from vascular endothelial cells with potential downstream effects (84, 85). Interestingly, unlike the marked pulmonary vascular remodeling that accompanies increased pulmonary blood flow from left-to-right shunts, pneumonectomy elicits only modest changes (61).

SUMMARY

Each year in the United States, approximately 60,000 noncardiac, thoracic surgical procedures are performed, largely for the treatment of cancer. During the last 20 years, patient outcome after lung resection has steadily improved; thus, even extensive resections such as pneumonectomy are now being offered to those with significant comorbidity and/or advanced age. Cardiac complications account for a large percentage of the perioperative morbidity associated with lung resection, in part because of the median age of 66 years and the prevalence of concomitant coronary vascular and/or heart valvular disease. Accordingly, specific clinical studies of cardiac sequelae after lung resection are influenced by the complexities of dissociating primary from secondary events. Nonetheless, clinical studies have consistently indicated postoperative RV dilation, which has been linked to changes in the capacity for cardiac compensation to perioperative stresses as well as postoperative exercise capacity and mortality. In turn, distension of the right atrium secondary to impaired RV ejection has been implicated in the development of supraventricular arrhythmias, which occur in as many as 35% of patients after lung resection.

Conventional wisdom holds that changes in RV mechanical function are the result of an increase in pulmonary vascular resistance (the contribution to afterload imposed predominantly by small vessels) secondary to the vascular disruption necessary for removing lung tissue. However, neither clinical nor experimental data overwhelmingly support this as the leading factor. Instead, it appears that the major effect of lung resection on RV afterload is the result of an increase in pulmonary vascular characteristic impedance, a component of afterload imposed primarily by large vessels. Clinical studies have also failed to demonstrate changes in intrinsic RV contractility after lung resection, although these investigations largely have been limited by methodology. In contrast, experimental study of RV mechanical function after both pneumonectomy and lobectomy in large animals has begun to indicate a progressive postoperative decline in contractility as defined by analysis of pressure-volume relations.

In regard to the long-term cardiac consequences of long resection, both the mechanism for and the magnitude of changes in postoperative exercise capacity remain somewhat controversial. Multiple studies support the prospect that a secondary exercise limitation is correlated with the magnitude of resection and is largely the result of a dampened RV capacity to increase stroke volume. In addition, data suggest that after pneumonectomy, reorientation of the heart within the mediastinum may influence the LV response to exercise as well. In contrast, other investigators contend that postoperative exercise limitation is primarily the result of respiratory, not cardiac, compromise and is not necessarily proportional to the amount of lung removed.

References

1. Reed CE: Physiologic consequences of pneumonectomy. Chest Surg Clin N Am 1999; 9:449–57.
2. Tanita T, Hoshikawa Y, Tabata T, Noda M, Handa M, Kubo H, Chida M, Suzuki S, Ono S, Fujimura S: Functional evaluations for pulmonary resection for lung cancer in octogenarians. Investigation from postoperative complications. Jpn J Thorac Cardiovasc Surg 1999; 47:253–61.
3. Mikami I, Koizumi K, Tanaka S: Changes in right ventricular performance in elderly patients who underwent lobectomy using

video-assisted thoracic surgery for primary lung cancer. Jpn J Thorac Cardiovasc Surg 2001; 49:153–9.

4. Okada M, Okada M, Ishii N, et al.: Right ventricular ejection fraction in the perioperative risk evaluation of candidates for pulmonary resection. J Thorac Cardiovasc Surg 1996; 112:364.

5. Ommen SR, Odell JA, Stanton MS: Atrial arrhythmias after cardiothoracic surgery. N Engl J Med 1997; 336:1429–34.

6. Amar D, Roistacher N, Burt M, et al.: Effects of diltiazem versus digoxin on dysrhythmias and cardiac function after pneumonectomy. Ann Thorac Surg 1997; 63:1374–82.

7. Jordan S, Mitchell JA, Quinlan GJ, Goldstraw P, Evans TW: The pathogenesis of lung injury following pulmonary resection. Eur Respir J 2000; 15:790–9.

8. Lases EC, Duurkens VA, Gerritsen WB, Haas FJ: Oxidative stress after lung resection therapy. Chest 2000; 117:999–1003.

9. Zeldin RA, Normandin D, Landtwing D, Peters RM: Postpneumonectomy pulmonary edema. J Thorac Cardiovasc Surg 1984; 87:359–365.

10. Waller DA, Gebitekin C, Saunders NR, Walker DR: Noncardiogenic pulmonary edema complicating lung resection. Ann Thorac Surg 1993; 55:140–143.

11. Kutlu CA, Williams EA, Evans TW, Pastorino U, Goldstraw P: Acute lung injury and acute respiratory distress syndrome after pulmonary resection. Ann Thorac Surg 1999; 69:376–80.

12. Mathisen DJ, Kuo EY, Hahn C, Moncure AC, Wain JC, Grillo HC, Hurford WE, Wright CD: Inhaled nitric oxide for adult respiratory distress syndrome after pulmonary resection. Ann Thorac Surg 1998; 66:1894–902.

13. Reed CE, Dorman BH, Spinale FG: Mechanisms of right ventricular dysfunction after pulmonary resection. Ann Thorac Surg 1996; 62:225–31.

14. Okada M, Ota T, Okada M, Matsuda H, Okada K, Ishii N: Right ventricular dysfunction after major pulmonary resection. J Thorac Cardiovasc Surg 1994; 108:503–11.

15. Lewis JW Jr, Bastanfar M, Gabriel F, Mascha E: Right heart function and prediction of respiratory morbidity in patients undergoing pneumonectomy with moderately severe cardiopulmonary dysfunction. J Thorac Cardiovasc Surg 1994; 108:169–75.

16. Hijazi OM, Ramanathan M, Estrera AS, Peshock RM, Hsia CC: Fixed maximal stroke index in patients after pneumonectomy. Am J Respir Crit Care Med 1998; 15:1623–9.

17. Fujisaki T, Gomibuchi M, Shoji T: Changes in left ventricular function during exercise after lung resection—study with a nuclear stethoscope. Nippon Kyobu Geka Gakkai Zasshi 1992; 40:1685–92.

18. Hsia CCW, Carlin JI, Cassidy SS, Ramanathan M, Johnson RL Jr: Hemodynamic changes after pneumonectomy in the exercising foxhound. J Appl Physiol 1990; 69:51–7.
19. Elzinga G, Piene H, DeJong JP: Left and right ventricular pump function and consequences of having two pumps in one heart: a study on the isolated cat heart. Circ Res 1980; 46:564–79.
20. Piene H: Matching between right ventricle and pulmonary bed. In: Yin FCP, ed: Ventricular/Vascular Coupling. New York, Springer-Verlag, 1987; 180–202.
21. Heerdt PM, Bachetta M, Port JL: Right ventricular function and TNF-α expression following pneumonectomy via open thoracotomy or a minimally invasive approach. Anesthesiology 2002; 97:A131.
22. Lucas CL, Murray GF, Wilcox BR, Shallal JA: Effects of pneumonectomy on pulmonary input impedance. Surgery 1983; 94:807–16.
23. Staněk V, Widimsky J, Hurych J, Petrikova J: Pressure, flow and volume changes during exercise within pulmonary vascular bed in patients after pneumonectomy. Clin Sci 1969; 37:11–22.
24. Johnson RL Jr, Hsia CCW, Cassidy SS, Carlin JI, Wagner PD, Ramanathan M. A postpneumonectomy comparison of cardiac output and gas exchange in humans and dogs during heavy exercise. In: Sutton JR, Coates G, Remmers JE, eds: Hypoxia: The Adaptations. Toronto, BC Decker, 1990; 148–54.
25. Groves BM., Reeves JT, Sutton JR, Wagner PD, Cymerman A, Malconian MK, Rock PB, Young PM, Houston CS: Operation Everest: II. Elevated high-altitude pulmonary resistance unresponsive to oxygen. J Appl Physiol 1987; 63:521–30.
26. Heerdt PM, Markov N: Disparity in the right ventricular inotropic response to conventional or minimally invasive pneumonectomy in swine (Abstract). Anesth Analg 2003; 96:A123.
27. Amar D, Burt ME, Roistacher N, Reinsel RA, Ginsberg RJ, Wilson RS: Value of perioperative Doppler echocardiography in patients undergoing major lung resection. Ann Thorac Surg 1996; 61:516–20.
28. Nugent AM, Steele IC, Carragher AM, McManus K, McGuigan JA, Gibbons JR, Riley MS, Nicholls DP: Effect of thoracotomy and lung resection on exercise capacity in patients with lung cancer. Thorax 1999; 54:334–8.
29. Kowalewski J, Brocki M, Dryjanski T, Kapron K, Barcikowski S: Right ventricular morphology and function after pulmonary resection. Eur J Cardiothorac Surg 1999; 15:444–8.
30. Heerdt PM, Blessios GA, Beach ML, Hogue CW: Flow dependency of error in thermodilution measurement of cardiac output during

acute tricuspid regurgitation. J Cardiothorac Vasc Anesth 2001; 15:183–7.

31. Burger W, Straube M, Behne M, Sarai K, Beyersdorf F, Eckel L, Dereser A, Satter P, Kaltenbach M: Role of pericardial constraint for right ventricular function in humans. Chest 1995; 107:46–9.

32. Takaki A, Sugi K, Sano T, Tanaka N, Matsuzaki M: Different responses of right and left ventricular diastolic function to pulmonary resection: echocardiographic study with leg elevation for preload augmentation. J Cardiol 2000; 36:241–9.

33. Ommen SR, Odell JA, Stanton MS. Atrial arrhythmias after cardiothoracic surgery. N Engl J Med 1997; 336:1429–34.

34. Krowka MJ, Pairolero PC, Trastek VF, Payne WS, Bernatz PE: Cardiac dysrhythmia following pneumonectomy. Clinical correlates and prognostic significance. Chest 1987; 91:490–5.

35. Amar D, Zhang H, Y Leung DH, Roistacher N, Kadish AH: Older age is the strongest predictor of postoperative atrial fibrillation. Anesthesiology 2002; 96:352–6.

36. Cardinale D, Martinoni A, Cipolla CM, Civelli M, Lamantia G, Fiorentini C, Mezzetti M: Atrial fibrillation after operation for lung cancer: clinical and prognostic significance. Ann Thorac Surg 1999; 68:1827–31.

37. Yue L, Feng J, Gaspo R, Li GR, Wang Z, Nattel S: Ionic remodeling underlying action potential changes in a canine model of atrial fibrillation. Circ Res 1997; 81:512–7.

38. Bode F, Katchman A, Woosley RL, Franz MR: Gadolinium decreases stretch-induced vulnerability to atrial fibrillation. Circulation 2000; 101:2200–5.

39. Van Wagoner DR, Nerbonne JM: Molecular basis of electrical remodeling in atrial fibrillation. J Mol Cell Cardiol 2000; 32:1101–17.

40. Amar D, Roistacher N, Burt M, Reinsel RA, Ginsberg RJ, Wilson RS: Clinical and echocardiographic correlates of symptomatic tachydysrhythmias after non-cardiac thoracic surgery. Chest 1995; 108:349–54.

41. Spach MS, Dolber PC: Relating extracellular potentials and their derivatives to anisotropic propagation at a microscopic level in human cardiac muscle. Evidence for electrical uncoupling of side-to-side fiber connections with increasing age. Circ Res 1986; 58:356–71.

42. Wei JY: Age and the cardiovascular system. N Engl J Med 1992; 327:1735–9.

43. Hsia CC: Coordinated adaptation of oxygen transport in cardiopulmonary disease. Circulation 2001;104:963–9.

44. Miyoshi S, Yoshimasu T, Hirai T, Hirai I, Maebeya S, Bessho T,

Naito Y: Exercise capacity of thoracotomy patients in the early postoperative period. Chest 2000; 118:384–90.

45. Nezu K, Kushibe K, Tojo T, Takahama M, Kitamura S: Recovery and limitation of exercise capacity after lung resection for lung cancer. Chest 1998; 113:1511–6.

46. Miyazawa M, Haniuda M, Nishimura H, Kubo K, Amano J: Long term effects of pulmonary resection on cardiopulmonary function. J Am Coll Surg 1999; 189:26–33.

47. Corris PA, Ellis DA, Hawkins T, Gibson GJ: Use of radionuclide scanning in the preoperative estimation of pulmonary function after pneumonectomy. Thorax 1987; 42:285–91.

48. Bolliger CT, Jordan P, Soler M, Stulz P, Tamm M, Wyser C, Gonon M, Perruchoud AP: Pulmonary function and exercise capacity after lung resection. Respir J. 1996; 9:415–21.

49. Pelletier C, Lapointe L, LeBlanc P: Effects of lung resection on pulmonary function and exercise capacity. Thorax 1990; 45:497–502.

50. DeGraff AC Jr, Taylor HF, Ord JW, Chuang TN, Johnson RL Jr: Exercise limitation following extensive pulmonary resection. J Clin Invest 1965; 44:1514–22.

51. Birath G, Malmberg R, Simonsson BG: Lung function after pneumonectomy in man. Clin Sci 1965; 29:59–72.

52. Johnson RL Jr, Taylor HF, DeGraff AC: Functional significance of a low pulmonary diffusing capacity for carbon monoxide. J Clin Invest 1965; 44:789–800.

53. Mossberg B, Bjork O, Holmgren A: Working capacity and cardiopulmonary function after extensive lung resections. Scand J Thorac Cardiovasc Surg 1976; 10:247–56.

54. Hsia CC, Ramanathan M, Estrera AS: Recruitment of diffusing capacity with exercise in patients after pneumonectomy. Am Rev Respir Dis 1992; 145(4 pt 1):811–6.

55. Calaghan SC, White E: The role of calcium in the response of cardiac muscle to stretch. Prog Biophys Mol Biol 1999; 71:59–90.

56. Swynghedauw B: Molecular mechanisms of myocardial remodeling. Pharmacol Rev 1999; 79:215–62.

57. Ogino K, Cai B, Gu A, Kohmoto T, Yamamoto N, Burkhoff D: Factors contributing to pressure overload-induced immediate early gene expression in adult rat hearts in vivo. Am J Physiol 1999; 277(1 pt 2):H380–7.

58. Bilich GL, Kiselev AA, Puzikov AO: Myocardial reaction of the right ventricle to lung resection. Arkh Anat Gistol Embriol 1988; 94:46–50.

59. Gnatiuk MS: Structural-functional changes in the myocardium of rats following pneumonectomy. Patol Fiziol Eksp Ter 1991; 4:39–40.

60. Gnatiuk MS: Morphometric research on the cardiomyocytes in cardiac hyperfunction Tsiologiia 1991; 33:51–60.
61. Smith M, Coates G, Kay JM, O'Brodovich H: The response of the pulmonary circulation to exercise during normoxia and hypoxia following pneumonectomy in the adult sheep. Can J Physiol Pharmacol 1989; 67:202–6.
62. Murray GF, et al.: Cardiopulmonary hypoxic response 5 years postpneumonectomy in beagles. J Surg Res 1986; 41:236–44.
63. Cagle PT, Thurlbeck WM: Postpneumonectomy compensatory lung growth. Am Rev Respir Dis 1988; 138:1314–26.
64. Cagle PT, Langston C, Thurlbeck WM: The effect of age on postpneumonectomy growth in rabbits. Pediatr Pulmonol 1988; 5:92–5.
65. Lakatta EG: Myocardial adaptations inn advanced age. Basic Res Cardiol 1993; 88(suppl 2):125–33.
66. Patel MB, Sonnenblick EH: Age-associated alterations in structure and function of the cardiovascular system. Am J Geriatr Cardiol 1998; 7:15–22.
67. Boldt J, Zickmann B, Thiel A, Dapper F, Hemplemann G: Age and right ventricular function during cardiac surgery. J Cardiothorac Vasc Anesth 1992; 6:29–32.
68. McCafferty WB, Edington DW: Skeletal muscle and organ weights of aged and trained male rats. Gerontologia 1974; 20:44–52.
69. Isoyama S, Wei JY, Izumo S, Fort P, Schoen FJ, Grossman W: Effect of age on the development of cardiac hypertrophy produced by aortic constriction in the rat. Circ Res 1987; 61:337–45.
70. Isoyama S, Grossman W, Wei JY: Effect of age on myocardial adaptation to volume overload in the rat. J Clin Invest 1988; 81:1850–7.
71. Florini JR, Saito Y, Manowitz EJ: Effect of age on thyroxine-induced cardiac hypertrophy in mice. J Gerontol 1973; 28:293–7.
72. Kuroha M, Isoyama S, Ito N, Takishima T: Effects of age on right ventricular hypertrophic response to pressure-overload in rats. J Mol Cell Cardiol 1991; 23:1177–90.
73. Sietsma K: Cardiovascular limitations in chronic pulmonary disease. Med Sci Sport Exerc 2001; 33:S656–61
74. Oswald-Mammosser M, Apprill M, Bachez P, Ehrhart M, Weitzenblum E: Pulmonary hemodynamics in chronic obstructive pulmonary disease of the emphysematous type. Respiration 1991; 58:304–10.
75. Matthay RA, Arroliga AC, Wiedemann HP, Schulman DS, Mahler DA: Right ventricular function at rest and during exercise in chronic obstructive pulmonary disease. 1992; 101(suppl 5):255S-62S.
76. Light RW, Mintz HM, Linden GS, Brown SE:. Hemodynamics of patients with severe chronic obstructive pulmonary disease during progressive upright exercise. Am Rev Respir Dis 1984; 130:391–5.

77. Takeda SI, Ramanathan M, Estrera AS, Hsia CC: Postpneumonectomy alveolar growth does not normalize hemodynamic and mechanical function. J Appl Physiol 1999; 87:491–7.
78. Takeda S, Hsia CC, Wagner E, Ramanathan M, Estrera AS, Weibel ER: Compensatory alveolar growth normalizes gas-exchange function in immature dogs after pneumonectomy. J Appl Physiol 1999; 86:1301–10.
79. Laros CD, Westermann CJ: Dilatation, compensatory growth, or both after pneumonectomy during childhood and adolescence. A thirty-year follow-up study. J Thorac Cardiovasc Surg 1987; 93:570–6.
80. Hsia CC, Herazo LF, Fryder-Doffey F, Weibel ER: Compensatory lung growth occurs in adult dogs after right pneumonectomy. J Clin Invest 1994; 94:405–12.
81. Hsia CC, Wu EY, Wagner E, Weibel ER: Preventing mediastinal shift after pneumonectomy impairs regenerative alveolar tissue growth. Am J Physiol Lung Cell Mol Physiol 2001; 281:L1279–87.
82. Landesberg LJ, Ramalingam R, Lee K, Rosengart TK, Crystal RG: Upregulation of transcription factors in lung in the early phase of postpneumonectomy lung growth. Am J Physiol Lung Cell Mol Physiol 2001; 281:L1138–49.
83. Dubaybo BA, Bayasi G, Rubeiz GJ: Changes in tumor necrosis factor in postpneumonectomy lung growth. J Thorac Cardiovasc Surg 1995; 110:396–404.
84. Leuwerke SM, Kaza AK, Tribble CG, Kron IL, Laubach VE: Inhibition of compensatory lung growth in endothelial nitric oxide synthase-deficient mice. Am J Physiol Lung Cell Mol Physiol 2002; 282:L1272–8.
85. McBride JT, Kirchner KK, Russ G, Finkelstein J: Role of pulmonary blood flow in postpneumonectomy lung growth. J Appl Physiol 1992; 73:2448–51.

David Amar, MD

Postthoracotomy
11 | Arrhythmias

Cardiac arrhythmias after thoracic surgical procedures were first reported in the early 1940s and have subsequently been well documented in the literature. The reported incidence of atrial tachyarrhythmias in this patient population ranges from 9% to 33%, with factors such as older age and extent of surgery markedly influencing the incidence (1–3). The major rhythm disturbance is atrial fibrillation (AF) and, less frequently, paroxysmal supraventricular tachycardia (SVT), atrial flutter, and multiform atrial tachycardia seen in patients who are acutely or in those with advanced pulmonary disease (1–4). The usual clinical presentation at the onset of AF is dyspnea, palpitations, dizziness, syncope, respiratory distress, and/or hypotension. Although usually well tolerated in younger patients, new-onset AF after thoracic surgery can be associated with life-threatening potential in elderly patients. We recently evaluated the incidence and outcome of ventricular arrhythmias after thoracic surgery and found a 15% incidence of nonsustained ventricular tachycardia (VT) (5). This chapter focuses on recent progress in the epidemiology, etiology, mechanisms, management, and prevention of common postoperative rapid atrial arrhythmias, and it concludes with a short discussion of ventricular arrhythmias after thoracic surgery.

EPIDEMIOLOGY

In patients undergoing major lung resection, the incidence of AF has been reported to be 12% to 25% after lobectomy, 20% to 30% after

Progress in Thoracic Anesthesia, edited by Peter Slinger,
Lippincott Williams & Wilkins, Baltimore © 2004.

pneumonectomy, and as high as 40% after extrapleural pneumonectomy for malignant pleural mesothelioma (1–3, 6). In our most recent experience, lobectomy in patients older than 60 years carries nearly the same risk of AF as that of pneumonectomy (7). The incidence of AF is less than 1% in patients undergoing minimal wedge or segment resection of lung tissue or in those undergoing exploratory thoracotomy only (1–3). An important prospective study of 4,181 patients (=50 years) in sinus rhythm scheduled for major noncardiac (including intrathoracic) surgery showed that supraventricular arrhythmia reported as being persistent or requiring treatment occurred in 2% of patients during and in 6.1% of patients after surgery (8). During the intraoperative period, the prevalence ratio of SVT to AF was 2:1, whereas the reverse was true after surgery (8). Using Medicare data, it is estimated that the total annual number of patients projected to be at risk for perioperative atrial tachyarrhythmias may be 1.2 million (9). The clinical symptoms, time of onset, and natural course of atrial arrhythmias are identical regardless of whether a patient has had cardiac, thoracic, or other surgery (1–3, 8–11). Onset of atrial arrhythmia peaks 2–3 days after surgery, with close to 85% of these episodes reverting to sinus rhythm with rate- or rhythm-control strategies during hospitalization (6, 12–15). The timing of onset of atrial arrhythmias is intriguingly similar to that of postoperative myocardial ischemia, and it is likely related to autonomic nervous system changes, perhaps associated with an inflammatory response (9, 16–19). Approximately 15% of patients have persistent AF on discharge from the hospital, and of these, 98% are free of AF at 2 months after surgery (6, 11, 14). Despite this good prognosis, patients with postoperative AF have a greater risk of stroke, especially when AF is persistent (6, 10, 11, 20).

In a series of 100 consecutive patients undergoing esophagectomy at Memorial Sloan-Kettering Cancer Center without a history of atrial arrhythmias or receiving antiarrhythmics, the effects of predefined risk factors, including history and pulmonary function, on the 30-day incidence of symptomatic postoperative SVT, need for admission to the intensive care unit, and mortality rate were evaluated (21). Symptomatic SVT occurred in 13 (13%) of the patients studied at a median of 3 days after operation, and it was accompanied by hypotension in 9 of 13 (69%). Univariate correlates of SVT were older age, perioperative use of theophylline, and a low carbon monoxide diffusion capacity on preoperative pulmonary function evaluation. On multivariate analysis, however, only greater age remained independently associated with SVT. Although patients in whom SVT developed had a higher rate of admission to the intensive care unit and a longer hospital stay, SVT was not the direct cause of death (21). This study was prospective and considered only clinically significant arrhythmias defined by electrocardiography (ECG) and their association with hemodynamic changes. It is possible that if continuous ECG monitoring was employed to detect asymptomatic arrhythmias, the overall incidence of SVT would be approximately 20%.

RISK FACTORS AND PROPOSED MECHANISMS

To date, the only consistent preoperative risk factor for an increased incidence of atrial arrhythmias after surgery has been an age of 60 years or older (Figure 11.1) (3–8, 22). It is well known that aging causes degenerative and inflammatory changes in atrial myocardium that lead to alterations in electrical properties of the sinoatrial and atrioventricular (AV) nodes and atria, including prolonged sinoatrial and AV nodal conduction times and shorter atrial effective refractoriness, all of which contribute to fragmentation of the propagating impulse (23, 24). We studied the effect of aging on supraventricular arrhythmias after right pneumonectomy in young and elderly dogs with the aim of better understanding potential age-related arrhythmogenic mechanisms (25). Electrocardiography was continuously recorded by an implantable telemetry system for 1 week after surgery. After pneumonectomy, seven of eight (88%) older animals developed a total of 23 episodes of

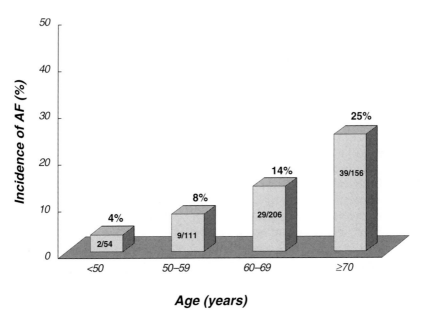

FIGURE 11.1 Incidence of postoperative atrial fibrillation (AF) by patient age. [From Amar et al. (22); with permission.]

sustained (>30 seconds) paroxysmal SVT, compared to zero of seven (0%) young dogs (25). Comparison of the heart rate and rhythm obtained in younger animals from the corresponding postoperative hour demonstrated that older animals developed significantly more atrial and ventricular premature contractions and episodes of nonsustained VT. Histologic examination of the atria showed interstitial fibrosis in old, but not in young, animals. In addition, four of eight (50%) elderly animals exhibited an inflammatory response within the atria consistent with acute myo- and epicarditis (Figure 11.2). We concluded that elderly dogs have a greater supraventricular arrhythmogenic potential than younger animals within the first week after pneumonectomy, perhaps because of increased atrial fibrosis and inflammation (25).

Until recently, it was proposed that an important mechanism responsible for the generation of AF after pulmonary resection was right-heart dilatation. Experimental (26) and clinical (27, 28) studies examining the effect of pulmonary resection on ventricular function suggest that significant right ventricular dilatation occurs in the immediate, early postoperative period. Reed et al. (27, 28), studying a small group of patients primarily undergoing lobectomy, demonstrated with right-heart ejection fraction catheters a mild increase in right ventricular end-diastolic volume on postoperative days 1 and 2 compared to baseline. Similarly, these investigators demonstrated a decrease in pulmonary vascular resistance on postoperative day 2 as well as a 15% decrease in right ventricular ejection fraction. The limitations of these studies are the small number of patients, the small changes seen in hemodynamic parameters, and the lack of correlation to clinical outcome. The reliability of right ventricular ejection fraction measurements in comparison to similar measurements obtained from cardiac catheterization needs to be established before clinical conditions may be defined in a small number of patients. A study of 47 patients undergoing lobectomy and 39 patients undergoing pneumonectomy was done at Memorial Sloan-Kettering Cancer Center using serial transthoracic echocardiograms to estimate right atrial and ventricular size and tricuspid regurgitation jet Doppler velocity to estimate right ventricular systolic pressure (29). Mild postoperative increases in right-heart pressure were noted only in patients undergoing pneumonectomy (Table 11.1) (29). These mild elevations in right ventricular systolic pressure were not associated with right atrial or right ventricular dilatation. Examination of two-dimensional echocardiograms revealed normal right ventricular systolic function in all the patients studied after surgery, despite some patients developing mild to moderate right ventricular enlargement in the setting of acute respiratory distress syndrome. In contrast to Reed et al. (28), our patients were ambulating early after surgery, did not have pulmonary artery catheters, and were studied with real-time echocardiography (29).

The concept of a pre-existing anatomic or electrophysiologic substrate for arrhythmias because of aging, which may be present at varying severity among individuals who are susceptible to AF, possibly explains why only some patients who undergo the exact same operation develop postoperative atrial arrhythmias (19, 24, 30). A prolonged P-wave signal averaged duration (a sign of delayed intra-atrial conduction) has been shown to be an independent predictor of AF after cardiac surgery (31, 32). An association between older age and prolonged P-wave duration was demonstrated in a nonsurgical population (33). The role of the signal-averaged P-wave duration to predict postoperative AF remains controversial (34, 35). In our previous experience, a prolonged signal-averaged P-wave duration did not differentiate patients who developed AF after thoracic surgery (35). Even among the workers who describe its usefulness as a predictor of postoperative AF, some propose a cutoff point of greater than 140 milliseconds and others greater than 155 milliseconds to indicate significant intra-atrial conduction delay and, hence, increased risk for arrhythmia occurrence (31, 32). In comparison to the 6.1% incidence of postoperative atrial arrhythmias among elderly patients who undergo major abdominal or peripheral surgery, the greater incidence of postoperative arrhythmias observed in elderly patients who undergo thoracic (20%) or cardiac (30% average for coronary artery bypass grafting and up to 65% for valvular repair or replacement) operations most likely corresponds to the amount of blunt or sharp surgical trauma to the atria and to sympathovagal fibers innervating the sinus node (8, 9, 30). Autonomic neural injury may then sensitize the atrial myocardium to catecholamines (denervation supersensitivity) to promote arrhythmias. Both AF and SVT often are initiated by an atrial premature contraction and later degenerate into one or more circuits that continuously re-enter themselves or one another (random re-entry) (9, 24). Once initiated, atrial tachyarrhythmias cause alterations in atrial electrical and structural properties (remodeling), including both rapid functional changes and slower alterations in ion-channel gene expression, which promote the maintenance of the arrhythmia and facilitate its reinitiation should it terminate (24). Recent studies have demonstrated acute downregulation of the lymphocyte β-adrenergic receptor system in response to thoracic or abdominal surgery on the first postoperative day that persists through the first postoperative week (36). These data suggest continued autonomic activation despite evidence showing that the plasma catecholamines during this period are not elevated. Although autonomic imbalance has also been implicated as a possible trigger of postoperative AF, some controversy exists regarding whether this is primarily vagal or sympathetic in nature (37, 38). Having a better understanding of the mechanisms of postoperative AF could lead to more targeted preventative or therapeutic interventions.

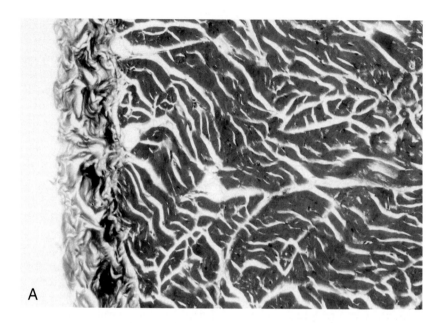

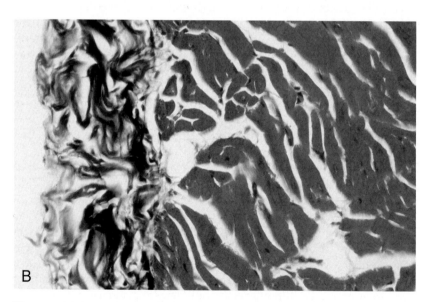

FIGURE 11.2   Transverse sections of the right atrium (Masson trichrome stain) from a representative young dog (*A* and *B*) and an old dog (*C* and *D*). Panel *D* shows moderate atrial fibrosis (large arrow) with accumulation of inflammatory mononuclear and polynuclear cells (small arrows) consistent with acute myo- and epicarditis. Original magnification × 200 (*A* and *C*) and × 400 (*B* and *D*). [From Amar et al. (25); with permission.]

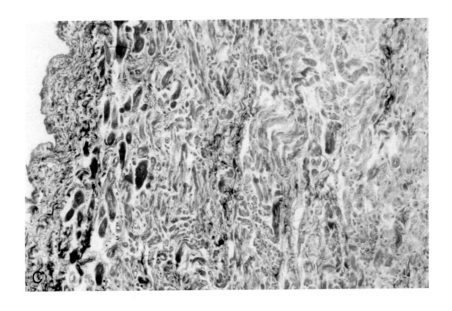

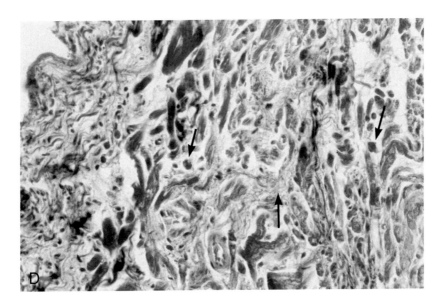

FIGURE 11.2 Continued

TABLE 11.1 Echocardiographic Findings in Patients Undergoing Lobectomy or Pneumonectomy

	Preoperative		Postoperative day 1		Postoperative days 2–6	
	Lobectomy (n)	Pneumonectomy (n)	Lobectomy (n)	Pneumonectomy (n)	Lobectomy (n)	Pneumonectomy (n)
Heart rate (beats/min)	80 ± 13 (47)	82 ± 13 (39)	92 ± 15 (47)	92 ± 15 (39)	92 ± 14 (47)	99 ± 14 (39)
Right atrial size (cm)	4.5 ± 0.6 (43)	4.4 ± 0.4 (37)	4.4 ± 0.4 (44)	4.5 ± 0.4 (26)	4.4 ± 0.5 (38)	4.5 ± 0.5 (32)
Left atrial size (cm)	4.7 ± 0.6 (46)	4.7 ± 0.5 (38)	4.9 ± 0.5 (45)	4.8 ± 0.6 (28)	4.9 ± 0.6 (39)	4.7 ± 0.7 (33)
Tricuspid regurgitation jet (m/sec)	2.2 ± 0.4 (37)	2.3 ± 0.5 (30)	2.2 ± 0.4 (41)	2.3 ± 0.5[a] (23)	2.2 ± 0.5 (37)	2.5 ± 0.61[a] (30)
Right ventricular systolic pressure (mm Hg)	24 ± 6 (37)	26 ± 11 (30)	25 ± 8 (41)	27 ± 9[b] (23)	25 ± 10 (37)	31 ± 15[b] (30)

Adapted from Amar (29); with permission.
Data are presented as the mean ±SD.
[a] $p < 0.05$, postoperative days 2–6 vs baseline (paired t-test).
[b] $p < 0.05$, pneumonectomy vs lobectomy (analysis of variance).

To gain insight regarding autonomic influences preceding postoperative AF, we recently compared time and frequency domain parameters of heart rate variability between 48 patients who developed this arrhythmia and 48 matched, postoperative controls without AF (39). In comparison to controls, patients who developed AF after major noncardiac thoracic surgery demonstrated significant changes in heart rate variability that were consistent with vagal resurgence competing in a background of increasing sympathetic activity as the primary autonomic mechanism responsible for triggering postoperative AF. To the best of my knowledge, these novel results represent the largest study using heart rate variability to understand autonomic influences preceding postoperative AF, and they suggest interventions that modulate both the sympathetic and parasympathetic nervous systems may be beneficial in suppressing postoperative AF (39). A current view of the pathophysiology underlying the genesis of perioperative atrial tachyarrhythmias is depicted in Figure 11.3.

PREVENTION OF POSTTHORACOTOMY ARRHYTHMIAS

A recent review summarized the results of numerous studies examining the efficacy of a variety of drugs to prevent postoperative atrial

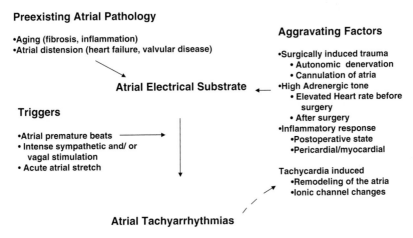

Pathophysiology of Perioperative Atrial Tachyarrhythmias

FIGURE 11.3 Proposed mechanisms for perioperative atrial tachyarrhythmias. [From Amar (9); with permission.]

arrhythmias (11). It is unclear whether prophylactic treatment against this complication improves clinical outcomes or shortens hospital stay and whether rate- or rhythm-control drugs should be employed for this purpose. Digoxin had been the drug of choice for the prevention of AF after thoracic surgery. However, its efficacy has not been proven in prospective trials, and its use may well be associated with untoward effects (40, 41). Although digoxin does directly affect atrial tissue and the AV node, this effect is minimal and is mediated by a secondary central nervous system effect to enhance vagal tone. This would explain digoxin's lack of efficacy after surgery, a period when vagal influences are lessened and adrenergic output is high (42). In our experience, diltiazem was shown to be more effective than digoxin in reducing the overall incidence of AF after standard or intrapericardial pneumonectomy (41). Because of the lack of proven efficacy of digoxin to prevent postoperative AF, its routine use should be discouraged. Because sympathetic activation is suspected in precipitating postoperative atrial arrhythmias in susceptible patients, β-adrenergic blocker prophylaxis has been studied extensively. β-Blockers are useful in this setting (43), but despite their administration, the rate of postoperative AF remains high (11, 44). Partial sympathectomy with epidural analgesia did not reduce AF in a well-designed study after cardiac surgery and only marginally attenuated the AF incidence in a small study after thoracic surgery (45, 46). We and others have found diltiazem to be effective in reducing AF and SVT after thoracic or cardiac surgery, respectively (6, 47). In our randomized, double-blind, placebo-controlled trial of 330 patients undergoing lobectomy or pneumonectomy, diltiazem given intravenously for 12 to 18 hours and then orally for 14 days after surgery reduced the incidence of clinically significant arrhythmias by nearly 50% in comparison to placebo-treated patients (6). Prophylactic amiodarone to reduce the incidence of postoperative AF has been safe and particularly effective when given orally for 1 week before cardiac surgery (11, 43, 48). Global use of intravenous amiodarone to prevent AF after cardiac surgery, however, is not recommended because of its high cost ($800 for a 48-hour course) and marginal efficacy unless used in older patients undergoing combined valvular and coronary surgery (49). Amiodarone is a Vaughan Williams class 3 drug, but it also has calcium-channel- and β-adrenergic blocking properties as well as class 1 and 4 actions. The cost, feasibility, and safety (ie, potential for proarrhythmia) of using amiodarone or other class 3 drugs for global prophylaxis of perioperative supraventricular arrhythmias deserves further study. Amiodarone is widely used and has a good overall safety record compared to other antiarrhythmic drugs, but it is not without cardiovascular or noncardiac toxicity (23, 50). Controversy exists regarding whether perioperative amiodarone causes severe pulmonary toxicity after cardiac and thoracic surgery (51–53). Unless hypomagnesemia is present, the prophylactic administration of magnesium during cardiac surgery did not reduce the incidence of postoperative supraventricular arrhythmias (54). The role of overdrive biatrial pacing for prophylaxis against postoperative AF after coronary artery bypass grafting has been well demonstrated (55). Its widespread use, however, will be limited by the availability of necessary specialized personnel and by complications related to lead failure.

TREATMENT OF POSTTHORACOTOMY ARRHYTHMIAS

When initiating specific drug therapy for rapid AF or SVT, one should assess and correct possible aggravating factors, such as respiratory failure or electrolyte imbalance. Only SVT (not AF) responds well to treatment with adenosine. Both arrhythmias, however, respond to rate-control drugs, such as β-blockers (eg, esmolol, metoprolol) or calcium-channel antagonists (eg, diltiazem, verapamil) (11, 23, 56). Calcium-channel blockers should be used with caution as single agents in patients with Wolff-Parkinson-White syndrome, because they can accelerate the ventricular rate with AF (4). Uniform or multiform atrial tachycardias usually respond to rate-control drugs but are not amenable to direct current cardioversion. Recent data suggest that once AF has occurred after cardiac surgery, rhythm control by pharmacologic means or direct current electrical cardioversion offers little advantage over a rate-control strategy (11–15, 23). Intuitively, the latter strategy may be associated with less risk of proarrhythmia. Similar studies have not been performed in patients after thoracotomy. Once sinus rhythm is restored, rate- or rhythm-control drugs may be discontinued at 4 to 8 weeks after surgery (11). A proposed algorithm for the treatment of recent-onset AF or SVT is presented in Figure 11.4. In general, however, digoxin may be used as a first-line drug only in patients with congestive heart failure, because it is not effective in high-adrenergic states, such as after surgery (23, 42) β-Blockers are preferred in patients with ischemic heart disease, but they may be relatively contraindicated in patients with proven bronchospastic potential, in those with congestive heart failure, and in those with severe sinus bradycardia or high-degree AV block (11, 23). Of the class 3 antiarrhythmic drugs, ibutilide has been used recently with moderate success to convert acute AF in 57% of patients after cardiac surgery; however, polymorphic VT was reported in 1.8% of patients and was attributed primarily to electrolyte imbalance (57). It is therefore recommended to correct potassium and magnesium levels before administration of ibutilide, to monitor patients for at least 4 hours afterward, and to have physicians who are trained to deliver defibrillatory shocks readily available. Although

Management of Perioperative Atrial Tachyarrhythmias

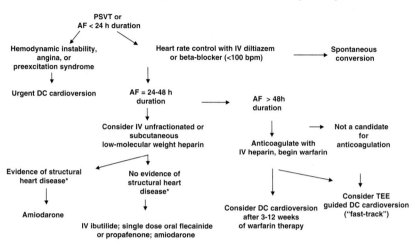

FIGURE 11.4   Management of perioperative atrial tachyarrhythmias. Structural heart disease (*) is defined as the presence of one of the following: left ventricular hypertrophy with wall thickness = 1.4 cm, mitral valve disease, coronary artery disease, or heart failure. AF = atrial fibrillation/flutter; bpm = beats per minute; DC = direct current; TEE = transesophageal echocardiography. [Adapted from Amar (9); with permission.]

commonly used for the acute management of postoperative AF, amiodarone can control the ventricular response; however, it has questionable superiority over placebo in the conversion of recent-onset AF unrelated to surgery (58). A recent meta-analysis concerning nonsurgical patients showed that the efficacy of amiodarone therapy for recent-onset AF was 56% at 6 to 8 hours and 82% at 24 hours, compared to 43% and 56%, respectively, with placebo (59). Efficacy studies of amiodarone versus placebo for the treatment (not prophylaxis) of acute postoperative AF are sparse. Furthermore, a growing body of evidence from studies that compared rate-control versus rhythm-control strategies for the management of acute AF after cardiac surgery shows no significant difference in time to conversion to sinus rhythm between the groups or in the proportion of patients free of AF at 48 hours (12–15). In patients with recent-onset AF but without structural heart disease (defined as the presence of one of the following: left ventricular hypertrophy with wall thickness = 1.4 cm, mitral valve disease, coronary artery disease, and heart failure), a single oral dose of the class 1c drugs flecainide (300 mg) or propafenone (600 mg) has been shown to be safe, with conversion rates at 8 hours of up to 91% and 76%, respectively (23). Although the chronic use of class 1c drugs is contraindicated in patients with coro-

nary artery disease, some clinicians would use them in a single dose to treat AF in patients recovering from cardiac surgery as long as there is no evidence of acute myocardial ischemia and the patients are continuously monitored with telemetry for at least 24 hours for detection of potentially harmful ventricular arrhythmias.

PREVENTION OF THROMBOEMBOLISM

The incidence of stroke after general surgery and anesthesia has been reported to be from 0.08% to 0.4% (60, 61). In a study of 330 patients undergoing noncardiac thoracic surgery, we found that of the 60 patients who developed AF, one (1.7%) sustained a stroke that was likely related to the arrhythmia (6). The risk of stroke or transient neurological injury of 1.6% to 3.3% for patients who develop postoperative AF after cardiac operations is consistently greater compared to those without AF (0.2–1.4%) (10, 11, 20). Risk factors for stroke in patients with AF unrelated to surgery include mitral stenosis, hypertension (including treated hypertension), previous transient ischemic attack or stroke, congestive heart failure, left ventricular dysfunction and an age of more that 75 years (23). Because the potential for thromboembolism with new-onset AF develops early (24–48 hours), prompt attempts to restore sinus rhythm within this period should be made (11, 23). If the arrhythmia persists beyond 24 to 48 hours, anticoagulant therapy should be considered after weighing the risk of postoperative bleeding. Antithrombotic therapy may range from no therapy (age < 60 years and no heart disease) to aspirin alone (age < 60 years with heart disease but no other risk factors, or age = 60 years with no risk factors), anticoagulation alone (age ≥ 60 years with diabetes mellitus or coronary artery disease, age ≥ 75 years, heart failure, left ventricular ejection fraction < 35%, thyrotoxicosis, hypertension, rheumatic heart disease with mitral stenosis, prosthetic heart valves, previous thromboembolism, and persistent atrial thrombus on transesophageal echocardiography), or their combination, depending on the patient's risk (23). The risks of anticoagulation and/or antiarrhythmic drugs must be weighed against the fact that 0% to 48% of patients with acute AF convert to sinus rhythm spontaneously (9, 23). In patients with multiple risk factors for thromboembolism who are not candidates for or do not wish to receive systemic anticoagulation, the "fast-track" approach to conversion of AF using transesophageal echocardiography is an acceptable and frequently used approach in settings where such services are available (Figure 11.4) (9, 23). Randomized, controlled trials assessing the perioperative use of intravenous heparin in patients with different indications for long-term anticoagulation would provide better data on which to base management decisions. Intravenous heparin may be initiated to maintain an activated partial thromboplastin time of 2- to 3-fold the control value but is discontinued if heparin-induced thrombocytopenia develops (platelet count falls by 30% from baseline or to <100,000 cells/mm^3) (9, 11, 23). Later, warfarin may be given to maintain an international normalized ratio between 2.0 and 3.0. Patients may then be considered for early cardioversion with the use of transesophageal echocardiography ("fast-track") or returned for cardioversion between 3 and 12 weeks after initiation of anticoagulant therapy (Figure 11.4) (9, 23). The prophylactic use of aspirin in postoperative AF has not been studied, but it can be used as recommended earlier for patients with AF unrelated to surgery (23).

POSTOPERATIVE VENTRICULAR ARRHYTHMIAS

Atrial arrhythmias are common after thoracic surgery, but the incidence and significance of ventricular arrhythmias early after such surgery are not well established. In 412 patients who had lobectomy ($n = 243$) or pneumonectomy ($n = 169$) and were continuously monitored with Holter recorders for 72 to 96 hours postoperatively, we determined the incidence and outcome of ventricular arrhythmias (5). The primary end point of the study was the occurrence of VT defined as three or more consecutive wide complexes. A total of 61 of 412 (15%) patients developed one or more episodes of VT. There were no episodes of sustained (>30 seconds) VT, and no patient required treatment for hemodynamic compromise associated with any VT episode. Patients with VT had a greater incidence of a preoperative left bundle branch block but did not differ in other clinical characteristics, operative data, or core temperature on arrival to the postanesthesia care unit when compared to those without VT. On multivariate logistic regression analysis, only postoperative AF occurrence was independently associated with VT (relative risk, 2.6; 95% confidence interval, 1.4 to 4.8) (5). Little data are available regarding whether repeated or frequent ventricular ectopy after noncardiac surgery is associated with poor long-term cardiovascular outcome. To date, only one study evaluated the relationship of the development of VT in patients without ischemia during hospitalization after noncardiac surgery, and it showed that VT was not associated with adverse long-term outcome (62). The incidence of sustained VT or fibrillation following cardiac surgery has been reported to be 0.5% to 1% from large observational studies of patients who were monitored postoperatively (63, 64). Attempts to prophylactically suppress nonsustained ventricular arrhythmias after cardiac surgery with lidocaine failed to show that such a strategy improves outcome (65). In the general population or after an acute myocardial infarction, electrophysiologic testing in patients with no symptoms or only mild ones related to frequent ventricular ectopy or nonsustained VT is now believed to be inappropriate because of the lack of evidence that therapeutic strategies for such events have improved outcome (66). Exceptions to these guidelines may be applied to patients with low ejection fraction, positive signal-averaged ECG of patients who are highly symptomatic.

CONCLUSIONS

In this cost-containment era, we need to better define the subgroup of patients at highest risk for morbidity related to postthoracotomy atrial arrhythmias to target the most aggressive pharmacologic therapies to these patients. This important step will lead to more useful studies to determine whether reduction of atrial arrhythmias among high-risk patients improves outcomes and shortens length of hospital stay. Finally, current data suggest that once postoperative AF has occurred, a rate-control strategy during the first 24 hours is reasonable, because nearly 80% of those episodes will resolve during this period. Beyond this period, a more aggressive approach utilizing class 1c or 3 antiarrhythmic drugs will hopefully reduce related drug toxicity and the number of patients who may require anticoagulation.

References

1. Amar D, Roistacher N, Burt M, Reinsel RA, Ginsberg RJ, Wilson RS: Clinical and echocardiographic correlates of symptomatic tachyarrhythmias after noncardiac thoracic surgery. Chest 1995; 108:349–54.
2. Curtis JJ, Parker BM, McKenney CA, Wagner-Mann CC, Walls JT, Demmy TL, Schmaltz RA: Incidence and predictors of supraventricular dysrhythmias after pulmonary resection. Ann Thorac Surg 1998; 66:1766–71.
3. Cardinale D, Martinoni A, Cipolla CM, Civelli M, Lamantia G, Fiorentini C, Mezzetti M: Atrial fibrillation after operation for lung cancer: clinical and prognostic significance. Ann Thorac Surg 1999; 68:1827–31.
4. Atlee JL: Perioperative cardiac arrhythmias. Diagnosis and management. Anesthesiology 1997; 86:1397–424.
5. Amar D, Zhang H, Roistacher N: The incidence and outcome of ventricular arrhythmias after noncardiac thoracic surgery. Anesth Analg 2002; 95:537–43.
6. Amar D, Roistacher N, Rusch VW, Leung DHY, Ginsburg I, Zhang H, Bains MS, Downey RJ, Korst RJ, Ginsberg RJ: Effects of diltiazem

prophylaxis on the incidence and clinical outcome of atrial arrhythmias after thoracic surgery. J Thorac Cardiovasc Surg 2000; 120:790–8.

7. Amar D, Zhang H, Heerdt PM, Park B, Rusch VW: Inflammatory markers and postoperative atrial fibrillation (abstract). Anesthesiology 2003; 99:A200.

8. Polanczyk CA, Goldman L, Marcantonio ER, Orav EJ, Lee TH: Supraventricular arrhythmia in patients having noncardiac surgery: clinical correlates and effect on length of stay. Ann Intern Med 1998; 129:279–85.

9. Amar D: Perioperative atrial tachyarrhythmias. Anesthesiology 2002; 97:1618–23.

10. Cresswell LL, Schuessler RB, Rosenbloom M, Cox JL: Hazards of postoperative atrial arrhythmias. Ann Thorac Surg 1993; 56:539–49.

11. Maisel WH, Rawn JD, Stevenson WG: Atrial fibrillation after cardiac surgery. Ann Intern Med 2001; 135:1061–73.

12. Lee JK, Klein GJ, Yee R, Krahn AD, Zarnke KB, Simpson CS, Skanes A, Spindler B: Rate control versus conversion strategy in postoperative atrial fibrillation: a prospective, randomized pilot study. Am Heart J 2000; 140:871–7.

13. Abordo M, Soucier R, Berns E, Silverman DI: Early antiarrhythmic therapy is no better than rate control therapy alone for suppression of atrial fibrillation after cardiac surgery. Ann Noninvas Electrocardiol 2000; 5:365–72.

14. Soucier RJ, Mizra S, Abordo MG, Berns E, Dalamagas HC, Hanna A, Silverman DI: Predictors of conversion of atrial fibrillation after cardiac operation in the absence of class I or III antiarrhythmic medications. Ann Thorac Surg 2001; 72:694–8.

15. Soucier R, Silverman D, Abordo M, et al.: Propafenone versus ibutilide for postoperative atrial fibrillation following cardiac surgery: neither strategy improves outcomes compared to rate control alone (the PIPAF study). Med Sci Monit 2003; 9:PI19–23.

16. Mangano DT: Perioperative cardiac morbidity. Anesthesiology 1990; 72:153–84.

17. Bruins P, Velthuis HT, Yazdanbakhsh AP, Jansen PGM, van Hardevelt FWJ, de Beaumont EMFH, Wildevuur CRH, Eijsman L, Trouwborst A, Hack CE: Activation of the complement system during and after cardiopulmonary bypass surgery. Postsurgery activation involves C-reactive protein and is associated with postoperative arrhythmia. Circulation 1997; 96:3542–8.

18. Amar D, Fleisher M, Zhang H: Elevated C-reactive protein but not troponin is associated with postoperative atrial fibrillation (abstract). Anesth Analg 2002; 94:S67.

19. Goette A, Juenemann G, Peters B, Klein HU, Roesner A, Huth C, Roecken C: Determinants and consequences of atrial fibrosis in patients undergoing open-heart surgery. Cardiovasc Res 2002; 54:390–6.

20. Stamou SC, Dangas G, Hill PC, Pfister AJ, Dullum MKC, Boyce SW, Bafi AS, Garcia JM, Corso PJ: Atrial fibrillation after beating heart surgery. Am J Cardiol 2000; 86:64–7.

21. Amar D, Burt ME, Bains MS, Leung DHY: Symptomatic tachydysrhythmias after esophagectomy: incidence and outcome measures. Ann Thorac Surg 1996; 61:1506–9.

22. Amar D, Zhang H, Leung DHY, Roistacher N, Kadish AH: Older age is the strongest predictor of postoperative atrial fibrillation. Anesthesiology 2002; 96:352–6.

23. Fuster V, Ryden LE, Asinger RW, Cannom DS, Crijns HJ, Frye RL, Halperin JL, Kay GN, Klein WW, Levy S, McNamara RL, Prystowsky EN, Wann LS, Wyse DG: ACC/AHA/ESC guidelines for the management of patients with atrial fibrillation: executive summary: a report of the American College of Cardiology/ American Heart Association Task Force on Practice Guidelines and the European Society of Cardiology Committee for Practice Guidelines and Policy Conferences (Committee to Develop Guidelines for the Management of Patients with Atrial Fibrillation). Circulation 2001; 104:2118–50.

24. Allessie MA, Boyden PA, Camm AJ, Kleber AG, Lab MJ, Legato MJ, Rosen MR, Schwartz PJ, Spooner PM, Van Wagoner DR, Waldo AL: Pathophysiology and prevention of atrial fibrillation. Circulation 2001; 103:769–77.

25. Amar D, Heerdt PM, Korst RJ, Zhang H, Nguyen H: The effects of advanced age on the incidence of supraventricular arrhythmias after pneumonectomy in dogs. Anesth Analg 2002; 94:1132–6.

26. Hsia CC, Carlin JI, Cassidy SS, et al.: Hemodynamic changes after pneumonectomy in the exercising foxhound. J Appl Physiol 1990; 69:51–7.

27. Reed CE, Spinale FG, Crawford FA Jr: Effect of pulmonary resection on right ventricular function. Ann Thorac Surg 1992; 53:578–82.

28. Reed CE, Dorman BH, Spinale FG: Assessment of right ventricular contractile performance after pulmonary resection. Ann Thorac Surg 1993; 56:426–31.

29. Amar D, Burt M, Reinsel RA, Roistacher N, Ginsberg RJ, Wilson RS: Value of perioperative Doppler echocardiography in patients undergoing major lung resection. Ann Thorac Surg 1996; 61:516–520.

30. Cox JL: A perspective of postoperative atrial fibrillation in cardiac operations. Ann Thorac Surg 1993; 56:405–9.

31. Steinberg JS, Zelenkofske S, Wong SC, Gelernt M, Sciacca R, Menchavez E: Value of the P-wave signal-averaged ECG for predicting atrial fibrillation after cardiac surgery. Circulation 1993; 88:2618–22.

32. Zaman AG, Archbold RA, Helft G, Paul EA, Curzen NP, Mills PG: Atrial fibrillation after coronary artery bypass surgery. A model for preoperative risk stratification. Circulation 2000; 101:1403–8.

33. Babaev AA, Vloka ME, Sadurski R, Steinberg JS: Influence of age on atrial activation as measured by the P-wave signal-averaged electrocardiogram. Am J Cardiol 2000; 86:692–5.

34. Frost L, Lund B, Pilegaard H, Christiansen EH: Re-evaluation of P-wave duration and morphology as predictors of atrial fibrillation and flutter after coronary artery bypass surgery. Eur Heart J 1996; 17:1065–71.

35. Amar D, Roistacher N, Zhang H, Baum MS, Ginsburg I, Steinberg JS: Signal averaged P-wave duration does not predict atrial fibrillation after thoracic surgery. Anesthesiology 1999; 91:16–23.

36. Amar D, Fleisher M, Pantuck CB, Shamoon H, Zhang H, Roistacher N, Leung DHY, Ginsburg I, Smiley RM: Persistent alterations of the autonomic nervous system after noncardiac surgery. Anesthesiology 1998; 89:30–42.

37. Dimmer C, Tavernier R, Gjorgov N, Nooten GV, Clement DL, Jordaens L: Variations of autonomic tone preceding onset of atrial fibrillation after coronary artery bypass grafting. Am J Cardiol 1998; 82:22–5.

38. Hogue CW, Domitrovich PP, Stein PK, et al.: RR interval dynamics before atrial fibrillation in patients after coronary artery bypass graft surgery. Circulation 1998; 98:429–34.

39. Amar D, Zhang H, Miodownik S, Kadish AH: Competing autonomic mechanisms precede the onset of postoperative atrial fibrillation. J Am Coll Cardiol 2003; 42:1262–8.

40. Ritchie AJ, Bowe P, Gibbons JRP: Prophylactic digitalization for thoracotomy: a reassessment. Ann Thorac Surg 1990; 50:86–8.

41. Amar D, Roistacher N, Burt M, Rusch VW, Bains MS, Leung DHY, Downey RJ, Ginsberg RJ: Effects of diltiazem versus digoxin on dysrhythmias and cardiac function after pneumonectomy. Ann Thorac Surg 1997; 63:1374–82.

42. Falk RH, Leavitt JJ: Digoxin for atrial fibrillation: a drug whose time has gone? Ann Intern Med 1991; 114:573–5.

43. Crystal E, Connolly SJ, Sleik K, Ginger TJ, Yusuf S: Interventions on prevention of postoperative atrial fibrillation in patients undergoing heart surgery. A meta-analysis. Circulation 2002; 106:75–80.

44. Mathew JP, Parks R, Savino JS, Friedman AS, Koch C, Mangano DT, Browner WS, for the Multicenter Study of Perioperative Is-

chemia Research Group: Atrial fibrillation following coronary artery bypass graft surgery: predictors, outcomes, and resource utilization. JAMA 1996; 276:300–6.

45. Jidéus L, Joachimsson P-O, Stridsberg M, Ericson M, Tydén H, Nilsson L, Blomström P, Blomström-Lundgvist C: Thoracic epidural anesthesia does not influence the occurrence of postoperative sustained atrial fibrillation. Ann Thorac Surg 2001; 72:65–71.

46. Oka T, Ozawa Y, Ohkubo Y: Thoracic epidural bupivacaine attenuates supraventricular tachyarrhythmias after pulmonary resection. Anesth Analg 2001; 93:253–9.

47. Seitelberger R, Hannes W, Gleichauf M, Keilich M, Christoph M, Fasol R: Effects of diltiazem on perioperative ischemia, arrhythmias, and myocardial function in patients undergoing elective coronary bypass grafting. J Thorac Cardiovasc Surg 1994; 107:811–21.

48. Giri S, White CM, Dunn AB, Felton K, Freeman-Bosco L, Reddy P, Tsikouris JP, Wilcox HA, Kluger J: Oral amiodarone for prevention of atrial fibrillation after open heart surgery, the atrial fibrillation suppression trial (AFIST): a randomized placebo-controlled trial. Lancet 2001; 357:830–6.

49. Mahoney EM, Thompson TD, Veledar E, Williams J, Weintraub WS: Cost-effectiveness of targeting patients undergoing cardiac surgery for therapy with intravenous amiodarone to prevent atrial fibrillation. J Am Coll Cardiol 2002; 40:737–45.

50. Connolly SJ: Evidence-based analysis of amiodarone efficacy and safety. Circulation 1999; 100:2025–34.

51. Van Miegham W, Coolen L, Malysse I, Lacquet L, Deneffe GJD, Demedts MGP: Amiodarone and the development of ARDS after lung surgery. Chest 1994; 105:1642–45.

52. Greenspon AJ, Kidwell GA, Hurley W, Mannion J: Amiodarone-related postoperative adult respiratory distress syndrome. Circulation 1991; 84(suppl III):III-407–15.

53. Rady MY, Ryan T, Starr NJ: Preoperative therapy with amiodarone and the incidence of acute organ dysfunction after cardiac surgery. Anesth Analg 1997; 85:489–97.

54. England MR, Gordon G, Salem M, Chernow B: Magnesium administration and arrhythmias after cardiac surgery. A placebo-controlled, double blind, randomized trial. JAMA 1992; 268:2395–402.

55. Daubert JC, Mabo P: Atrial pacing for the prevention of postoperative atrial fibrillation. How and where to pace? J Am Coll Cardiol 2000; 35:1423–7.

56. Balser JR, Martinez EA, Winters BD, Perdue PW, Clarke AW, Huang W, Tomaselli GF, Dorman T, Campbell K, Lipsett P, Breslow MJ, Rosenfeld BA: β-Adrenergic blockade accelerates conver-

sion of postoperative supraventricular tachycardia. Anesthesiology 1998; 89:1052–9.

57. VanderLugt JT, Mattioni T, Denker S, Torchiana D, Ahern T, Wakefield LK, Perry KT, Kowey PR, for the Ibutilide Investigators: Efficacy and safety of ibutilide fumarate for the conversion of atrial arrhythmias after cardiac surgery. Circulation 1999; 100:369–75.

58. Galve E, Rius T, Ballester R, Artaza MA, Arnau JM, Garcia-Dorado D, Soler-Soler J: Intravenous amiodarone in treatment of recent-onset atrial fibrillation: results of a randomized, controlled study. J Am Coll Cardiol 1996; 27:1079–82.

59. Chevalier P, Durand-Dubief A, Burri H, Cucherat M, Kirkorian G, Touboul P: Amiodarone versus placebo and class Ic drugs for cardioversion of recent-onset atrial fibrillation: a meta-analysis. J Am Coll Cardiol 2003; 41:255–62.

60. Forrest JB, Rehder K, Cahalan MK, Goldsmith CH: Multicenter Study of General Anesthesia. III. Predictors of severe perioperative adverse outcomes. Anesthesiology 1992; 76:3–15.

61. Parikh S, Cohen JR: Perioperative stroke after general surgical procedures. N Y State J Med 1993; 93:162–5.

62. Mangano DT, Browner WS, Hollenberg M, et al.: Long-term cardiac prognosis following noncardiac surgery. JAMA 1992; 268:233–9.

63. Topol EJ, Lerman BB, Baughman KL, et al.: De novo refractory ventricular tachyarrhythmias after coronary revascularization. Am J Cardiol 1986; 57:57–9.

64. Stamou SC, Hill PC, Stample GA, et al.: Prevention of atrial fibrillation after cardiac surgery. The significance of postoperative oral amiodarone. Chest 2001; 120:1936–41.

65. Johnson RG, Goldberger AL, Thurer RL, et al.: Lidocaine prophylaxis in coronary revascularization patients: a randomized prospective trial. Ann Thorac Surg 1993; 55:1180–4.

66. Zipes DP, DiMarco JP, Gillette PC, et al.: Guidelines for clinical intracardiac electrophysiological studies and catheter ablation procedures. A report of the American College of Cardiology/American Heart Association Task Force on Practice Guidelines. Circulation 1995; 92:673–91.

Rebecca Jacob, MD, DA

Challenges in the Practice of Thoracic Anesthesia in
12 | Developing Countries

Anesthesia for lung surgery is a specialty with problems of its own. This area has a great scope for lateral thinking, and any problem can always be tackled in several ways. No attempt has been made here to describe all the methods that can be used. I hope, however, that the methods described to meet the peculiar challenges of thoracic anesthesia in developing countries will be of value to the reader.

Conditions or "degrees of development" vary both from country to country and within each country in the developing world, so that at least in parts of a country, the environment in which hospital medicine is practiced may, in many respects, be little different from that in developed nations. A few major differences, however, are found in the practice of thoracic anesthesia. In general, patients in developing countries are more anemic and undernourished, and they tend to present later out of fear, ignorance, superstition, isolation, or lack of communication. Infectious diseases of pyogenic origin, tuberculosis, and hydatid disease, not malignancy, are the predominant reasons for their pulmonary disease In addition, maintenance and servicing of a wide range of equipment as well as drugs for providing quality anesthesia care are not always available.

In this chapter, I will present a number of common conditions seen in our setting and will let the patients and their problems speak for themselves. I will then present a general discussion on problems and challenges as well as cover the ways we have found of circumventing or overcoming them.

Progress in Thoracic Anesthesia, edited by Peter Slinger,
Lippincott Williams & Wilkins, Baltimore © 2004.

CASE 1

This 12-year-old girl presented with a bulge in the right anterior chest wall and no other symptoms. Radiologically, a large anterior mediastinal mass showing cystic and calcific changes was seen (Fig. 12.1). A diagnosis of mediastinal teratoma was made, and the mass was removed via a median sternotomy under general anesthesia. Biopsy proved the tumor to be a benign teratoma.

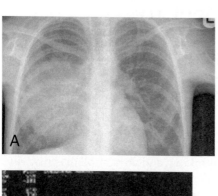
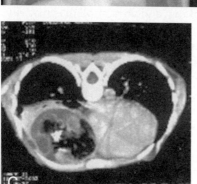
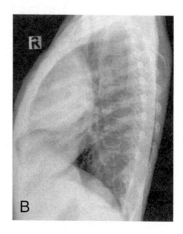

FIGURE 12.1 Chest x-ray (A and B) and CT scan (C) showing a large anterior mediastinal mass with cystic and calcific changes.

CASE 2

This 5-year-old boy presented with respiratory distress. Radiology revealed a right thoracic "white out" (Fig. 12.2A), which was initially diagnosed as an empyema. However, because no pus was found on aspiration, a computed tomographic (CT) scan was done. This showed a solid tumor filling the right hemithorax (Fig. 12.2B) A needle biopsy showed a rhabdomyosarcoma. Chemotherapy was followed by surgery under general anesthesia and an endotracheal tube (ETT). The tumor recurred, however, and the boy died 6 months later.

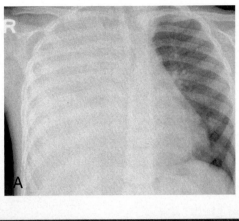

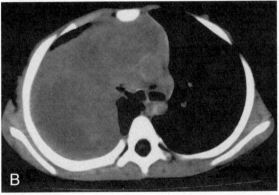

FIGURE 12.2 Chest x-ray (A) showing "white-out" of right hemithorax. CT scan (B) shows solid tumors filling right hemithorax.

CASE 3

An otherwise healthy preteen boy presented to the emergency department with a history of sudden onset of cough. During examination, he developed a cardiorespiratory arrest. He was resuscitated, recovered completely, but was admitted to the intensive care unit for observation. He had a similar episode the next day, and the surgeons were called in. A review of the chest radiograph (Fig. 12.3) showed a faintly opaque shadow in the right main bronchus. Rigid bronchoscopy under general anesthesia revealed a pebble, which was removed.

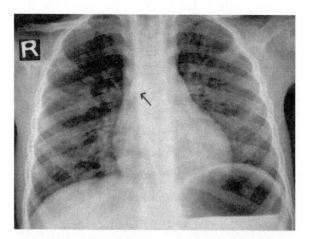

FIGURE 12.3 Chest x-ray showing a faint radioopaque shadow in right main bronchus.

CASE 4

This 8-year-old girl presented with a history of loss of weight, chronic fatigue, and cough. A chest radiograph revealed an empyema with thick pus filling the left hemithorax with a shift of the mediastinum (Fig 12.4), which had been drained at a peripheral hospital under local anesthesia. She required definitive surgery under general anesthesia A left thoracotomy and a decortication of the lung were performed. Perioperative pain relief was with an infusion of 0.1% bupivacaine and 1 μg/mL of fentanyl via an epidural catheter.

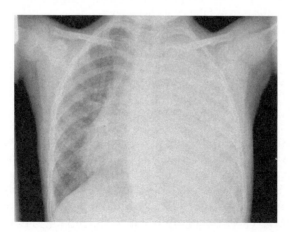

FIGURE 12.4 Chest x-ray showing empyema thoraces of the left hemithorax with a shift of the mediastinum.

CASE 5

This 6-year-old boy presented with a chronic cough, ill health, severe anemia, and clubbing. Chest radiography (Fig. 12.5) revealed a chronic empyema with entrapment of the right lung, contracted hemithorax, and scoliosis. It required decortication of the lung under general anesthesia with an ETT and steep head-down tilt.

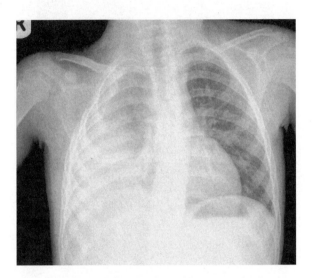

FIGURE 12.5   Chest x-ray showing chronic empyema, with lung entrapment, contrasted with hemithorax and scoliosis.

CASE 6

An emaciated 12-year-old girl presented with chronic ill health, cough, and clubbing. Radiography and CT (Fig. 12.6) showed a destroyed right lung and bilateral bronchiectasis. A right pneumonectomy was planned. The first time that general anesthesia was attempted, the child became severely hypoxic and bradycardic on mask ventilation. Perhaps this was due to aspiration of pus into the left lung. The surgery was postponed to a week later, when the child was preoxygenated and an ETT passed into the left main bronchus. Because this still could not ensure protection to the left lung (see Intraoperative Challenges and Lung Isolation Techniques [Especially in Pediatrics] page 276), the surgery was done in the supine position through an anterolateral thoracotomy through the bed of the fourth rib. The hilar dissection and isolation of the bronchus was done before the lung was handled. Although residual bronchiectasis was seen on the left side, the child has made a remarkable recovery.

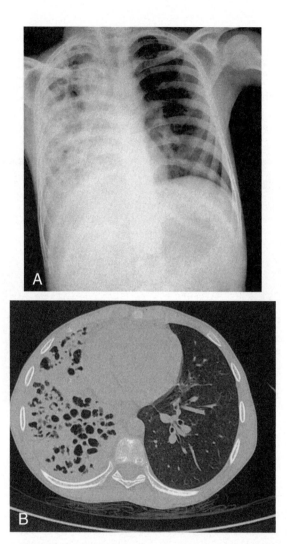

FIGURE 12.6 Chest x-ray (A) and CT scan (B) showing bilateral bronchiectasis and a destroyed right lung.

CASE 7

This 4-year-old girl presented with pneumonia (Fig. 12.7A) not resolving with antibiotics and increasing respiratory distress. Subsequent radiography showed a large intrapulmonary air fluid level (Fig 12.7B). A diagnosis of lung abscess was made, which was confirmed by CT scan (Fig 12.7C). A Malecot tube was placed as a drain under local anesthesia as an emergency measure (Fig 12.7D). Recovery was complete.

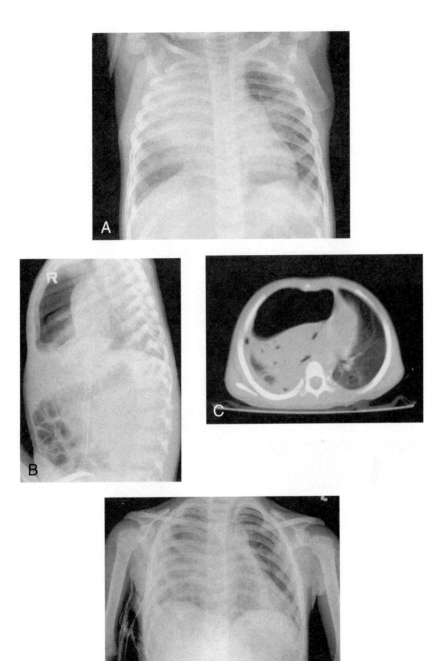

FIGURE 12.7   Serial chest x-rays showing pneumonia (A) developing into lung abscess with mediastinal shift (B and D) confirmed by CT scan (C).

CASE 8

This 5-year-old girl presented with respiratory distress. Radiography showed a large air fluid level and a diagnosis of lung abscess was made (Fig. 12.8A). A chest drain was placed in the abscess as an emergency measure under oxygen, sedation, and local anesthesia (Fig. 12.8B). The drain was placed to relieve tension in the cyst and to prevent rupture into the pleura or bronchus. The parents then found a radiograph taken 3 years earlier that also shows a cyst, although much smaller in size (Fig 12.8C). Definitive surgery showed a large sequestration involving the left lower lobe, with large feeder vessels from the thoracic aorta. (Single-lumen ETT with surgery was performed in the steep head-down position.)

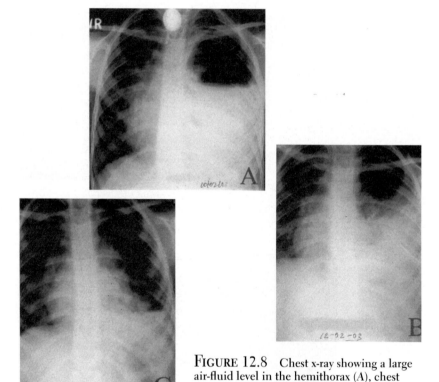

FIGURE 12.8   Chest x-ray showing a large air-fluid level in the hemithorax (A), chest drain inserted (B). And earlier x-ray (C) shows a much smaller cyst.

CASE 9

This 11-year-old girl presented with chronic cough, ill health, anemia, emaciation, and clubbing. She also had a history of a tracheo-esophageal fistula repaired at birth in another center. Radiography (Fig. 12.9 *Top*) showed severe bronchiectasis. Barium swallow showed recurrent fistulae just below the anastomotic site (Fig. 12.9 *Bottom*). Preliminary flexible bronchoscopy identified the fistula, which was cannulated under spontaneous ventilation. The fistula was then repaired through a right thoracotomy under controlled ventilation with an ETT.

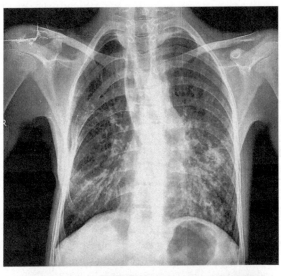

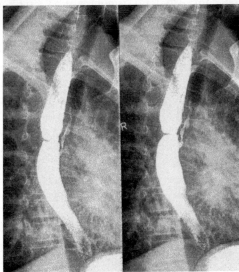

FIGURE 12.9 (*Top*) Chest x-ray showing severe bronchiectasis. (*Bottom*) Barium swallow showing recurrent fistula just below the anastomotic site.

INTRAOPERATIVE CHALLENGES AND LUNG ISOLATION TECHNIQUES (ESPECIALLY IN PEDIATRICS)

Isolation of the diseased or nondependent lung is advocated to prevent blood or purulent secretions from soiling the "good lung," to ventilate only the uninvolved lung in case of bronchopleural fistula (BPF), or to improve surgical exposure for intrathoracic procedures. In adults, this is commonly achieved with double-lumen endobronchial tubes or bronchial blockers, the position of which is confirmed with a fiberoptic scope. Bronchial blockers and fiberoptic scopes of the appropriate sizes, however, are not commonly available in all centers. Most commonly used are the red-rubber, reusable, autoclavable double-lumen endo-bronchial tubes, with clinical judgement and experience being heavily relied on. This, of course, is not practical in children (1–3). Univent tubes are expensive and not freely available in all sizes. Selective endo-bronchial intubation with an ETT long enough to reach the bronchus but small enough in diameter to enter the bronchus atraumatically is sometimes advocated. In case of right mainstem intubation, ventilation of the right upper lobe may be a problem. Location of the "Murphy's eye" may solve this. If not, cut a hole in the tube at approximately the level required. Check upper lobe ventilation to verify accurate placement of the endobronchial tube. Having tried it for a number of years, I am personally dissatisfied with this technique. The problems I encountered include the fact that the endobronchial tube is not really a tight fit, may move during surgery, does not provide complete isolation and protection to the dependent lung, and does not prevent inflation of the upper lung (Fig. 12.10A). It just lulls us into a false sense of security. Another problem is that the tube used is much smaller than an ETT, and suction of blood clots and purulent material is much more difficult. I therefore advocate use of the largest ETT, a steep head-down tilt, and frequent suction of the ETT (Fig. 12.10B). (Of course, this is not advisable in large BPF.)

If after locating the tube down one lung or in the trachea you are still afraid of spill and soiling of the "good lung," the procedure may be done in the supine head-down position through an anterolateral thoracotomy, with the hilum being dissected first and the bronchus clamped before the lung is handled as in Case 6. Very few surgeons, however, are comfortable with this technique.

Lung separation may also be achieved with an ETT and a bronchial blocker placed in the mainstem bronchus of the diseased side. The bronchial blocker can be placed using a rigid bronchoscope, with the ETT being placed later. The position of the blocker may be confirmed with a fiberoptic bronchoscope if one (of the appropriate size) is available. Accidental dislodgment of the blocker can prove catastrophic, be-

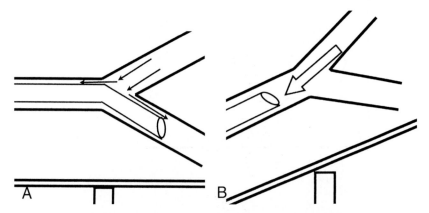

FIGURE 12.10 (A) Small endobronchial tube down the dependent "good" lung provides inadequate protection. (B) Larger endotracheal tube with the steep head-down tilt, though still not foolproof, provides better protection and facility for suction.

cause ventilation of the dependent lung may be impossible (2, 3). Proper anchoring of the ETT is essential, because the airway may be virtually inaccessible once the patient is positioned.

Postoperative pain relief can be a problem. The interpleural technique for regional analgesia is useful, especially in centers with t no drug infusion pumps and/or close monitoring facilities (eg, one-on-one nursing) to ensure safety (4, 5). How does an interpleural block (IPB) work? Essentially, when the local anesthetic agent is placed in the paravertebral gutter, it diffuses through the parietal pleura and the innermost intercostal muscles to block more than one intercostal nerve. It then goes further medially to block the sympathetics, as is seen by Horner's syndrome developing in high blocks. Because this is unilateral, hypotension is not associated with this block. This block may be used for any case requiring analgesia in dermatomes T2 to T12.

In 1991, we (6) did a study using IPB in both adults and children. We were not impressed by the "single shots," because they appeared to be on par with opioids and intercostals blocks. However, we found that intermittent "top up" of IPB with catheters was especially effective in thoracotomies in children. A 5- or 8-French infant-feeding tube (relatively inexpensive) is now used as the interpleural catheter, placed in a hole other than the drain hole to ensure an airtight fit (Fig. 12.11A). A three-way tap is fixed to its outer end, which makes top ups cleaner and safer and prevents air entrainment.

I have found that bupivacaine in a dose of 0.5 mg/kg given every 4 hours as a 0.25% solution is very effective; do not wait for pain to set in. Some authors, using a continuous infusion of local anaesthetic agent, have stated that IPB is ineffective. This may be the result of drug loss via

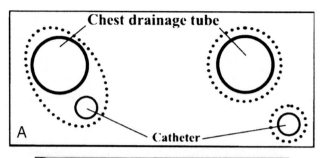

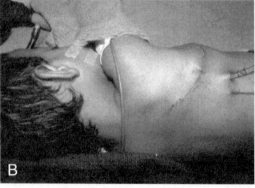

FIGURE 12.11 (A and B) Positioning of interpleural catheter in a hole other than that of the chest drain.

the chest drain or of dilution with blood, so that an insufficient quantity of the drug is at the effector site at any one time. I would recommend the following regime for postthoracotomy pain relief: Place the patient lateral, with the diseased side up (Fig. 12.11*B*), and then clamp the chest drain, give the required drug dose as described above, and keep the chest drain clamped for 20 to 30 minutes. Children like this position of "diseased-side up," unlike "diseased-side down," as in epidural top ups, with its attendant pain and discomfort . This regime is not possible in patients with a large air leak or significant chest drainage. Complications mentioned in the literature (7) include pneumothorax, catheter displacement, and infection, all of which fortunately are rare and can be avoided by meticulous attention to detail.

CASE 10

This case demonstrates, in some measure, how equipment and methods may be modified to fit unusual circumstances without going to great expense.

As background, hydatid disease of the lung is common in some countries, such as India. These cases have been managed conventionally by various techniques, including simple extirpation, suture closure of bronchial communications, capitonage, lobectomy, and pneumonectomy (8–11). Very often, multiple bronchial openings are seen in the wall of the residual cavity. This is caused by pressure necrosis on the bronchial wall from the expanding cyst. Some of these openings are very large. Conventional methods, such as simple suture closure, may not always be effective in sealing them, or their closure may compromise airflow to other parts of the lung. When such lesions are left in situ, bronchial leaks develop, resulting in BPF with resultant lung collapse and pyopneumothorax. The unexpanded lung is not conducive to spontaneous closure of the BPF, and a vicious cycle results that is poorly tolerated, especially in patients with bilateral lung disease. The pneumonostomy technique, on the other hand, electively creates a bronchoatmospheric fistula (BAF) and prevents formation of BPF. The pleural cavity is sealed off from the pulmonary cavity, and lung expansion is encouraged, allowing natural healing of the lesion. Although BAF presents no problems during spontaneous ventilation, excessive air leak can occur during intermittent positive-pressure ventilation (IPPV). This can be managed optimally by increasing the airflow resistance via the pneumonostomy tube by increasing the water level in the water-seal drainage bottle (12, 13),

In this case, the patients was a 12-year-old, thin, anemic, and undernourished boy who presented with a history of cough and fever of 1 months' duration. He had one episode of hemoptysis along with ex-

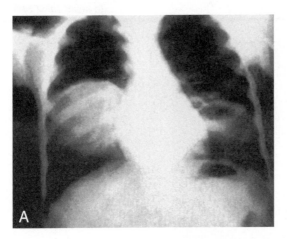

FIGURE 12.12   (A) Chest x-ray showing bilateral rounded opacities in mid zones. (B) CT scan. Bilateral rounded opacities with the left one communicating with the bronchus. (C) Creation of a bronchoatmospheric fistula (BAF). (D) Patient with Malecot catheter draining the BAF connected to a urine bag.

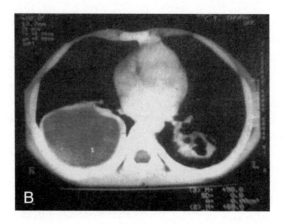

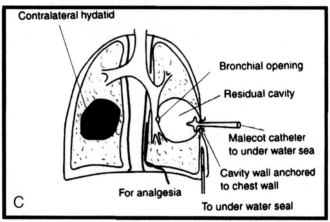

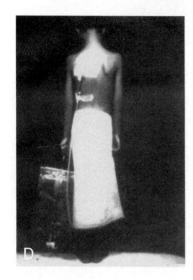

FIGURE 12.12 Continued

pectoration of thick, whitish sputum. Diminished air entry in the midzones, a packed cell volume of 29%, and bilateral rounded opacities in the midzones on the chest radiograph were findings of relevance (Fig. 12.12*A*). A CT scan of the chest confirmed the radiographic findings, with the added information that the cyst on the left was communicating with the bronchus (Fig. 12.12*B*).

An ultrasound of the abdomen revealed no abnormality. A provisional diagnosis of an hydatid cyst lung was made, and the patient was posted for a left thoracotomy. An iv access was obtained, as were pulse oximetry and electrocardiography. Noninvasive blood pressure monitoring was also established (invasive monitoring was established after the child was asleep). Anesthesia was induced with oxygen and halothane, with nitrous oxide (50%) being introduced after confirmation of adequate oxygenation and ventilation. Vecuronium bromide was given to help intubate the trachea. This was done with an ETT (inner diameter, 6.5 mm), and the patient was placed in the right lateral, steep head-down position. The chest was opened via a seventh rib bed posterolateral incision, the adhesions dissected, the cyst isolated with 1% cetrimide packs, the ectocyst opened, and the hydatid endocyst removed. At this stage, we found that it was impossible to ventilate the patient because of large bronchial communications at the medial end of the cyst cavity; occlusion by the surgeon's finger permitted us to resume ventilation. The bronchial openings were very large, and it was felt that suturing these would compromise airflow to the lower lobe. Therefore, a 20-gauge Malecot catheter was inserted into the cyst cavity and brought out through a separate wound in the chest, and the edges were sutured to the chest wall at this site. The Malecot catheter was connected to an underwater seal drain. This effectively isolated the cavity to the atmosphere without producing a BPF, and the underwater seal provided a mild resistance to ventilation. (Fig. 12.12*C*). After 3 days, this drain was connected to a collapsible plastic urine drainage bag containing a nonreturn valve that allowed free egress of air on expiration but prevented indrawing of air in inspiration (Fig. 12.12*D*). It was hoped that granulation of the cyst cavity would thus occur over time.

Another interpleural drain that had been inserted and connected to another underwater seal drain was removed on the second postoperative day. Pain relief intraoperatively was with fentanyl and postoperatively via an 8-French feeding tube placed in the interpleural space. The child returned for surgery on the right lung 3 weeks later. Although the child was comfortable with the left-sided pneumonostomy tube attached to the urine bag, we anticipated problems during IPPV, remembering that the "good lung" would this time be the one with the appreciable air leak. We circumvented this by inducing the child with oxygen, nitrous oxide, and halothane and then maintaining him on spontaneous ventilation until the pneumonostomy tube was connected to an underwater seal. With gentle positive pressure, we gauged the amount of air leak. Addition of water to the bottle increased the resistance to airflow via this route (the BAF). When we felt reasonably comfortable with the ventilation and hemodynamic status of the patient, we administered muscle relaxants and intubated him as before. He was operated on un-eventfully in the left lateral, steep head-down position, and pneu-monostomy tubes and interpleural catheters were placed as described above. The patient was discharged with the BAF pneumonostomy tubes in situ; these were removed 3–4 weeks after surgery.

There was resolution of the cavities and good expansion of the lungs.

CASE 11

A 48-year-old man presented with progressive stridor over 7 years. He was most comfortable when sitting up and bending forward. He also gave a history of hemoptysis on three occasions. He was a moderately built man, with no clubbing, cyanosis, or engorgement of neck veins. No tracheal shift was noted. Scattered rhonchi were heard in the right lung fields. Other systems were normal.

Rigid bronchoscopy, performed under local anesthesia, showed multiple polypoid masses, more in the anterior aspect of the trachea 7 cm below the vocal cords. At biopsy, a diagnosis of benign lipoan-giomatous tumor of the trachea was made.

At surgery, airway nerve blocks and oral spray of 10% lignocaine were administered. Oral fiberoptic bronchoscopy was performed after inhalational induction of anesthesia with oxygen, nitrous oxide, and halothane. Having visualized the lesion, a J-wire was introduced through the side port of the fiberoptic bronchoscope by the side of the tumor to pass beyond the lesion. Threading of a Patil Tube Changer (PTC) beyond the lesion followed this. The J-wire was removed and anesthesia maintained, with the patient breathing spontaneously through the PTC (Fig.12.13C).

A PTC (inner diameter, 3.4 mm) has two pieces, which are detach-able (Fig. 13, *A* and *B*). An ETT connector may be attached to either piece. In this case, we detached the proximal piece and used the distal piece only so that less resistance was encountered during spontaneous ventilation.

Anesthesia was thus maintained through this tube changer, with the patient breathing oxygen, nitrous oxide, and halothane spontaneously. A rigid bronchoscope (Karl Storz, 7.5 mm ID, 43 cm in length) was passed alongside the PTC, and the tumors were visualized (Fig. 12.13C). The patient was then placed in a steep head-down position. Local anesthesia was applied, the pedicles fulgurated using a colonoscopy cautery loop, and

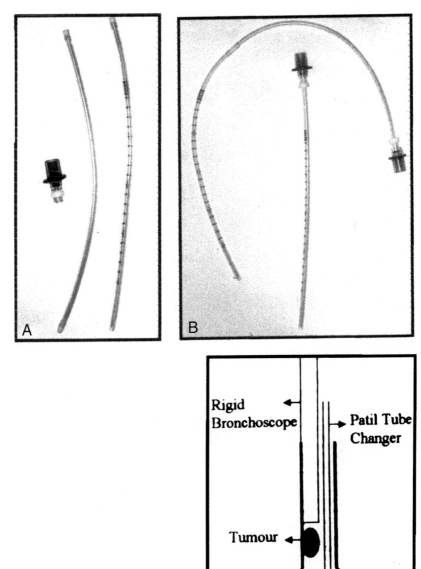

FIGURE 12.13 (A) Patil tube changes (PTC) dismantled. (B) PTC in its entirety and distal piece only connected to the universal connector. (C) Diagrammatic representation of relative position of the tumor, PTC, and bronchoscope.

the tumor removed piecemeal. A colonoscopy cautery loop was used for this purpose, because it could be easily introduced and manipulated through the rigid bronchoscope. The oxygen saturation and hemodynamic parameters remained stable throughout the procedure. The patient was extubated after achieving hemostasis. No residual stridor was noted. At 1-year of follow up, this case showed no residual lesion (14). This technique avoided major surgery involving a thoracotomy, transection of the trachea, and/or cardiopulmonary bypass to gain access to the trachea.

CONCLUSION

Patients present to us with a variety of problems. In developing countries, it is not always possible to have access to sophisticated equipment or diagnostic tools. Postoperative management often is not highly specialized and, thus, is not optimal. Maintaining the safety of the patient while treating them within the bounds of our resources is a continuing challenge. It allows plenty of scope for lateral thinking and innovation while providing us with a great deal of satisfaction.

ACKNOWLEDGMENTS

To Dr. Sudipta Sen, one of the most innovative and knowledgeable surgeons I know; Dr. Usha Gajbhiye, for her help in collecting the data presented; Dr. Paul Wilson, for his computer wizardry; and Dr. J. Jellsingh, for his ability to find a solution to most of the problems I encountered in trying to write this manuscript.

References

1. Haynes SR, Bonner S: Anaesthesia for thoracic surgery in children. Paediatr Anaesth 2000; 10:237–51.
2. Cooper MG: Bronchial blocker placement in infants—a technique and some considerations. Paediatr Anaesth 1994; 4:73–4.
3. Tobias JD: Anaesthetic implications of thoracoscopic surgery in children. Paediatr Anaesth 1999; 9:103–10.
4. Murphy DF: Interpleural analgesia. Br J Anaesth 1993; 71:426–34.
5. Downs CS, Cooper MG: Continuous extrapleural intercostal nerve block for post thoracotomy analgesia in children. Anaesth Intens Care 1997; 25:390–7.

6. Jacob R, Soundaravalli B: Analgesic effect of interpleural bupivacaine after thoracic and upper abdominal surgery. Indian J Anaesth 1994, 42:321–8.
7. Stromskag KE, Minor B, Steen PA: Side effects and complications related to interpleural analgesia: an update. Acta Anaesthesiol Scand 1990, 34:473–7.
8. Burgos L, Baquerizo A, Munoz W, et al.: Experience in surgical management of 331 patients with pulmonary hydatidosis. J Thorac Cardiovasc Surg 1991; 102:427–30.
9. Halezeroglu S, Celik M, Uysal A, et al.: Giant hydatid cysts of the lung. J Thorac Cardiovasc Surg 1997; 113:712–7.
10. Sarsam A: Surgery of pulmonary hydatid cysts. J Thorac Cardiovasc Surg 1971; 62:663–8.
11. Wolcott MW, Harris SH, Briggs JN: Hydatid disease of the lung. J Thorac Cardiovasc Surg 1971, 62:465–9.
12. Anand V, Sen S, Jacob R, et al.: Pneumonostomy in the surgical management of bilateral hydatid cysts of the lung. Paediatr Surg Int 2001; 17:29–31.
13. Jacob R, Sen S: The anaesthetic management of a deliberately created bronchoatmospheric fistula in bilateral pulmonary hydatids. Paediatr Anaesth 2001; 11:733–6.
14. Jacob R, Subash PN, Saravanavel S, et al.: Other uses of tube changers. Ann Cardiac Anaesth 1998; 2:72–8.

Rajiv Jhaveri, MD
Roger Johns, MD

Metabolic and Hormonal Functions of the Lung

13

INTRODUCTION

In addition to their function of gas exchange, the lungs play a central role in maintaining cardiovascular homeostasis through their metabolic activity. Because the entire cardiac output traverses the lungs, they are able to modulate the chemical composition of blood by removing, metabolizing, or activating compounds in the circulation. Furthermore, a variety of vasoactive and immunoregulatory substances are released in the circulation, where they elicit localized or systemic effects. This chapter briefly presents these metabolic and hormonal functions of the lungs. In addition, some physiologic and pathophysiologic conditions that either influence or are influenced by the metabolic and hormonal activities of the lungs are also described.

CELLULAR COMPONENTS INVOLVED IN METABOLIC AND SECRETORY FUNCTIONS

Although each lung contains more than 40 different cell types, only a small proportion of these cells are involved in its metabolic and hormonal activity. The most important of these cells include the vascular endothelial cells, the type II pneumocytes, neuroendocrine cells, Clara cells, and mast cells.

Progress in Thoracic Anesthesia, edited by Peter Slinger,
Lippincott Williams & Wilkins, Baltimore © 2004.

Vascular Endothelium

The pulmonary capillary bed is the largest capillary bed in the body, with a surface area of 50 to 70 m^2 at rest (1). Projections and invaginations (caveolae) on the endothelial cell surface further increase the surface area (Fig. 13.1). The pulmonary endothelium is exposed to the entire cardiac output. The total perfused endothelial area is actively controlled, with areas that normally are poorly perfused being recruited in response to physiological and pathophysiological changes in the milieu. Rate of blood flow and, therefore, the transit time affect the uptake and surface metabolism of compounds in the blood. It is relevant to note that the pulmonary capillary flow can increase from 4 L/min at rest to 40 L/min during exercise.

Endothelial cells make up approximately 30% of the cellular structure in the lung parenchyma, and they perform both metabolic and secretory functions (2). These functions include removal of compounds such as norepinephrine and 5-hydroxytryptamine (5-HT) from the blood, synthesis and release of prostaglandin (PG) I_2 and nitric oxide (NO), and metabolism of compounds such as adenine nucleotides (3–5). The endothelium is also responsible for conversion of the inactive peptide angiotensin I to the active metabolite angiotensin II and for inactivation of bradykinin (6, 7). In addition, pulmonary vascular endothelium is involved in the metabolism of xenobiotics (foreign substances, including drugs and environmental pollutants) via metabolic enzyme systems, including cytochrome P450 mono-oxygenases (8). The pulmonary cytochrome P450 mono-oxygenases may also be important in production of endogenous vasoactive substances (9).

The pulmonary endothelial cells are joined by tight intracellular junctions to form a continuous lining in the pulmonary vessels (10, 11). The endothelial lining in the larger pulmonary vessels possess gap junctions, but the capillaries are devoid of gap junctions (12), thus providing a physical barrier between the blood and the outside environment—the so-called alveolar-capillary membrane.

Type II Pneumocytes (Alveolar Epithelial Type II Cells)

Type II pneumocytes are smaller and more cuboidal than the type I cells. They comprise 60% of the alveolar epithelial cells by number, but they provide only 4% of the alveolar epithelial cell surface area (13). Type II pneumocytes are primarily responsible for synthesis, secretion, recycling of surface-active material, and repair after alveolar epithelial injury. In addition, these cells are involved in metabolism of xenobiotics, prevent transalveolar movement of water, and participate in providing

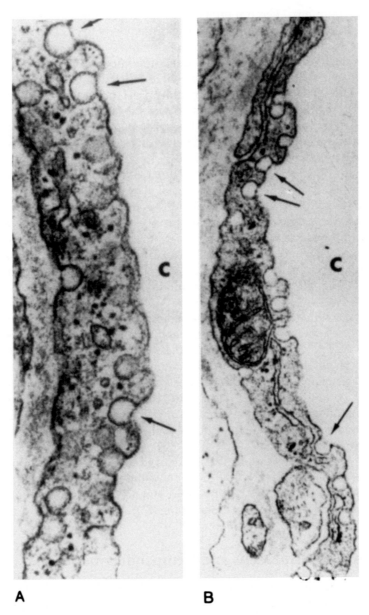

A   **B**

FIGURE 13.1 The caveolae of pulmonary artery endothelial cells are demonstrated using transmission-electron microscopy. A delicate membrane composed of a single lamella (in contrast to bilamellar cell membranes) spans the luminal stoma of the caveolae (arrows). C = capillary lumen. Magnification $\times$ 68,000 (A) and $\times$ 44,000 (B). [From Ryan and Ryan (170); with permission.]

innate immunity. The importance of type II pneumocytes in maintenance of a functional alveolar unit has caused them to be called the "defender of the alveolus" (14).

Type II cells are the primary source of pulmonary surfactant, which
is synthesized and stored in the lamellar bodies within the pneumocytes
(15). The surfactant is largely made of the phospholipid dipalmi-
toylphosphatidylcholine, which is responsible for reducing surface tension at the air-liquid interface and for preventing alveolar collapse at the
end of expiration (16). In addition, the surfactant also contains four proteins, two of which are hydrophilic (SP-A and SP-D) and two of which
are hydrophobic (SP-B and SP-C) (17). Of these proteins, SP-B is mainly
responsible for reduction of surface tension by increasing to 150-fold the
rate of adsorption of phospholipids to the air-water interface (18). It is
indispensable for lung function and survival of the newborn. However,
reduction of surface tension is not the only function of the surfactant
proteins. They are also responsible for provision of innate immunity
(SP-A and SP-D), protection against oxygen-induced pulmonary toxicity (SP-C), and regulation of surfactant turnover and metabolism (SP-D)
(19–21).

Type II pneumocytes have the ability to proliferate and are capable
of both self-maintenance and terminal differentiation into type I pneumocytes. Type I pneumocytes form the epithelial component of the air-
blood barrier. Furthermore, type II pneumocytes remove apoptotic type
II cells by phagocytosis. Thus, these cells are of central importance in the
repair of epithelial injury after acute lung injury (ALI) and in the
restoration of normal lung architecture (22). Hyperplasia and altered
expression of type II pneumocytes in pathological conditions may lead
to pulmonary fibrosis.

Type II pneumocytes are also involved in the metabolism of xenobiotics through cytochrome P450 mono-oxygenases. In addition, they
keep the alveoli free of fluid by rapid and active transport of sodium
and water across the plasma membrane (23).

Neuroendocrine Cells and Neuroendocrine Bodies

Neuroendocrine cells are specialized basal epithelial cells in the lung
that are derived from APUD (amine precursor, uptake, and decarboxy-
lation) cells. These cells may be found either singly or in groups, in
which case they are referred to as neuroendocrine bodies. They are localized most frequently in subsegmental bronchi, primarily at or near
bifurcation points and at the site of transition from terminal bronchioles
to respiratory bronchioles (17). Nonmyelinated afferent and efferent

nerve endings are found in close synaptic contact with neuroendocrine cell clusters (>3 cells) (24). In humans and other species, neuroendocrine cells and bodies are most prevalent in the fetal lung, and they decrease with age in adults (17, 24).

Neuroendocrine cells are believed to contain a number of peptides (bombesin, leu-enkephalin, somatostatin, and calcitonin), 5-HT, catecholamines, and acetylcholinesterase (24–27). Because these cells are predominantly located at the bifurcations of the airways, it has been suggested that they may serve as chemoreceptors, sensitive to changes in the intraluminal environment and responding by releasing bioactive substances. For example, airway hypoxia (but not arterial hypoxemia) causes neuroendocrine cell degranulation and release of 5-HT (17, 28, 29). The neuroendocrine cells may be involved in maintaining hypoxic pulmonary vasoconstriction (HPV) during intrauterine life (29).

Neuroendocrine cells may also be involved in a number of pulmonary disorders, such as small-cell lung tumors and carcinoid tumor of the lung (30). Excessive production of bombesin-like peptides by the neuroendocrine cells may be responsible for bronchopulmonary dysplasia (31).

Clara Cells

Clara cells are nonciliated, columnar cells that line the terminal bronchioles and may project into the airway lumen. These nonmucous, nonserous secretory cells are highly active metabolically. They act as progenitor cells for bronchial epithelial cells and are responsible for regeneration of the epithelial lining after injury (32). Clara cells secrete a number of proteins, with the major protein being Clara cell 10-kDa (CC10) protein. The primary role of this protein is poorly understood, but it may modulate airway inflammation by influencing production and/or activity of phospholipase A_2, proinflammatory cytokines, and chemokines. Secretion of CC10 protects the respiratory tract against inflammation and oxidative injury. Reduced levels of CC10 protein are found in patients who smoke (33, 34) and in patients with nonsmall-cell lung tumors (35). Higher levels are demonstrated in survivors after ALI.

Clara cells are the primary site of cytochrome P450-dependent metabolism in the lung. Cytochrome P450 isozymes are involved in oxidative metabolism of xenobiotics, leading to detoxification but also, in some cases, production of metabolites more toxic than the parent compound. Thus, Clara cells may also be the initial site of parenchymal injury from agents such as paraquat, carbon tetrachloride, or bleomycin.

Mast Cells

Mast cells develop from bone marrow-derived progenitor cells, and they mature and differentiate in the peripheral tissue. In the respiratory tract, the mast cells are located in the airway lumen, submucosa, the connective tissue surrounding small airways and capillaries, and subpleurally (36). The mast cells contain a vast array of biologically active compounds through which they play a central role in immune surveillance and host defense (36–38). Mast cells produce a complex inflammatory reaction in response to a variety of stimuli, including antigens, superoxides, complement proteins, neuropeptides, and lipoproteins. Mast cells, along with T cells, produce the cytokines that modulate airway smooth muscle tone and vascular permeability, and the cytokines induce many of the changes observed in inflammatory diseases, such as asthma, rhinitis, urticaria, and anaphylaxis. Mast cells also play a role in development of fibrosis and may be implicated in such fibrotic diseases as sarcoidosis, farmer's lung disease, cryptogenic fibrosing alveolitis, and histiocytosis (39).

METABOLIC PROCESSES WITHIN THE LUNG

The lung is intimately involved in the metabolism of humoral substances, either at the cell surface or after their uptake into the cells. In addition, synthesis and release of bioactive agents in the lung produces effects both locally and further afield. These activities occur mainly (but not exclusively) in the pulmonary endothelium, which is in intimate contact with the blood traversing the pulmonary vasculature.

Metabolism at the Cell Surface

The luminal surface of the pulmonary endothelial cells contains several enzyme systems that are associated with metabolism of the adenine nucleotides, bradykinin, and angiotensin I. The enzymes, ATPase, ADP-ase, and 5'-nucleotidase, which handle the adenine nucleotides, are located solely in the endothelial caveolae (11, 40, 41). On the other hand, angiotensin-converting enzyme (ACE), carboxypeptidase N, and carbonic anhydrase are more widely distributed, both in the caveolae and on the endothelial projections (Fig. 13.2) (42). The ACE-inhibitor drugs captopril, enalapril, and lisinopril prevent the conversion of angiotensin I to angiotensin II (and the inactivation of bradykinin) by ACE.

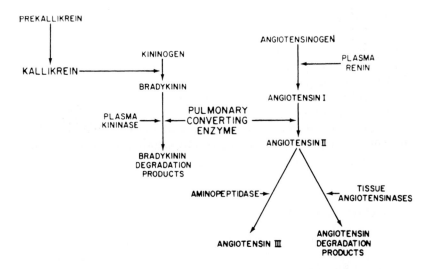

FIGURE 13.2 An example of synthesis and degradation of important metabolites by the lung endothelium. In this case, angiotensin-converting enzyme inactivates bradykinin and also produces the active angiotensin II from angiotensinogen. [From Block and Stalcup (171); with permission.]

Metabolism after Active Transport

Norepinephrine, a polar molecule that does not diffuse rapidly through lipoprotein membranes, and 5-HT, which is lipid insoluble, both require carrier-mediated, active transport by the pulmonary endothelium before their metabolism (43). The active-transport mechanisms of these compounds are saturable, energy-dependent processes that require the Na,K-ATPase, are temperature sensitive, and are not inhibited by one another (43, 44). Uptake of norepinephrine occurs mainly in the pre- and postcapillary vessels and in the pulmonary veins, with 30% of the agent being cleared from the lungs during a single passage (45). Uptake of 5-HT, on the other hand, occurs primarily in the arterioles and capillaries (46). Approximately 65% of 5-HT is cleared during a single passage through the lung (43). The intracellular enzyme, monoamine oxidase, metabolizes these agents. Norepinephrine is then further metabolized by catechol-O-methyltransferase (6).

Adenosine, a by-product of ADP metabolism at the endothelial cell surface, is also actively transported and then metabolized. Dipyridamole inhibits this cellular uptake (47). In the cell, adenosine is partly converted to inosine, and the rest is reincorporated into intracellular AMP, ADP, and ATP.

Prostaglandin A, PGB, and PGI_2 traverse through the lung largely unchanged. In contrast, PGE_1, PGE_2, and $PGF_{2\alpha}$ are almost completely removed during a single passage through the lung. This clearance requires active transport and is followed by intracellular metabolism by 15-hydroxyprostaglandin dehydrogenase (43, 48).

Cortisone, cortisol, and some androgens are actively transported into bronchial epithelial cells. 11α-Hydroxysteroid dehydrogenase type II converts cortisol to the inactive compound cortisone in fetal lungs (49). Inhaled steroids may exert their anti-inflammatory action through glucocorticoid receptors in the bronchial epithelial cells (50).

Synthesis and Release of Compounds

A number of humoral agents are synthesized and released from the lung and then act either locally (paracrine function) or at a distant site (endocrine function). Examples include 5-HT, histamine, thromboxane (TX), leukotrienes (LTs), platelet-activating factor, kinins, PGI_2, and angiotensin II. Compounds such as NO, endothelium-derived hyperpolarizing factor (EDHF), adenosine, and endothelium-derived contracting factor (EDCF) are released from the lung and play a role in regulating pulmonary circulation.

Eicosanoids

Eicosanoids are a group of agents derived from the metabolism of the membrane lipid arachidonic acid (icosatetraenoic acid). Low levels of eicosanoids are produced constitutively under basal conditions. Larger amounts are released from the cell membrane in response to a wide variety of stimuli. After release, arachidonic acid is metabolized via one of three major pathways: the cyclo-oxygenase pathway (producing PGs, TX, and prostacyclin), the lipoxygenase pathway (producing the LTs, midchain hydroxyeicosatetraenoic acids [HETEs], and lipoxins), or the cytochrome P450 mono-oxygenase pathway (producing midchain and ω-terminal HETEs and *cis*-epoxyeicosatrienoic acids [EETs]) (Fig. 13.3) (9). These metabolic products produce an array of effects, including dilation or constriction of pulmonary vessels and bronchi and regulation of pulmonary immune responses. Many of the cell types in the lung are capable of both synthesizing and inactivating these compounds. Thus, the lung is capable of finely regulating the levels of various eicosanoids in the cardiovascular system, and the lung may even use these compounds to regulate its own perfusion.

In addition to being enzymatically metabolized, arachidonic acid can undergo nonenzymatic peroxidation, either in its free form or while

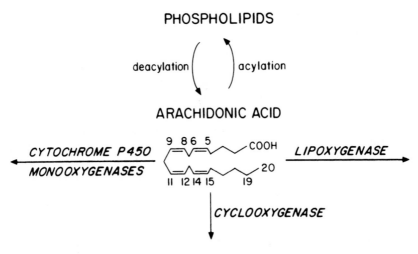

FIGURE 13.3 Arachidonic acid, dynamically exchanging with membrane phospholipids through acylation and deacylation, is enzymatically metabolized to a number of active products through three major pathways: cyclo-oxygenase (prostanoids), lipoxygenase (leukotrienes, lipoxins, hydroxyeicosatetraenoic acids [HETEs], and di-HETEs), and cytochrome P450 (epoxides, HETEs, and di-HETEs). [From Johns and Peach (9); with permission.]

still esterified to the lipid membrane. This type of reaction leads to the production of isoprostanes, which have effects on virtually every cell type in the lung (51).

Cyclo-oxygenase pathway

The metabolism of arachinoid acid via this pathway leads to the production of PGs, TX, and prostacyclin. These are potent eicosanoids that elicit a wide range of often opposing actions that affect both the pulmonary vasculature and the airways. They may induce pulmonary vasoconstriction (TXA_2, $PGF_{2\alpha}$, PGE_2, and PGD_2) or vasodilatation (PGI_2 and PGE_1), promote (TXA_2) or inhibit (PGI_2) platelet aggregation, or elicit bronchoconstriction ($PGF_{2\alpha}$, $PGD_{2\alpha}$, and TXA_2) or bronchodilation (PGE_2 and PGI_2) (52–55).

Although pulmonary vascular endothelial cells are capable of synthesizing all the PGs and TX, they primarily produce PGI_2 (prostacyclin) (56). The PGI_2 is continuously released from the lung, with up-regulation during conditions causing increased pulmonary blood flow and faster respiratory rate (57, 58).

Metabolism of the products of the cyclo-oxygenase pathway occurs in the cell and requires active transport. During a single passage through the lung, PGE_1, PGE_2, and $PGF_{2\alpha}$ are almost entirely removed, whereas PGA_1, PGA_2, and PGI_2 traverse the pulmonary circulation essentially unchanged (59, 50). Thromboxane A_2, which is highly unstable, undergoes hydrolysis to TXB_2 in circulation, which is extracted in the lung by a different active-transport mechanism than that responsible for the removal of other PGs (61). Further details of their intracellular metabolism are currently unclear.

Lipoxygenase Pathway

Arachidonic acid metabolism via the lipoxygenase pathway leads to the production of LTs and lipoxins (9).

Leukoktrienes

Arachidonic acid is converted to 5-hydroxyperoxyeicosatetraenoic acid (5-HPETE) via the action of cytosolic 5-lipoxygenase. Further enzymatic action generates the unstable intermediate LTA_4, which may then be converted to LTB_4 or to the cysteinyl leukotrienes LTC_4, LTD_4, and LTE_4 (previously known as slow-reacting substance of anaphylaxis [SRS-A]) (9). Monocytes, alveolar macrophages, and neutrophils are mainly involved in the production of LTB_4, whereas eosinophils, basophils, mast cells, and alveolar macrophages produce cysteinyl leukotrienes. In addition, platelets and vascular endothelium convert LTA_4 derived from circulating neutrophils to LTC_4.

Leukotrienes are proinflammatory agents that act through specific receptors. The LTB_4 is chemotactic and chemokinetic for leukocytes, especially for neutrophils, and also causes neutrophil degranulation (62, 63); it has no effect on bronchomotor tone (64). Cysteinyl leukotrienes LTC_4 and LTD_4 are potent pulmonary vasoconstrictors, with preferentially greater effect on the pulmonary veins (65–67). Cysteinyl leukotrienes (LTC_4, LTD_4, and LTE_4) are also potent bronchoconstrictors, with approximately 1,000-fold greater potency than histamine. They increase endothelial membrane permeability, leading to airway edema and increased mucous production (68). Leukotrienes are important mediators in asthma (69). Specific LT-receptor antagonists (eg, montelukast and zafirlukast) and 5-lipoxygenase-inhibitor agents (eg, zileuton) have now been established as effective treatment of asthma (70, 71). Leukotrienes may also play a role in a variety of respiratory conditions, including acute respiratory distress syndrome (ARDS), HPV, and persistent pulmonary hypertension of the neonate (72–75).

The LTB_4 is inactivated in pulmonary neutrophils. Cysteinyl leukotrienes, on the other hand, are inactivated extracellularly by myeloperoxidases to form sulfoxides (76, 77).

Lipoxins

Lipoxin A_4 and lipoxin B_4 are formed by sequential actions of 15-lipoxygense and 5-lipoxygenase or 5-lipoxygenase and 12-lipoxygenase (78). Alveolar macrophages, monocytes, eosinophils, and epithelial cells contain 15-lipoxygenase, whereas neutrophils and monocytes contain 5-lipoxygenase. The 12-lipoxygenase is found in platelets. Thus, lipoxin production involves transcellular and cell-to-cell interactions.

Lipoxins are anti-inflammatory and counterbalance the proinflammatory activities of the LTs. In fact, LT production is blocked at the 5-lipoxygenase level during lipoxin synthesis (78). Lipoxins inhibit neutrophil and eosinophil chemotaxis, transmigration, and adhesion at the inflammation site, and they also inhibit neutrophil adhesion to epithelial and endothelial cell surfaces (79, 80). They also inhibit natural killer cell activation, thus preventing cytotoxicity. Lipoxins stimulate chemotaxis of monocytes. Furthermore, lipoxins possess potent vasodilatory effects on both the aorta and pulmonary artery. The vasodilatation is endothelium dependent, and it may be mediated by stimulating release of prostacyclin or NO by the endothelial cells (81, 82).

Lipoxins are rapidly taken up by circulating monocytes and inactivated (78).

Cytochrome P450 mono-oxygenase pathway

Cytochrome P450 (CYP) enzymes metabolize arachidonic acid in a number of organ systems in the body, including the lung, liver, kidney, gastrointestinal tract, and cerebral and coronary vasculature. Three major pathways have been recognized and lead to the production of HETEs and di-HETEs. In the lung, several isoforms of CYP enzymes exist in different cell types. The CYPA4 subfamily is contained in the peripheral lung microsomes and produces 20-HETE. The CYP2J subfamily, on the other hand, is found in both ciliated and nonciliated airway epithelial cells, in bronchial and vascular smooth muscle cells, endothelium, and alveolar macrophages. The isoforms are expressed constitutively, and they also are induced by xenobiotics.

The HETEs and the unstable EETs decrease bronchomotor and pulmonary vascular tone (83, 84). The 20-HETE may reduce acute HPV. The HETEs and EETs also possess anti-inflammatory properties, prevent platelet aggregation, and protect the endothelium during reperfusion.

Platelet-Activating Factor

Platelet-activating factor (PAF) is a family of structurally related, acetylated phospholipids released from the cell membrane by phospholipase

A$_2$. It increases pulmonary vascular and bronchial smooth muscle tone, increases airway reactivity, and causes inflammatory cell accumulation and airway edema (85). It may be one of the many mediators released in patients with chronic obstructive airway disease and asthma (86).

Peptides

A myriad of bioactive peptides are present in the lung, but these peptides are not unique to the lung. They are also present in the nervous system and the gastrointestinal tract.

Adrenocorticotrophic hormone

Adrenocorticotrophic hormone, which is present in the normal lung, plays an important role in lung maturation and surfactant production. Its effect on surfactant biosynthesis is independent of corticosteroids. It is increased in patients with bronchial tumors and in long-term smokers (87, 88). It inhibits ACE and, thus, may play a role in regulating angiotensin metabolism in the lung.

Angiotensin

Angiotensin I is converted to the active compound angiotensin II during a single passage through the lung by the action of ACE located within both the pinocytic vesicles and the endothelial surface projections (Fig. 13.3) (89). Angiotensin II passes unchanged through the lung and has wide-ranging effects on the cardiovascular system. These effects include vasoconstriction (in both the large arteries and the resistance vessels), smooth muscle proliferation, myocardial hypertrophy, and altered ventricular remodeling (90). In addition, it stimulates nonosmotic release of arginine vasopressin, causing increased renal water absorption. Stimulation of angiotensin receptors on the vascular endothelium induces release of NO and prostacyclin (91, 92). Furthermore, angiotensinogen and angiotensin II are expressed by the myofibroblasts in fibrotic lung. Thus, locally produced angiotensin II may play a role in regulation of apoptosis of pulmonary endothelial cells and in pulmonary fibrosis (93). The importance of the renin-angiotensin system in the pathophysiology of congestive heart failure is highlighted by the clinical improvement and increased survival of these patients with the use of ACE inhibitor and angiotensin-receptor blocking agents (94–96).

Bradykinin

Bradykinin is a nonapeptide that is produced through metabolism of plasma and tissue kininogens. It is also inactivated by ACE. In contrast to angiotensin II, bradykinin is a potent endothelium-dependent pulmonary vasodilator. However, it produces vasoconstriction when the endothelium is denuded or damaged (97). Bradykinin also stimulates metabolism of arachidonic acid and release of different eicosanoids (98, 99). Bradykinin has minimal effect on isolated bronchial smooth muscle, yet in patients with asthma, it causes bronchoconstriction (100).

Atrial natriuretic peptide

Atrial natriuretic peptide (ANP) is mainly produced by the atrial myocytes in response to increased atrial stretch (as in heart failure), and it plays a role in maintaining circulating blood volume and blood pressure. Its primary physiologic role appears to be the prevention of sodium and fluid retention and hypertension (101). Although the cardiac atria are the main source of the circulating ANP, significant amounts of its prohormone as well as the active form are found in lungs. The *ANP* gene is expressed in pulmonary veins as well as in the pneumocytes (102). Thus, lungs are an important source of extracardiac ANP. In addition, lungs clear 20% to 25% of circulating ANP during a single passage. Pulmonary production of ANP is stimulated by glucocorticoids, hypoxia, and water overload and is inhibited by dehydration (102).

The ANP is an endothelium-independent vasodilator, with greater effect on pulmonary arteries than on veins (103). It is a weak bronchodilator, especially in the presence of bronchospasm (104). Under some conditions, ANP increases capillary permeability, leading to leakage of water and proteins into alveolar space. However, it also appears to protect against oxidant-induced endothelial damage (105, 106). Probably the most important effect of ANP is its ability to suppress the renin-angiotensin-aldosterone system at three separate points: suppression of renin release, reduction ACE activity, and blockade of aldosterone secretion from the adrenals (107). These actions promote sodium and water loss via the kidneys. Although ANP ameliorates the hypoxic pulmonary vasoconstrictor response and its secretion is increased in hypoxic conditions and in pulmonary hypertension, its precise role in these conditions remains unclear (108).

Vasoactive intestinal peptide

Vasoactive intestinal peptide (VIP) is contained in the nerve fibers and nerve terminals in the tracheobronchial tree, bronchial and pulmonary blood vessels, bronchial smooth muscle, and bronchial submucosal glands and is also present in the mast cells in the lung (109). It is a pulmonary vasodilator (110). It also relaxes bronchial smooth muscle independent of adrenergic- and cholinergic-receptor activity or cyclo-oxygenase activity (111). Reduced VIP activity may be implicated in the pathophysiology of cystic fibrosis and asthma. The VIP may ameliorate ALI by preventing death of alveolar epithelial cells and endothelial cells (112).

Endothelins

Endothelins (ETs) are 21-amino acid peptides that are produced from their precursor proteins, prepro-ET and pro-ET. Enzymatic cleavage of the precursors leads to an inactive intermediate, big ET, which is then further processed by the ET-converting enzyme to produce the active enzyme. Three distinct isoforms of ETs (ET-1, ET-2, and ET-3) have been described. Endothelins and their precursors are also found in the airway epithelial cells and submucosal glands, but only ET-1 is synthesized by the vascular endothelial cells (113). Production of ET is stimulated by epinephrine, angiotensin II, arginine vasopressin, transforming growth factor (TGF)-α, thrombin, and interleukin (IL)-1 and by mechanical and physical factors, such as hypoxia, ischemia, and shear stress (114).

Endothelins act through four different types of receptors, ET_A, ET_B, ET_C, and ET_{AX} (115). The ET_A receptors, which are present in the vascular smooth muscle, have a high affinity for ET-1 and ET-2. In contrast, ET_B receptors, which are found in both endothelial and smooth muscle cells, bind all the ETs equally. Acting through ET_A receptors, ET-1 causes pulmonary and systemic vasoconstriction and enhances mitogenesis in vascular and airway smooth muscle cells and fibroblasts (116). Stimulation of ET_B receptors causes release of PGI_2 and NO, with resultant vasodilatation of the peripheral resistance vessels (117). In addition, ET_B receptors are responsible for the removal of almost 50% of circulating ET-1 during pulmonary transit, for promoting reuptake of ET-1 by the endothelial cells, and for inhibition of ET-converting enzyme (118–120). In the pulmonary circulation, ET response is dependent on the initial vascular tone (117, 121). When the basal tone is normal, ET causes pulmonary vasoconstriction. However, in the presence of high initial vascular tone, ET infusion has a dual response, with early vasodilatation followed by vasoconstriction. The ET-1 causes bronchoconstriction via ET_B receptors in both patients with and patients without asthma (122). Endothelins and ET receptors play a significant role in the pathophysiology of primary and secondary pulmonary hypertension, both through their pulmonary vasoconstrictor activity and through stimulation of smooth muscle cell proliferation, which leads to vascular remodeling. Production of ET-1 is up-regulated, and its clearance is impaired in patients with pulmonary hypertension. Increased circulating levels of ET-1 correlate with pulmonary arterial pressures in patients with primary pulmonary hypertension (123). A number of selective ET_A or combined

ET_A/ET_B-receptor blocking agents are in the advanced stages of clinical evaluation for treatment of pulmonary hypertension (124, 125). Endothelins are also believed to play a role in many other pulmonary diseases, including ALI, lung infections, asthma, pulmonary hypertension, and ischemia-reperfusion injury (117, 126, 127).

Cytokines

Cytokines are small, extracellular signaling proteins that are produced by a wide array of both resident and inflammatory cells, including endothelial cells, epithelial cells, monocytes, eosinophils, activated macrophages, T-helper (Th) cells, and platelets. A bewildering number of cytokines have been identified: Interleukins (IL-2, -3, -4, -5, -13, -15, -16, and -17), proinflammatory cytokines (IL-1, IL-6, IL-11, tumor necrosis factor, granulocyte-macrophage colony-stimulating factor, stem cell factor), anti-inflammatory cytokines (IL-10, IL-1ra, IL-12, IL-18, and interferon-α,), chemotactic cytokines or chemokines (regulated upon activation, normal T expressed and secreted [RANTES]; monocyte chemoattractant protein [MCP]-1, -2, -3, -4, -5; macrophage inflammatory protein [MIP]-1α; IL-8; and eotaxin), and growth factors (platelet-derived growth factor, TGF-α, fibroblast growth factor, epidermal growth factor, insulin-like growth factor) (128). Many of these cytokines possess overlapping functions. Because they also stimulate release of the same or other cytokines, it is difficult to assign specific effects to individual cytokines (128). Cytokines play an integral role in co-ordinating the inflammatory response in chronic inflammatory conditions. They activate target cells, induce cellular proliferation, chemotaxis, immunomodulation, cell differentiation, and apoptosis. Through release of mediators, such as histamine and cysteinyl leukotrienes, cytokines cause bronchial hyperreactivity, bronchoconstriction, and airway remodeling. Chemokines recruit and activate leukocytes and cause smooth muscle proliferation and fibrogenesis. Chemokines also maintain airway hyperreactivity.

Summary of the biological actions of peptides in the lung

The peptides found in the lung influence and regulate pulmonary vascular and bronchomotor tone, increase pulmonary vascular permeability, and stimulate bronchial secretions. Pulmonary vascular tone may be increased (angiotensin II, spasmogenic lung peptide, substance P, and ETs) or decreased (VIP and ANP). The bronchial tone may be increased by ETs, substance P, and spasmogenic lung peptide, or it may be decreased by VIP. Substance P and VIP increase bronchial secretions. Increased capillary permeability, leading to airway or pulmonary edema, may be caused by ANP, ETs, and some cytokines. Kinins are produced in the lung during immunoglobulin E-mediated allergic responses. Chemokines, through their chemotactic action on eosinophils and granulocytes, are involved in anaphylaxis and acute inflammatory conditions.

Nonpeptide Agents
Catecholamines

Norepinephrine is released from the autonomic neurons as well as from the neuroendocrine cells around the tracheobronchial tree. Its uptake and metabolism were discussed earlier.

5-Hydroxytryptamine

Enterochromaffin cells in the gastrointestinal mucosa produce the bulk of the 5-HT that is released in the peripheral circulation. However, only traces of 5-HT from this source reach the pulmonary circulation, with most of it being taken up by platelets in the portal circulation. In the lung, 5-HT is released from the mast cells and the neuroendocrine cells and bodies. The uptake and metabolism of 5-HT in the lung were discussed earlier.

Histamine

Histamine differs from norepinephrine and 5-HT in that it passes largely unchanged through the lung because of an absence of an uptake mechanism in the lung (129, 130). This inability of the lung to inactivate histamine leaves the pulmonary vasculature and the airways vulnerable to the actions of endogenous histamine.

Adenine nucleotides

Adenine nucleotides (ATP, ADP, and AMP) are metabolized at the cell surface by the 5′-nucleotidase and ATPase located in the endothelial caveolae (40, 131). The endothelium-dependent vasodilators ATP and ADP are thus converted to the endothelium-independent vasodilators AMP and adenosine. Adenosine produced by this process is then taken up by the endothelial cells, where it is recycled to produce intracellular nucleotides, mainly ATP (40, 131). Either by removing adenine nucleotides and adenosine from the circulation or by producing additional quantities of adenosine in response to stimuli such as hypoxia, the endothelium helps to regulate vascular tone.

Endothelium-derived relaxing, hyperpolarizing, and contracting factors

Nitric oxide

Furchgott and Zawadzki (132) demonstrated that acetylcholine and other muscarinic agonist agents required an intact endothelium for their vasodilatory effects on the strips of rabbit aorta. Ignarro et al (133) and Furchgott et al (134) subsequently established the similarities between the endothelium-derived relaxing factor and NO. Since then, NO has been one of the most intensely investigated molecules in every medical specialty.

Nitric oxide is produced from L-arginine by the enzyme NO synthase (NOS). Three isoforms of NOS exist: neuronal NOS, which is expressed constitutively in central and peripheral neurons; inducible NOS, which is induced by certain inflammatory mediators; and endothelial NOS, which is expressed constitutively in the endothelial cells in the presence of calcium-calmodulin complex. Nitric oxide activates soluble guanylyl cyclase, leading to increased intracellular cyclic GMP (cGMP) and vasodilatation. It is also capable of producing vasodilatation by cGMP-independent mechanisms, such as activation of Ca^{2+}-dependent K^+ channels and regulation of angiotensin II receptors (134, 135) After release, NO rapidly binds to hemoglobin, for which it has a 1,500-fold greater affinity than carbon monoxide. Both oxy- and deoxy-hemoglobins can bind with NO to produce nitrosylhemoglobin and methemoglobin. Rapid binding with hemoglobin is responsible for NO's short half-life (2–30 seconds) and for the selective pulmonary vasodilatation that occurs when it is inhaled as a therapeutic agent.

In the human lungs, synthesis of NO occurs in pulmonary vessels as well as in alveolar cells and the airway. In addition, NO is detectable in a number of cellular components of the lung, such as macrophages, mast cells, neutrophils, fibroblasts, smooth muscle cells, platelets, and endothelial and epithelial cells. Within the cells, NOS is detectable in a number of cellular elements, including the nucleus, Golgi apparatus, mitochondria, plasma membrane, and endoplasmic reticulum (136).

In the lungs, NO has effects on vascular, airway, and inflammatory events. It is a potent pulmonary vasodilator, with greater effect on the precapillary resistance vessels compared to larger vessels (137). Vasoconstrictor stimuli, such as hypoxia, angiotensin II, and ET-1, up-regulate NO production, modulating the effects of these stimuli on the pulmonary vascular tone. In patients with primary or secondary pulmonary hypertension, expression of NOS and production of NO are depressed, although the significance of this finding is unclear. Along with prostacyclin, NO prevents endothelial thrombus formation by inhibiting platelet aggregation and platelet recruitment by a platelet thrombus and by breaking up platelet aggregates that are formed (138, 139). Nitric oxide is also produced by the inhibitory nonadrenergic, noncholinergic neurons, and it relaxes bronchial smooth muscle.

Production of NO is affected in a number of pathological conditions, such as ALI and ischemia-reperfusion injury. Endogenous or exogenous inhaled NO may reduce ALI through its ability to reduce leukocyte adhesion and activation, reduce production of inflammatory mediators, and prevent intravascular thrombosis. The precise role of NO in many disease conditions remains to be elucidated.

A number of endogenous agents (eg, bradykinin, histamine, substance P, VIP, ATP, ADP, thrombin, calcitonin gene-related peptide, arachidonic acid, and trypsin) require an intact endothelium for their vasodilatory effect. The therapeutic agent sodium nitroprusside is an NO analogue and acts as an NO donor to produce vasodilatation. Furthermore, vasoconstrictors, such as norepinephrine, 5-HT, and vasopressin, also stimulate NO release from the endothelium to modulate their direct effect on the vascular smooth muscle.

Endothelium-dependent hyperpolarizing factor

Acetylcholine and bradykinin produce both systemic and pulmonary vasodilatation that is dependent on endothelium but is independent of NO and prostacyclin (140, 141). This vasorelaxation is achieved through hyperpolarization of the vascular smooth muscle cell membrane by activation of calcium-sensitive potassium channels and production of a putative transmitter, EDHF (142). Neither the precise nature of EDHF nor its role in the regulation of vascular tone has been determined.

Endothelium-derived contracting factor

Vascular endothelium also produces several vasoconstrictor agents, such as ETs, TX, and PGs. These were discussed previously.

Modulation of smooth muscle growth

In addition to the production of factors that modulate vascular smooth muscle tone, endothelium also influences smooth muscle growth (143). Under basal conditions, endothelium produces heparin-like factors that inhibit smooth muscle proliferation (144). In disease conditions, such as chronic hypoxia or hyperoxia, or when endothelium is injured, such as during ALI, growth factors (eg, platelet-derived growth factor and epidermal growth factor) are released, whereas the antiproliferative factors are inhibited. These factors may influence the development of vascular smooth muscle hypertrophy and hyperplasia that lead to pulmonary hypertension.

Metabolism of Xenobiotics

Xenobiotics are foreign substances that are carried to the lung either through blood (eg, drugs such as sympathomimetic agents, antihistamines, opioids, tricyclic antidepressants, and local anesthetics) or through inhalation from the environment (eg, tobacco smoke, anesthetic gases, inhaled bronchodilators, and organic solvents). They are removed and metabolized, or they accumulate in the lung. If the agent is stored in the lung, it may potentially produce pulmonary toxicity. Metabolism of the xenobiotics involves several cell types (Clara cells, type II pneumocytes, and endothelium) that are rich in the CYP enzyme family. Metabolism by the CYP isozymes may inactivate the xenobiotic, thereby protecting against the agent. Thus, lung injury produced by exposure to xenobiotics is reduced by the induction of CYP enzymes (145). In some instances, however, metabolism leads to generation of products that can cause pulmonary toxicity. For example, pulmonary toxicity from paraquat, nitrofurantoin, and mitomycin C involves metabolism by CYP (146).

Some of the drugs that are removed by the lung may require carrier-mediated uptake (eg, amphetamine, metaraminol, and isoproterenol). Others are removed by nonspecific mechanisms and are dependent on their physicochemical properties. In general, drugs that are basic amines (pKa > 8), are lipophilic, and possess a charged cationic group at physiologic pH are effectively removed by the lung (147). Examples of such drugs include bupivacaine, lidocaine, fentanyl, and meperidine (148–150).

PHYSIOLOGIC AND PATHOPHYSIOLOGIC CONDITIONS WITH IMPACT ON PULMONARY FUNCTION

Hypoxic Pulmonary Vasoconstriction

Unlike the systemic circulation, where hypoxia produces vasorelaxation, alveolar hypoxia leads to pulmonary vasoconstriction. This response is termed HPV and is responsible for closely matching pulmonary perfusion to ventilation by directing blood away from poorly ventilated areas of the lung. Von Euler and Liljestrand (151) first described HPV in 1946. The HPV response is independent of endothelium;

however, endothelium helps to modulate the response through release of factors, including EDCFs, NO, and EDHF (152, 153). Damage to endothelium may occur in some pathological conditions, leading to reduced production of NO that in turn may cause an augmented HPV response. During acute hypoxia, voltage-gated potassium (Kv) channels close, resulting in an inhibition of potassium current, changes in the resting membrane potential, and opening of the voltage-dependent calcium channels, which leads to an influx of calcium into the cells (154). Increased intracellular calcium causes arterial smooth muscle cell contraction and development of HPV. Redirection of blood during acute hypoxia is beneficial, but sustained pulmonary vasoconstriction during chronic hypoxic conditions results in vascular remodeling, pulmonary hypertension, and eventually, right ventricular dysfunction.

ALI and ARDS

Acute lung injury and its ultimate manifestation, ARDS, can result from direct pulmonary injury (eg, aspiration of stomach contents or smoke inhalation) as well as various systemic processes (eg, sepsis, acute pancreatitis, and severe trauma). The clinical manifestations include acute bilateral pulmonary infiltrates, with normal left atrial pressure and hypoxemia. The alveoli are flooded with protein-rich edematous fluid because of increased capillary endothelial permeability, which allows fluid exudation in the absence of an increase in hydrostatic pressure (155). In addition to damage to the endothelium, epithelial injury is present and, in fact, is a determinant of outcome after ALI and ARDS (156). Disruption of the epithelial barrier allows alveolar flooding. Injury to the type II alveolar cell causes reduced clearance of alveolar fluid, decreased production and turnover of surfactant, and impairment of innate immunity, which in turn increases susceptibility to bacterial infections. Furthermore, type II pneumocytes are involved in the cellular repair and restoration of cellular architecture. Damage to these cells leads to a disorganized epithelial repair and fibrosis (Fig. 13.4) (157).

   Sequestration and activation of neutrophils in the pulmonary vasculature are consistent findings in ALI and ARDS. The "early response" cytokines (IL-1β, α tumor necrosis factor, and CXC group of chemokines) initiate recruitment of neutrophils (157, 158). The sequestered neutrophils are then activated by the adhesion molecules, IL-8, and platelet-activating factor (157). A complex response involving pro- as well as anti-inflammatory cytokines, arachidonic acid metabolites, eicosanoids, LTs, ETs, and endothelium-derived relaxing factor ensues. The resulting inflammatory reaction leads to endothelial and epithelial injury, which in

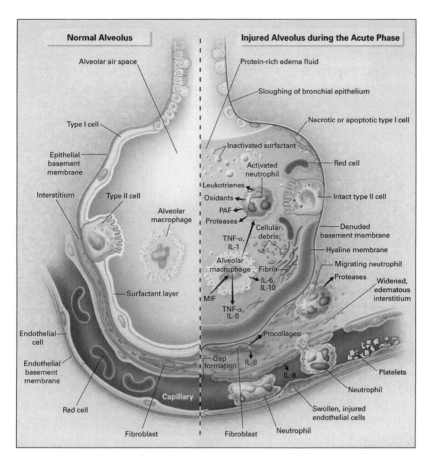

FIGURE 13.4 During acute respiratory distress syndrome, bronchial and alveolar epithelial cells are shed while a protein-rich hyaline membrane forms on the denuded basement membrane. Neutrophils and macrophages migrate through the interstitium into the air space, which becomes filled with a protein-rich edematous fluid that inactivates surfactant. The macrophages secrete cytokines, including interleukins (IL)-1, -6, -8, and -10 and tumor necrosis factor (TNF-)α, which stimulate chemotaxis and activate neutrophils. Neutrophils release oxidants, proteases, leukotrienes, and other proinflammatory molecules. MIF = macrophage-inhibitory factor; PAF = platelet-activating factor. [From Ware and Matthay (157); with permission.]

turn affects a number of metabolic activities of the lung. The overall physiologic effects depend on the balance of contradictory functions of the variety of mediators that are released. Thus, the increase in bronchial muscle tone may be partially mitigated by the bronchodilatory influences of VIP. Prostacyclin-induced pulmonary vasorelaxation may counteract the vasoconstriction caused by the LTs. In addition, prostacyclin inhibits neutrophil and platelet aggregation, and it prevents pulmonary vascular permeability and pulmonary hypertension.

In the reparative phase following the acute injury, the type II alveolar cells are involved with regeneration of type I cells and development of fibrosis (159). In the pulmonary vasculature, loss of precapillary units and hypertrophy of vascular smooth muscle cells have been observed (160).

Asthma

Asthma is characterized by airway inflammation, bronchial hyperresponsiveness, and reversible airflow obstruction. Airway inflammation is the hallmark of the disease, and it is detectable even in patients with only mild or intermittent symptoms. Antigenic exposure incites inflammatory cell infiltration in the mucosa and submucosa with mast cells, eosinophils, and T lymphocytes, with resultant release of many inflammatory mediators. Furthermore, epithelial cells, endothelial cells, fibroblasts, and smooth muscle cells undergo phenotypic transformation to release inflammatory mediators (161, 162).

The CD4+ Th lymphocytes are primarily responsible for orchestrating the inflammatory response. The Th-2 cells have been detected in the bronchoalveolar fluid as well as in the airway biopsies of asthmatics. The Th-2 lymphocytes produce IL-4, -5, -9, and -13 (Th-2 cytokines). Activation of eosinophils and release of immunoglobulin E leads to production of cysteinyl leukotrienes and IL-5. The cysteinyl leukotrienes increase bronchomotor tone, causing bronchoconstriction, and increase membrane permeability, leading to airway edema and increased mucus production.

Many of the inflammatory mediators (TGF-α, IL-1, and IL-6) induce hypertrophy and hyperplasia of the airway smooth muscle cells (163, 164). Furthermore, epithelial damage, thickened basement, increased bronchial capillary bed airway edema, and goblet cell hyperplasia, which occur in asthma, also lead to an increase in airway wall thickness (165). These changes lead to the bronchial hyperresponsiveness characteristic of asthma.

Steroids reduce airway infiltration with CD4+ Th-2 cells and decrease mRNA for many cytokines, thus reducing the airway inflammation (166). In addition, anti-LT agents produce symptomatic relief in many phenotypes of asthma. The anti-LT agents may inhibit LT synthesis by blocking the 5-lipoxygenase enzyme (eg, zileuton) or the LT receptors (eg, zafirlukast [Accolate®, AstraZeneca] or montelukast [Singulair®, Merck]) (70, 167).

Markers of Pulmonary Disease Processes

Decreased uptake or clearance of peptides, such as 5-HT, PGE_1, or nor-epinephrine, which normally are cleared during passage through the lungs, may serve as an early indication of disease processes that cause endothelial damage (168). More recently, researchers have focused on the constituents of exhaled breath as markers of inflammation and oxidative processes in the lung. For example, increased levels of exhaled NO are detected in normal individuals with "subclinical" asthma as well as in patients with asthma. Thus, exhaled NO may be useful as an early indicator of asthmatic exacerbation. Exhaled NO levels are also altered in many other diseases: They are decreased in chronic obstructive pulmonary disease, chronic bronchitis, cystic fibrosis, and Kartagener's syndrome, whereas they are increased in bronchiectasis, fibrosing alveolitis, sarcoidosis, and some forms of lung carcinomas. Products of NO metabolism are inversely correlated with pulmonary artery pressure in patients with primary pulmonary hypertension, and their levels increase after prostacyclin therapy (169). Exhaled NO levels may also provide early, noninvasive warning of obliterative bronchiolitis or acute rejection after lung transplantation. In ARDS, exhaled levels of NO are low, despite up-regulation of NOS and increased production of NO.

Carbon monoxide in exhaled breath has also been studied as a marker of pulmonary disease. Elevated levels are detected in bronchiectasis, cystic fibrosis, interstitial pulmonary fibrosis, scleroderma, and allergic rhinitis.

Other agents, including hydrocarbons, prostanoids, isoprostanes, cytokines, vasoactive amines, and ammonia, have been investigated for their possible role as markers of pulmonary processes.

CONCLUSION

The lung is an important site of extensive metabolic and hormonal activity, which produces a wide range of local and remote effects. A number of agents are produced, activated, modified, and/or metabolized in the lung. Other compounds are removed while coursing through the lung. Through these bioactive compounds, the lung influences pulmonary and systemic vascular tone as well as bronchial smooth muscle tone, modulates immune responses, and removes xenobiotics. In a number of physiologic and pathophysiologic conditions, the complex balance between the bioactive compounds is altered in a way that influences the clinical course of these conditions. During the past three decades, our understanding of these processes has improved a great deal. In turn, this has led to better management of many diseases and development of new classes of drugs that have become the mainstay of treatment in many instances (eg asthma and pulmonary hypertension). Further expansion of our knowledge bodes well for the future.

References

1. Weibel ER, Gomez DM: The architecture of the human lung. Science 1962; 137:577–85.
2. Crapo JD, et al: Cell number and cell characteristics of the normal human lung. Am Rev Respir Dis 1982; 126:332–7.
3. Ryan US, Grantham CJ: Metabolism of endogenous and xenobiotic substances by pulmonary vascular endothelial cells. Pharmacol Ther 1989; 42:235–50.
4. Gryglewski R., Korbut R, Dietkiewicz A: Generation of prostacyclin by lungs in vivo and its release into the arterial circulation. Nature 1978; 273:765–7.
5. Ignarro LJ, Buga GM, Chaudhuri G: EDRF generation and release from perfused bovine pulmonary artery and vein. Eur J Pharmacol 1988; 149:79–88.
6. Said SI: Metabolic functions of the pulmonary circulation. Circ Res 1982; 50:325–33.
7. Ryan JW, Ryan US: Pulmonary endothelial cells. Federation Proceedings 1977; 36:2683–91.
8. Serabjit-Singh CJ, et al: The distribution of cytochrome P450 monooxygenase in cells of the rabbit lung: an ultrastructural immunocytochemical characterization. Mol Pharmacol 1988; 33:279–88.
9. Johns RA, Peach MJ: Metabolism of arachidonic acid and release of endothelium-derived relaxing factors. In: M VP, ed: Relaxing and Contracting Factors. Clifton, NJ: Humana, 1988.
10. Simionescu M: Cell organization of the alveolar-capillary unit: structural-functional correlations. In: Said SI, ed: The Pulmonary Circulation and Acute Lung Injury. Mount Kisco, NY: Futura, 1985; 13–36.
11. Smith U, Ryan JW: Electron microscopy of endothelial and epithelial components of the lungs: correlations of structure and function. Federation Proceedings 1973; 32:1957–66.
12. Ryan JW, Ryan US: Metabolic functions of the pulmonary vascular endothelium. Adv Vet Sci Comp Med 1982; 26:79–98.
13. Crapo JD, et al: Morphometric characteristics of cells in the alveolar region of mammalian lungs. Am Rev Respir Dis 1983; 128(2 Pt 2):S42–6.
14. Mason RJ, Williams MC: Type II alveolar cell: defender of the alveolus. Am Rev Respir Dis 1977; 115:81–91.

15. Askin FB, Kuhn C: The cellular origin of pulmonary surfactant. Lab Invest 1971; 25:260–8.
16. Van Rozendaal BA, van Golde LM, Haagsman HP: Localization and functions of SP-A and SP-D at mucosal surfaces. Pediatr Pathol Mol Med 2001; 20:319–39.
17. Scheuermann DW: Morphology and cytochemistry of the endocrine epithelial system in the lung. Int Rev Cytol 1987; 106:35–88.
18. Griese M: Pulmonary surfactant in health and human lung diseases: state of the art. Eur Respir J 1999; 13:1455–76.
19. LeVine AM, et al: Surfactant protein-A-deficient mice are susceptible to *Pseudomonas aeruginosa* infection. Am J Respir Cell Mol Biol 1998; 19:700–8.
20. Crouch E, Wright JR: Surfactant proteins A and D and pulmonary host defense. Annu Rev Physiol 2001; 63:521–54.
21. Hawgood S, Poulain FR: The pulmonary collectins and surfactant metabolism. Annu Rev Physiol 2001; 63:495–519.
22. Sutherland LM, Edwards YS, Murray AW: Alveolar type II cell apoptosis. Comp Biochem Physiol A Mol Integr Physiol 2001; 129:267–85.
23. Goodman BE, Fleischer RS, Crandall ED: Evidence for active Na^+ transport by cultured monolayers of pulmonary alveolar epithelial cells. Am J Physiol 1983; 245:C78–88.
24. Cutz E: Neuroendocrine cells of the lung. An overview of morphologic characteristics and development. Exp Lung Res 1982; 3(3–4):185–208.
25. Cutz E, Chan W, Track NS: Bombesin, calcitonin, and leu-enkephalin immunoreactivity in endocrine cells of human lung. Experientia 1981; 37:765–7.
26. Becker KL, Monaghan KG, Silva OL: Immunocytochemical localization of calcitonin in Kulchitsky cells of human lung. Arch Pathol Lab Med 1980; 104:196–8.
27. Dayer AM, De Mey J, Will JA: Localization of somatostatin-, bombesin-, and serotonin-like immunoreactivity in the lung of the fetal rhesus monkey. Cell Tissue Res 1985; 239:621–5.
28. Youngson C, et al: Oxygen sensing in airway chemoreceptors. Nature 1993; 365(6442):153–5.
29. Lauweryns JM, Cokelaere M: Hypoxia-sensitive neuro-epithelial bodies. Intrapulmonary secretory neuroreceptors, modulated by the CNS. Z Zellforsch Mikrosk Anat 1973; 145:521–40.
30. Gail DB, L'enfant CJM: Cells of the lung: biology and clinical implications. Am Rev Respir Dis 1983; 127:366–87.
31. Sunday ME, Yoder BA, Cuttilta F, et al: Bombesin-like peptide mediates lung injury in a baboon model of bronchopulmonary dysplasia. J Clin Invest 1998; 102:584–94.

32. Hook GE, et al: Repopulation of denuded tracheas by Clara cells isolated from the lungs of rabbits. Exp Lung Res 1987; 12:311–29.
33. Shijubo N, et al: Serum and BAL Clara cell 10-kDa protein (CC10) levels and CC10-positive bronchiolar cells are decreased in smokers. Eur Respir J 1997; 10:1108–14.
34. Andersson O, et al: Clara cell secretory protein. Levels in BAL fluid after smoking cessation. Chest 2000; 118:180–2.
35. Linnoila RI, et al: The role of CC10 in pulmonary carcinogenesis: from a marker to tumor suppression. Ann N Y Acad Sci 2000; 923:249–67.
36. Friedman MM, Kaliner MA: Symposium on mast cells and asthma: human mast cells and asthma. Am Rev Respir Dis 1987; 135:1157–64.
37. Wasserman SI: The lung mast cell: its physiology and potential relevance to defense of the lung. Environ Health Perspect 1980; 35:153–64.
38. Krishnaswamy G, et al: The human mast cell: functions in physiology and disease. Front Biosci 2001; 6:D1109–27.
39. Pesci A, et al: Mast cells in fibrotic lung disorders. Chest 1993; 103:989–96.
40. Ryan JW, Smith U: Metabolism of adenosine 5'-monophosphate during circulation through the lungs. Trans Assoc Am Physicians 1971; 84:297–306.
41. Smith U, Ryan JW: Pinocytolic vesicles of the pulmonary endothelial cells. Chest 1971; 59:125–55.
42. Ryan US, Frokjaer-Jensen J: Pulmonary endothelium and processing of plasma solutes: structure and function. In: Vane J, ed: The Pulmonary Circulation and Acute Lung Injury. Mount Kisco, NY: Futura, 1985; 37–60.
43. Fishman AP, Pietra GG: Handling of bioactive materials by the lung. N Engl J Med 1974; 291:953–9.
44. Alabaster VA, Bakhle YS: Removal of 5-hydroxytryptamine in the pulmonary circulation of rat isolated lungs. Br J Pharmacol 1970; 40:468–82.
45. Nicholas TE, et al: Site and mechanism of uptake of ^{3}H-1-norepinephrine by isolated perfused rat lungs. Circ Res 1974; 35:670–80.
46. Fisher AB, Pietra GG: Comparison of serotonin uptake from the alveolar and capillary spaces of isolated rat lung. Am Rev Respir Dis 1981; 123:74–8.
47. Fitzgerald GA: Dipyridamole. N Engl J Med 1987; 316:1247–57.
48. Piper PJ, Vane JR, Wyllie JH: Inactivation of prostaglandins by the lungs. Nature 1970; 225:600–4.
49. Suzuki T, et al: 11α-Hydroxysteroid dehydrogenase type 2 in hu-

man lung: possible regulator of mineralocorticoid action. J Clin Endocrinol Metab 1998; 83:4022–5.

50. LeVan TD, et al: Pharmacological characterization of glucocorticoid receptors in primary human bronchial epithelial cells. Biochem Pharmacol 1999; 57:1003–9.

51. Janssen LJ: Isoprostanes: an overview and putative roles in pulmonary pathophysiology. Am J Physiol Lung Cell Mol Physiol 2001; 280:L1067–82.

52. Hanley SP: Prostaglandins and the lung. Lung 1986; 164:65–7.

53. Kadowitz PJ, Spannhake EW, Hyman AL: Prostaglandins evoke a whole variety of responses in the lung. Environ Health Perspect 1980; 35:181–90.

54. Kadowitz PJ, et al: Action and metabolism of prostaglandins in the pulmonary circulation. In: Oates JA, ed: Prostaglandins and the Cardiovascular System. New York: Raven, 1982; 333–56.

55. Ogletree ML: Pharmacology of prostaglandins in the pulmonary microcirculation. Ann N Y Acad Sci 1982; 384:191–206.

56. Robinson C, Hardy CC, Holgate ST: Pulmonary synthesis, release, and metabolism of prostaglandins. J Allergy Clin Immunol 1985; 76:265–71.

57. Frangos JA, et al: Flow effects on prostacyclin production by cultured human endothelial cells. Science 1985; 227:1477–9.

58. Reeves JT, et al: Prostacyclin production and lung endothelial cell shear-stress. Prog Clin Biol Res 1983; 136:125–31.

59. Ferreira SH, Vane JR: Prostaglandins. Their disappearance from and release into the circulation. Nature 1967; 216:868–73.

60. Hammond GL, et al: Fate of prostaglandins E_1 and A_1 in the human pulmonary circulation. Surgery 1977; 81:716–22.

61. Hoult JRS, Robinson C: Selective inhibition of thromboxane B_2 accumulation and metabolism in perfused guinea-pig lung. Br J Pharmacol 1983; 78:85–8.

62. Bakhle YS, Ferreira SH: Lung metabolism of eicosanoids: prostaglandins, prostacyclin, thromboxane, and leukotrienes. In: Fisher AB, ed: Handbook of Physiology. Bethesda, MD: American Physiological Society, 1985; 365–86.

63. Garcia JGN, et al: Leukotrienes and the pulmonary microcirculation. Am Rev Respir Dis 1987; 136:161–9.

64. Nicosia S, Capra V, Rovati GE: Leukotrienes as mediators of asthma. Pulm Pharmacol Ther 2001; 14:3–19.

65. Ohtaka H, et al: Comparative effects of leukotrienes on porcine pulmonary circulation in vitro and in vivo. J Appl Physiol 1987; 63:582–8.

66. Hand JM, Will JA, Buckner CKJ: Effects of leukotrienes on isolated guinea-pig pulmonary arteries. Eur J Pharmacol 1981; 76:439–42.

67. Schellenberg RR, Foster A: Differential activity of leukotrienes upon human pulmonary vein and artery. Prostaglandins 1984; 27:475–82.
68. Dahlen SE, et al: Leukotrienes are potent constrictors of human bronchi. Nature 1980; 288:484–6.
69. Wenzel SE: Arachidonic acid metabolites: mediators of inflammation in asthma. Pharmacotherapy 1997; 17:3S-12S.
70. Meltzer SS, et al: Inhibition of exercise-induced bronchospasm by zileuton: a 5-lipoxygenase inhibitor. Am J Respir Crit Care Med 1996; 153:931–5.
71. Israel E, et al: The pivotal role of 5-lipoxygenase products in the reaction of aspirin-sensitive asthmatics to aspirin. Am Rev Respir Dis 1993; 148:1447–51.
72. Stephenson A, et al: Increased concentrations of leukotrienes in bronchoalveolar lavage fluid of patients with ARDS or at risk for ARDS. Am Rev Respir Dis 1988; 138:714–9.
73. Voelkel NF: Mechanisms of hypoxic pulmonary vasoconstriction. Am Rev Respir Dis 1986; 133:1186–95.
74. Stenmark KR, et al: Leukotriene C_4 and D_4 in neonates with hypoxemia and pulmonary hypertension. N Engl J Med 1983; 309:77–80.
75. Pearl RG, Prielipp RC: Leukotriene synthesis inhibition and receptor blockade do not inhibit hypoxic pulmonary vasoconstriction in sheep. Anesth Analg 1991; 72:169–76.
76. Brom J, et al: Characterization of leukotriene B_4-omega-hydroxylase activity within human polymorphonuclear granulocytes. Scand J Immunol 1987; 25:283–94.
77. Hammarstrom S, Orning L, Bernstrom K: Metabolism of leukotrienes. Mol Cell Biochem 1985; 69:7–16.
78. Serhan CN: Lipoxins and novel aspirin-triggered 15-epi-lipoxins (ATL): a jungle of cell-cell interactions or a therapeutic opportunity? Prostaglandins 1997; 53:107–37.
79. Soyombo O, Spur BW, Lee TH: Effects of lipoxin A_4 on chemotaxis and degranulation of human eosinophils stimulated by platelet-activating factor and N-formyl-L-methionyl-L-leucyl-L-phenylalanine. Allergy 1994; 49:230–4.
80. Raud J, Palmertz U, Dahlen SE, et al: Lipoxins inhibit microvascular inflammatory actions of leukotriene B_4. Adv Exp Med Biol 1991; 314:185–92.
81. Brezinski ME, et al: Lipoxins stimulate prostacyclin generation by human endothelial cells. FEBS Lett 1989; 245(1–2):167–72.
82. Bratt J, Gyllenhammar H: The role of nitric oxide in lipoxin A_4-induced polymorphonuclear neutrophil-dependent cytotoxicity to human vascular endothelium in vitro. Arthritis Rheum 1995; 38:768–76.

83. Jacobs ER, Zeldin DC: The lung HETEs (and EETs) up. Am J Physiol Heart Circ Physiol 2001; 280:H1–10.
84. Birks EK, et al: Human pulmonary arteries dilate to 20-HETE and endogenous eicosanoid of lung tissue. Am J Physiol Lung Cell Mol Physiol 1997; 272:L823–9.
85. McManus LM, Deavers SI: Platelet-activating factor in pulmonary pathobiology. Clin Chest Med 1989; 10:107–17.
86. Page CP: The role of platelet-activating factor in asthma. J Allergy Clin Immunol 1988; 81:144–52.
87. Yalow RS, et al: Plasma and tumor ACTH in carcinoma of the lung. Cancer 1979. 44:1789–92.
88. Gerwitz G, Yalow RS: Ectopic ACTH production in carcinoma of the lung. J Clin Invest 1974; 53:1022–32.
89. Ryan JW, et al: Metabolism of angiotensin I in the pulmonary circulation. Biochem J 1970; 120:221–3.
90. Lee MA, et al: Tissue renin-angiotensin systems. Their role in cardiovascular disease. Circulation 1993; 87:IV7–13.
91. Seyedi N, Xu X, Nasjletti A, et al: Coronary kinin generation mediates nitric oxide release after angiotensin receptor stimulation. Hypertension 1995; 26:164–70.
92. Lin L, Nasjletti A: Role of endothelium-derived prostanoid in angiotensin-induced vasoconstriction. Hypertension 1991; 18:158–64.
93. Filippatos G, et al: Regulation of apoptosis by angiotensin II in the heart and lungs. Int J Mol Med 2001; 7:273–80.
94. The Consensus Trial Study Group: Effects of enalapril on mortality in severe congestive heart failure. Results of the Cooperative North Scandinavian Enalapril Survival Study (CONSENSUS). N Engl J Med 1987; 316:1429–35.
95. The SOLVD Investigators: Effect of enalapril on mortality and the development of heart failure in asymptomatic patients with reduced left ventricular ejection fractions. N Engl J Med 1992; 327:685–91.
96. The SOLVD investigators: Effect of enalapril on survival in patients with reduced left ventricular ejection fractions and congestive heart failure. N Engl J Med 1991; 325:293–302.
97. Chand N, Altura BM: Acetylcholine and bradykinin relax intrapulmonary arteries by acting on endothelial cells: role in lung vascular diseases. Science 1981; 213(4514):1376–9.
98. Schlemper V, Calixto JB: Mechanisms underlying the contraction induced by bradykinin in the guinea pig epithelium-denuded trachea. Can J Physiol Pharmacol 2002; 80:360–7.
99. Barst RJ, Stalcup SA, Mellins RB: Bradykinin-induced changes in circulating prostanoids in unanesthetized sheep. Federation Proceedings 1983; 42:302.

100. Farmer SG: Role of kinins in airway disease. Immunopharmacology 1991; 22:1–20.
101. Nicholls MG: Minisymposium: the natriuretic peptide hormones. Introduction, editorial, and historical review. J Intern Med 1994; 235:507–14.
102. Di Nardo P, Peruzzi G: Physiology and pathophysiology of atrial natriuretic factor in lungs. Can J Cardiol 1992; 8:503–8.
103. Ignarro IJ, et al: Atriopeptin II relaxes and elevated cGMP in bovine pulmonary artery but not vein. J Appl Physiol 1986; 60:1128–33.
104. Hulks G, et al: Bronchodilator effect of atrial natriuretic peptide in asthma. BMJ 1989; 299(6707):1081–2.
105. Valentine JP, Ribstein J, Mimran A: Effect of nicardipine and atriopepin on transcapillary shift of fluid and proteins. Am J Physiol 1989; 257:174–9.
106. Lofton CE, et al: Atrial natriuretic peptide inhibits oxidant-induced increases in endothelial permeability. J Mol Cell Cardiol 1991; 23:919–27.
107. Struthers AD: Ten years of natriuretic peptide research: a new dawn for their diagnostic and therapeutic use? British Medical Journal 1994; 308:1615–9.
108. Rogers TK, Thompson JS, Morice AH: Inhibition of hypoxic pulmonary vasoconstriction in isolated rat resistance arteries by atrial natriuretic peptide. Eur Respir J 1997; 10:2061–5.
109. Cutz E, et al: Release of vasoactive intestinal polypeptide in mast cells by histamine liberators. Nature 1978; 275(5681):661–2.
110. Saga T, Said SI: Vasoactive intestinal peptide relaxes isolated strips of human bronchus, pulmonary artery, and lung parenchyma. Trans Am Assoc Physicians 1984; 97:304–10.
111. Matsuzaki Y, Hamasaki Y, Said SI: Vasoactive intestinal peptide: a possible transmitter of nonadrenergic relaxation of guinea pig airways. Science 1980; 210:1252–3.
112. Said SI, Dickman KG: Pathways of inflammation and cell death in the lung: modulation by vasoactive intestinal peptide. Regul Pept 2000; 93:21–9.
113. Marciniak SJ, et al: Localization of immunoreactive endothelin and proendothelin in the human lung. Pulm Pharmacol 1992; 5:175–82.
114. Boulanger C, Luscher TF: Release of endothelin from the porcine aorta. Inhibition by endothelium-derived nitric oxide. J Clin Invest 1990; 85:587–90.
115. Masaki T, Vane JR, Vanhoutte PM: International Union of Pharmacology nomenclature of endothelin receptors. Pharmacol Rev 1994; 46:137–42.

116. Haynes WG, Webb DJ. Endothelin as a regulator of cardiovascular function in health and disease. J Hypertens 1998; 16:1081–98.
117. Boscoe MJ, Goodwin AT, Amrani M, et al: Endothelins and the lung. Int J Biochem Cell Biol 2000; 32:41–62.
118. Fukuroda T, et al: Clearance of circulating endothelin-1 by ETB receptors in rats. Biochem Biophys Res Commun 1994; 199:1461–5.
119. Dupuis J, Stewart DJ: Human pulmonary circulation is an important site for both clearance and production of endothelin-1. Circulation 1996; 94:1578–84.
120. Ozaki S, et al: ETB-mediated regulation of extracellular levels of endothelin-1 in cultured human endothelial cells. Biochem Biophys Res Commun 1995; 209:483–9.
121. MacLean MR, Mackenzie JF, Docherty CC: Heterogeneity of endothelin-B receptors in rabbit pulmonary resistance arteries. J Cardiovasc Pharmacol 1998; 31:S115–8.
122. Goldie RG, et al: Endothelin-1 receptor density, distribution, and function in human isolated asthmatic airways. Am J Respir Crit Care Med 1995; 152:1653–8.
123. Rubens C, et al: Big endothelin-1 and endothelin-1 plasma levels are correlated with the severity of primary pulmonary hypertension. Chest 2001; 120:1562–9.
124. Luscher TF, Barton M: Endothelins and endothelin receptor antagonists: therapeutic considerations for a novel class of cardiovascular drugs. Circulation 2000; 102:2434–40.
125. Williamson DJ, et al: Hemodynamic effects of Bosentan, an endothelin receptor antagonist, in patients with pulmonary hypertension. Circulation 2000; 102:411–8.
126. Druml W, et al: Endothelin-1 in adult respiratory distress syndrome. Am Rev Respir Dis 1993; 148:1169–73.
127. Dupuis J, et al: Reduced pulmonary clearance of endothelin-1 in pulmonary hypertension. Am Heart J 1998; 135:614–20.
128. Chung KF, Barnes PJ: Cytokines in asthma. Thorax 1999; 54:825–57.
129. Vane JR: Metabolic activities of the lung. Excerpta Medica 1980; 78:1–10.
130. Junod AF: 5-Hydroxytryptamine and other amines in the lungs. In: Fisher AB, ed: Handbook of Physiology. Bethesda, MD: American Physiological Society, 1985; 337–49.
131. Pearson JD, Gordon JL: Nucleotide metabolism by endothelium. Annu Rev Physiol 1985; 47:617–27.
132. Furchgott RF, Zawadzki JV: The obligatory role of endothelial cells in the relaxation of arterial smooth muscle by acetylcholine. Nature 1980; 288:373–6.

133. Ignarro LJ, Buga GM, Wood KS, et al: Endothelium-derived relaxing factor produced and released from artery and vein is nitric oxide. Proc Natl Acad Sci U S A 1987; 184:9265–9.

134. Bolotina VM, Najibi S, Palacino JJ, et al: Nitric oxide directly activates calcium-dependent potassium channels in vascular smooth muscle. Nature 1994; 368:850–3.

135. Hernandez I, et al: Role of angiotensin II in modulating the hemodynamic effects of nitric oxide synthesis inhibition. Am J Physiol 1999; 277:R104–11.

136. Michel T, Feron O: Nitric oxide synthases: which, where, how, and why? J Clin Invest 1997; 100:2146–52.

137. Ferrario L, Amin HM, Sugimori K, et al: Site of action of endogenous nitric oxide on pulmonary vasculature in rats. Pflugers Arch 1996; 432:523–7.

138. Freedman JE, Loscalzo J, Barnard MR, et al: Nitric oxide released from activated platelets inhibits platelet recruitment. J Clin Invest 1997; 100:350–6.

139. Radomski MW, Palmer RM, Moncada S: The antiaggregating properties of vascular endothelium: interactions between prostacyclin and nitric oxide. Br J Pharmacol 1987; 92:639–46.

140. Feletou M, Vanhoutte PM: Endothelium-dependent hyperpolarization of anine coronary smooth muscle. Br J Pharmacol 1988; 93:515–24.

141. Chen G, et al: Hyperpolarization of arterial smooth muscle induced by endothelial humoral substances. Am J Physiol 1991; 260(6 pt 2):H1888–92.

142. Fulton D, MuGiff JC, Quilley J: Role of K^+ channels in the vasodilator response to bradykinin in the rat heart. Br J Pharmacol 1994; 113:954–8.

143. Campbell JH, Campbell GR: Endothelial cell influences on vascular smooth muscle phenotype. Annu Rev Physiol 1986; 48:295–306.

144. Clowes AW, Karnovsky MJ: Suppression by heparin of smooth muscle cell proliferation in injured arteries. Nature 1977; 265(5595):625–6.

145. Mansour H, et al: Protection of rat from oxygen toxicity by inducers of cytochrome P450 system. Am Rev Respir Dis 1988; 137:688–94.

146. Serabjit-Singh CJ, et al: Cytochrome P450: localization in rabbit lung. Science 1980; 207:1469–70.

147. Pietra GG, et al: Transcapillary movement of cationized ferritin in the isolated perfused rat lung. Lab Invest 1983; 49:54–61.

148. Jorfeldt L, et al: Lung uptake of lidocaine in healthy volunteers. Acta Anaesth Scand 1979; 23:567–84.

149. Jorfeldt L, et al: Lung uptake of lidocaine in man as influenced by anaesthesia, mepivacaine infusion or lung insufficiency. Acta Anaesth Scand 1983; 27:5–9.

150. Roerig DL, et al: First pass uptake of fentanyl, meperidine, and morphine in the human lung. Anesthesiology 1987; 67:466–72.

151. Von Euler US, Liljestrand G: Observations on the pulmonary arterial blood pressure in the cat. Acta Physiol Scand 1946; 12:301–20.

152. Madden JA, Dawson CA, Harder DR: Hypoxia-induced activation in small isolated pulmonary arteries from the cat. J Appl Physiol 1985; 59:113–8.

153. Murray TR, et al: Hypoxic contraction of cultured pulmonary vascular smooth muscle cells. Am J Respir Cell Mol Biol 1990; 3:457–65.

154. Yuan XJ: Voltage-gated K^+ currents regulate resting membrane potential and $(Ca^{2+})i$ in pulmonary arterial myocytes. Circ Res 1995; 77:370–8.

155. Pugin J, et al: The alveolar space is the site of intense inflammatory and profibrotic reactions in the early phase of acute respiratory distress syndrome. Crit Care Med 1999; 159(suppl):A694.

156. Matthay MA, Wiener-Kronish JP: Intact epithelial barrier function is critical for the resolution of alveolar edema in humans. Am Rev Respir Dis 1990; 142:1250–7.

157. Ware LB, Matthay MA: The acute respiratory distress syndrome. N Engl J Med 2000; 342:1334–49.

158. Strieter RM, et al: Chemokines in lung injury. Chest 1999; 116:103S-110S.

159. Bitterman PB: Pathogenesis of fibrosis in acute lung injury. Am J Med 1992; 92:39S-43S.

160. Jones R, Zapol WM, Reid L: Pulmonary arterial wall injury and remodeling by hyperoxia. Chest 1983; 83(Suppl 5):40S–42S.

161. Barnes PJ, Page C: Mediators of asthma: a new series. Pulm Pharmacol Ther, 2001; 14:1–2.

162. Vignalo AM, Gagliardo R, et al: New evidence of inflammation in asthma. Thorax 2000; 55(suppl 2):S59-S60.

163. Cohen MD, Ciocca V, Panettieri RAJ: TGF-â₁ modulates human airway smooth-muscle cell proliferation induced by mitogens. Am J Respir Cell Mol Biol 1997; 16:85–90.

164. De S, et al: IL-1α and IL-6 induce hyperplasia and hypertrophy of cultured guinea pig airway smooth muscle cells. J Appl Physiol 1995; 78:1555–63.

165. Brusasco V, Crimi E, Pellegrino R: Airway hyperresponsiveness in asthma: not just a matter of airway inflammation. Thorax 1998; 53:992–8.

166. Ray A, Cohn L: The cells and GATA-3 in asthma: new insights into the regulation of airway inflammation. J Clin Invest 1999; 104:985–93.

167. Israel E, et al: The effects of a 5-lipoxygenase inhibitor on asthma induced by cold, dry air. N Engl J Med 1990; 323:1740–4.

168. Dawson CA, Roerig DL, Linehan JH: Evaluation of endothelial injury in the human lung. Clin Chest Med 1989; 10:13–24.
169. Kaneko FT, et al: Biochemical reaction products of nitric oxide as quantitative markers of primary pulmonary hypertension. Am J Respir Crit Care Med 1998; 158:917–23.
170. Ryan US, Ryan JW: Correlations between the fine structure of the alveolar-capillary unit and its metabolic activities. In: Bakhle YS, Vane JR, eds: Metabolic Functions of the Lung. New York: Marcel Dekker, 1977; 197–242.
171. Block ER, Stalcup SA: Today's practice of cardiopulmonary medicine: metabolic functions of the lung: of what clinical relevance? Chest 1982; 81:215–23.

Peter J. Papadakos, MD, FCCM
Younsuck Koh, MD, PhD
Burkhard Lachmann, MD, PhD

14 | Respiratory Pharmacology

A large number of patients who present for thoracic surgery will be on medications that are modulating their lung function. The lung contains a large surface area for both the absorption and function of medications and gases. During the last 10 years, an explosion has occurred in the development of pharmacologic agents that not only modulate bronchodilation and bronchoconstriction but that also affect lung function and gas exchange in respiratory failure. These therapeutic agents and aerosols have greatly added to our understanding of how the lung functions during both normal and pathologic states.

We are challenged each day by patients with complex lung diseases who present for elective and emergent surgery and care. The importance of a rapid, comprehensive work-up, including a comprehensive history and physical examination, along with specific tests, including an arterial blood gas, cannot be overemphasized. All too often, patients are cared for without proper information being collected. The preoperative and postoperative course in patients with pulmonary diseases will be facilitated if the pulmonary diagnosis and severity of pulmonary dysfunction are established before surgery. It is wise to record at least a preoperative blood gas and to collect measurements of lung volumes and flow rates to ascertain the degree of functional impairment and the baseline pulmonary function. However, any preoperative laboratory data can reliably predict postoperative lung complications. For optimal lung care, we must become experts in the function of many drugs and

Progress in Thoracic Anesthesia, edited by Peter Slinger,
Lippincott Williams & Wilkins, Baltimore © 2004.

treatment modalities that will act on the physiology of the lung. With both proper and early intervention, we can improve outcome in the care of both baseline disease states and acute lung diseases.

AIRWAY STRUCTURE AND FUNCTION

A basic understanding of the airway anatomy and function will help us understand the pharmacologic actions of treatment modalities. Gas enters the thorax via the mouth, nose, or artificial airway into the trachea, which divides into the right and left mainstem bronchi. The airways continue to branch, and each division results in two daughter branches that are unequal in diameter, length, and takeoff (1). The primary function of these airways is to conduct gas through the airway to the gas-exchange zones. The increasing cross-sectional area of the airway leads to a reduction in airflow resistance as gas moves to the periphery, thus facilitating mass flow of gas. In respiratory bronchioles and alveolar ducts, gas diffusion is more important than mass gas flow and is facilitated by the large cross-referenced area.

The airway wall consists of layers of mucosa and smooth muscle and, finally, a connective tissue sleeve. Bronchi and small bronchi contain cartilage within the wall, whereas bronchioles contain no cartilage. Respiratory bronchioles contain alveoli that increase in number with each branching such that only alveoli line the alveolar ducts and sacs. In the bronchi, the mucosal layer contains tall, ciliated epithelial cells as well as mucus-producing glands, goblet cells, and Clara cells (2). In the periphery, the mucosal layer thins, and the ciliated cells become more cuboidal. In the bronchioles, glands disappear, and goblet cells decrease in number and finally disappear as the number of Clara cells increases. The Clara cells decrease and also finally disappear within the respiratory bronchioles and alveolar ducts, which are lined with epithelial cells (3).

The smooth muscle layer is continuous from the trachea to the alveolar ducts. The smooth muscle bundles encircle the airways in an oblique course. Contraction results in airway narrowing as well as shortening (1). In the alveolar ducts, the muscle bundles occur in the alveolar entrance rings (1).

The pulmonary blood supply from the right and left arteries follows the mainstem bronchi into the lung parenchyma. Both the arteries and the bronchi then follow the branching pattern to the level of the respiratory bronchiole ($\approx$17–23 orders or generations). The arteries give rise to arteriolar and capillary networks within the walls of the alveolar ducts and alveoli (4). These vessels produce a massive surface area: The pulmonary arteries and arterioles comprise a surface area of approximately 2.5 m^2 and , the capillary surface area is estimated at 50–150 m^2.

This large surface area provides a location where drugs can be absorbed into the circulation.

Airway caliber and tone are regulated by the parasympathetic and sympathetic divisions of the autonomic nervous system (5, 6). The vagally mediated mechanisms of the parasympathetic nervous system are the primary determinants of normal bronchomotor tone and bronchial submucosal gland secretion (5, 7). On stimulation of vagal efferent nerves, the neurotransmitter acetylcholine is released from the presynaptic nerve terminal. The acetylcholine then diffuses through the synaptic cleft and binds to muscarinic cholinergic receptors found throughout the respiratory tree. Stimulation of the cholinergic receptors results in an increase in the intracellular levels of cyclic $3',5'$-guanosine monophosphate (cGMP) in the cytoplasm (7). These acetylcholine receptors are located in or adjacent to the respiratory epithelium submucosal glands, mast cells, and smooth muscle (5, 6, 8). Stimulation of these acetylcholine receptors in the lung triggers bronchoconstriction, decreased airway caliber, and activation of mast cell degranulation and increase in glandular secretion (9).

Direct sympathetic nervous system innervation of the respiratory tree is sparse; nevertheless, the bronchial smooth muscle cells, especially those in the small airways, are well-populated with noninnervated β_2-adrenergic receptors (10). β_1-Adrenergic receptors are also present but have only a minimal role in lung physiology. β_2-Adrenergic receptors are stimulated by adrenergic agonists, both endogenous (the presynaptic neurotransmitter norepinephrine or epinephrine released by the adrenal medulla) or exogenous (pharmacologic agents). This stimulation results in activation of membrane-bound adenylate cyclase to catalyze the conversion of adenosine triphosphate to cyclic $3',5'$-adenosine monophosphate (cAMP) (11). Activation of an enzymatic cascade then occurs, resulting in bronchodilation and, possibly, increased secretion of mucus.

α-Adrenergic receptors are also found in the lung (8). Stimulation of these receptors, which are located predominantly in the bronchial and vascular smooth muscle and submucosal glands, causes bronchoconstriction and increased mucous secretion. In the lung, α_2-receptors are located on the postsynaptic nerve terminal, although they are also located presynaptically elsewhere in the body. Presynaptic α_2-receptors regulate the release of nonepinephrine from the presynaptic nerve terminal (12).

A third nonadrenergic, noncholinergic (NANC) system of the lung has been demonstrated in the airways all the way to the small bronchi (13). A major component of this system appears to be the principal inhibitor system in human airways, causing bronchodilation when stimulated. The neurotransmitter involved is a vasoactive intestinal polypeptide that is more potent than isoproterenol. An excitatory component to the NANC system also exists and is probably mediated by a peptide, substance P, that when stimulated causes bronchoconstriction. The exact function of the NANC system continues to be an active avenue of investigation.

Various endogenous substances, such as histamine, prostaglandins, platelet-activating factor, bradykinin, and various leukotrienes, also have documented inflammatory effects on smooth muscle tone that cause bronchoconstriction (15).

The alveolar macrophages, when stimulated by systemic inflammatory response, also modulate a cascade that releases various leukotrienes and cytokines that will act both locally and in the systemic circulation (16). During the last few of years, we have also discovered that the alveolar surfactant system may be involved in protecting the lung against its own mediators (eg, angiotensin II) and in protecting the cardiocirculatory system against mediators and cytokines produced by the lung (16).

BRONCHODILATORS AND BRONCHOACTIVE DRUGS

The basic way to think about bronchodilator drugs is based on their action. This leads to their classification within three groups:

1. Direct respiratory smooth muscle relaxants (theophylline and related salts).
2. β-Adrenergic agonists (isoetharine isoproterenol, epinephrine, metaproterenol, albuterol, terbutaline, bitolterol, and pirbuterol).
3. Anticholinergics (atropine, glycopyrrolate, and ipratropium).

Their site of action is depicted in Figure 14.1, which was summarized by Kelly (17).

Theophylline

Theophylline, a naturally occurring methylxanthine that is closely related to caffeine and is found in tea, has been used to treat bronchospasm for more than 100 years (18). At one time, it was the most widely used drug in the treatment of reactive airway disease; however, because of conflicting reports regarding its efficacy and safety, theophylline use in the treatment of acute bronchospasm remains controversial (19). Still, theophylline has become one of the most extensively prescribed drugs for the treatment of reversible airway obstruction around the world. The development of methods to monitor serum theo-

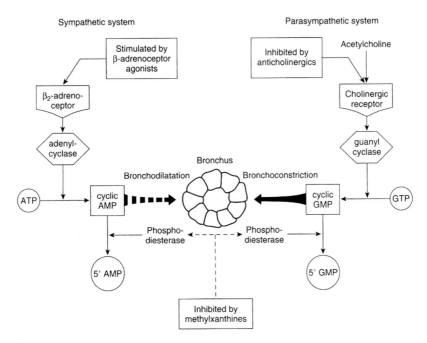

FIGURE 14.1 The mechanism of action of bronchodilator drugs.

phylline concentrations in patients has contributed to the safe and effective clinical use of this drug in this era.

Pharmacology

The exact mechanism by which theophylline exerts its pharmacologic effect is not entirely clear (20). It is well-established that theophylline competitively inhibits the activity of cytoplasmic phosphodiesterase, the enzyme that catalyzes the degradation of cAMP and cGMP to their inactive 5'-mononucleotides: 5'-AMP and 5'-GMP (21). Previously, this was thought to be the mechanism of action; however, the in vitro doses used to achieve phosphodiesterase inhibition appear to be too high to be achieved clinically (22).

In guinea pig and dog trachea muscle preparations, the theophylline levels achievable in humans had no effect on cAMP or cGMP but did increase calcium ion uptake and redistribution, consistent with a decrease of myoplasmic calcium ion and calcium sequestration in the mitochondrion (22). Other postulated mechanisms of action include prostaglandin inhibition (23), indirect β-adrenergic stimulation via release of catecholamines(24), and increased binding of cAMP to cAMP-binding protein (25). Adenosine-receptor antagonism has been proposed as the primary mediator of the pharmacologic and therapeutic actions of methylxanthines; however, the exact cellular mechanisms underlying bronchial smooth muscle relaxation remain to be clarified.

Regardless of its mechanism of action, theophylline is a direct bronchial smooth muscle relaxant. If bronchospasm is not present, the effects of theophylline on airflow and respiratory mechanics are minimal. The drug also acts by decreasing mucosal edema and by reducing the production of excessive secretions (26). Theophylline seems to have anti-inflammatory and immunomodulatory actions (27) in addition to stimulating the respiratory drive (28). Other effects of theophylline include direct augmentation of myocardial inotrophy and chronotrophy; stimulation of respiratory muscle contractility; dilation of the coronary, pulmonary, renal, and systemic arterioles and veins; diuresis; stimulation of epinephrine and nonepinephrine synthesis and release by the adrenal medulla; stimulation of the medullary respiratory center; and decreased cerebral blood flow. In normal patients, theophylline causes a chronotropic effect, a decrease in coronary artery blood flow, an increase in myocardial oxygen extraction, and a decrease in left ventricular ejection time (29). In patients with chronic obstructive pulmonary disease (COPD) and cor pulmonale, increased heart rate, stroke volume, and cardiac output as well as decreased right ventricular end-diastolic pressure, left ventricular end-diastolic pressure, wedge pressure, and systemic vascular resistance can occur (29).

Side Effects

Use of theophylline has declined especially in patients with bronchial asthma because of concerns related to its narrow therapeutic window in addition to the introduction of newer, potent bronchodilators. The most common side effects of theophylline involve the gastrointestinal tract and include nausea, vomiting, and anorexia (30). Adverse gastrointestinal affects associated with oral use can be minimized by administering the drug with food. Effects on the central nervous system include headache, irritability, restlessness, nervousness, dizziness, and seizures (19). Theophylline-induced seizures are often unresponsive to standard anticonvulsive therapy, and the mortality rate is very high (in the range of 50%) (31). Theophylline may cause a number of cardiovascular side effects that are often poorly tolerated by patients who are critically ill. These side effects include palpitations, arrhythmias (eg, tachycardia, extrasystoles, and multifocal atrial tachycardia), and ventricular arrhythmias; other cardiovascular effects can include hypotension and circulatory collapse. Rapid intravenous injection of aminophylline and theophylline may increase the incidence of side effects; therefore, slow intravenous titration or use of an infusion pump is suggested. Cardiac arrest may follow the rapid bolus dosage of aminophylline. Other side effects may include dizziness, palpitations, flushing, hypotension, and profound bradycardia.

An important point to consider is the pharmacologic preparation of theophylline. Before 1983, the only parental form of theophylline was aminophylline. Aminophylline is theophylline compounded with ethylenediamine, which confers water solubility to the insoluble theophylline molecule. This ethylenediamine contributes to the respiratory and cardiac stimulatory effects of theophylline. Also of great importance is that ethylenediamine can induce hypersensitivity reactions characterized by urticaria, generalized pruritus, angioedema, and bronchospasm (30).

Pharmacokinetics

Theophylline is manufactured as a variety of salts for oral, rectal, and parenteral administration. Rectal use of theophylline mixtures is no longer recommended because of its erratic absorption. Liquid and plain-tablet forms of theophylline are rapidly and completely absorbed (32). Slow-release preparations now dominate the market. The intravenous forms of theophylline are limited primarily to hospitalized patients and use in emergent cases.

The pharmacokinetics are well-described. Once absorbed, the drug is distributed rapidly throughout the body water, but more in the extracellular than in the intracellular body water (30). Theophylline binds to serum proteins, principally albumin, at a rate varying from 50% to 60%, which increases as the serum pH increases. Theophylline can freely pass into the breast milk and cross into the placenta. Theophylline achieves a volume of distribution of 0.3 to 0.7 L/kg in children and adults (31). Oral standard, non-time release preparations give a peak serum level within 1 to 2 hours after administration. In contrast, extended- and slow-release tablets release theophylline over a longer period of time, and peak levels are reached approximately 4 hours after administration.

Administration of theophylline by intravenous infusion produces the highest and most rapidly achieved peak serum concentration. In healthy, nonsmoking adults, a standard infusion of 5 mg/kg over 30 minutes produces an average peak serum concentration of 10 mg/mL (30).

Hepatic metabolism of theophylline is via the cytochrome P-450 system, which is also its principal method of elimination. Approximately 10% is eliminated unchanged through the kidney. Metabolism can be affected by ingestion of other drugs, however. The half-life of theophylline is increased in patients using cimetidine, ranitidine, erythromycin, allopurinol, propranolol, mexiletine, oral contraceptives, quinolones, verapamil, and diltiazam. Disease states, especially liver disease, can also affect and lengthen the half-life of theophylline. Patients who smoke either cigarettes or marijuana have a much shorter average elimination half-life (in the range of 4–5 hours). In contrast, patients with congestive heart failure, cor pulmonale, COPD, or liver disease have a markedly prolonged elimination half-life (in some cases, >12 hours) (30).

Great care must be taken in the administration of theophylline because of its low therapeutic ratio, but with close monitoring of levels, the drug can be given safely. When used with appropriate caution, theophylline should cause few cardiovascular side affects and no convulsions or deaths. Theophylline endured a bad reputation during with 1970s and 1980s, before the time of rational dosage schedules and widespread monitoring.

A therapeutic range for theophylline is frequently cited as between 10 and 20 mg/mL in plasma. Marked inter- and intrapatient variability exists for dose-response curves. Therefore, the ideal way to use the drug is to titrate serum levels to the optimal drug level to achieve maximal bronchodilation within the therapeutic range.

Clinical use of theophylline is for the prevention of bronchospasm in patients with hyperactive airway disease. No theophylline products are currently used for the initial treatment of acute bronchospasm. Rather, they are used as second-line drugs (ie, only if an inhaled â-adrenergic agonist gives a suboptimal effect). In these patients, 5 mg/kg is administered as a loading dose over 30 minutes if they have not received the drug within 24 hours. In patients taking theophylline, the dosage is lowered to half. Subsequent intravenous infusions are administered to clinical effect with very close monitoring. The majority of patients now on theophylline are undergoing prophylaxis for chronic bronchospasm.

β-Adrenergic Receptor Agonists

The introduction of inhaled β_2-agonists has greatly improved the care of patients with pulmonary diseases. The β_2-agonists are the most effective bronchodilators currently available, and they have gained widespread use both in maintenance therapy and in the acute care of patients.

β_2-Adrenergic receptor stimulation activates adenyl cyclase, which produces an increase in intracellular cAMP, which in turn induces airway relaxation through phosphorylation of muscle regulatory proteins and decreases the unbound intracellular calcium concentration (33). Selective β_2-adrenergic receptor agonist has antiallergic activity by suppressing the immunoglobulin E (IgE)-mediated release of mediators from lung mast cells and basophils. These mediators increase in mucociliary clearance and inhibit pulmonary vascular leakage (34). β_2-Adrenergic stimulation also activates Na^+/K^+-adenosine triphosphatase (ATPase), produces gluconeogenesis, and enhances insulin secretion, thereby producing a mild to moderate decrease in serum potassium concentration by driving potassium intracellularly. All β-adrenergic receptor agonists act by binding β_1 and β_2 cell membrane receptors. This action induces a relaxation of bronchial and vascular smooth muscle. These agents may also induce increased mucociliary transport of respiratory secretions. In addition, stimulation of these receptors affects mast cells and inhibits release of the mediators of bronchospasm, such as histamine and the slow-reacting substance of anaphylaxis.

These sympathomimetic bronchodilators have been used widely for many years to induce bronchodilation. Figure 14.2 displays the structures of the sympathomimetic drugs. The inhalational use of β_2-adrenergic receptor stimulators has more advantage than oral administration in terms of efficacy and side effects. Regular use of these drugs has raised concern, however, regarding increased asthma morbidity and mortality rates; thus, these drugs are recommended for use on an "as-needed" basis for symptomatic relief (35, 36, 37, 38).

Epinephrine

Epinephrine (adrenaline) is a naturally occurring catecholamine that is synthesized, stored, and released from the adrenal medulla and certain adrenergic nerve terminals. Because of its broad stimulation of adrenergic receptors, epinephrine is the drug of choice in systemic hypersensitivity reactions and is usually given in a subcutaneous dose of 0.3 to 1.0 mL of a l:l,000 aqueous solution. Similar doses can be used to treat acute bronchospasm. Subcutaneous epinephrine in a dose of 0.3 to 0.5 mL of a 1:1,000 aqueous solution can be used for acute wheezing. It is an excellent drug and appears to have no more cardiovascular side effects than subcutaneous terbutaline, but it has a shorter (1–2 hours vs 2–4 hours) duration of action than terbutaline (35). The usual way to deliver epinephrine in its racemic form is by metered dose inhaler (MDI) or in solution delivered by a nebulizer.

In many cases, epinephrine is still used to break highly resistant bronchospasm. Norepinephrine, a weak β_2-agonist, has little utility in the treatment of airway and lung disease.

Isoproterenol and Isoetharine

Isoproterenol is the most potent β_1- and β_2-agonist. It is currently available in an MDI or as a solution for use in a handheld or gas-powered

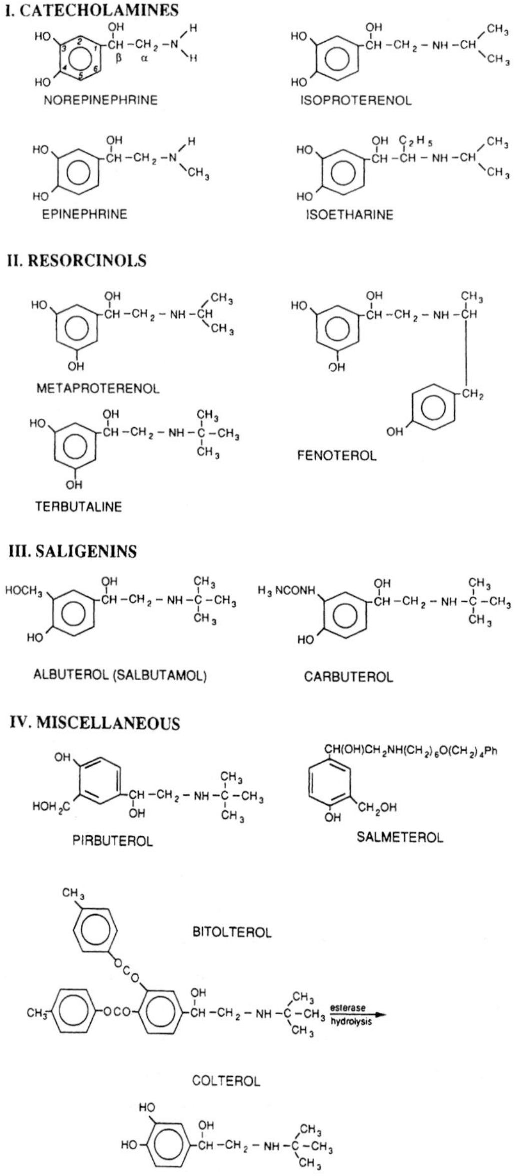

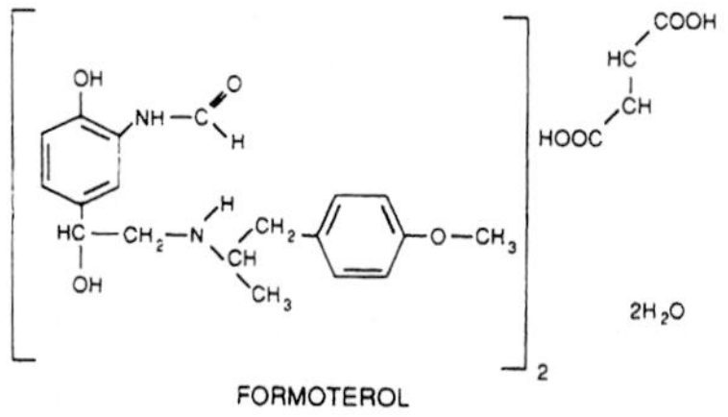

FIGURE 14.2 The chemical structures of sympathomimetic drugs.

nebulizer. However, because of its cardiovascular effects, its use has been largely replaced by the more specific agents.

Isoetharine has one-tenth the potency of isoproterenol and a duration of action of up to 3 hours. It is available as an MDI and in solution for use in a nebulizer. The aerosolized dose is 0.25 to 0.5 mL diluted in 1 mL of sterile water or saline, or 0.68 mg (two puffs) from an MDI. It, too, has been replaced by more selective β_2-agonists.

Terbutaline

Terbutaline is a slightly less potent bronchodilator than isoproterenol, but it has far fewer cardiovascular side effects, with a duration of action of up to 6 or 7 hours, when given orally or by aerosol. Given subcutaneously, the incidence of cardiovascular side effects is similar to that of epinephrine, even though the duration of bronchodilation is longer. The oral dose range is from 1.25 to 5.0 mg every 6 hours.

The MDI dose of terbutaline is 200 μg/puff, and the usual dosage is two puffs every 4 to 6 hours. The injectable form of terbutaline can be nebulized by being diluted to a total volume of 2 to 3 mL by sterile water or saline. The usual dose is 1 mg every 4 to 6 hours. It is a very popular drug.

Albuterol (Salbutamol)

Albuterol is the most commonly used agent. It has the fewest cardiovascular side-effects of the sympathomimetic bronchodilators. Given orally or by aerosol, its peak action occurs within 2 hours, and its duration of action is up to 6 hours (34, 36).

Oral doses range from 1 to 8 mg every 6 hours for the standard, short-acting preparation to 4 to 8 mg every 12 hours for the sustained-release preparation. Clinical studies have shown similar improvements in pulmonary function with the sustained-release preparations given every 12 hours as compared to the standard product given four times daily.

The MDI dose is 0.18 mg (two puffs) every 4 hours. The nebulizer dose is up to a maximum of 3.0 mg. The frequency of administration depends on the severity of bronchospasm and wheezing every 30 minutes to 1 hour for acute, severe asthma to every 4 to 6 hours for stable airway disease.

Pirbuterol

Pirbuterol is a relatively selective β-agonist, but it demonstrates both bronchodilator and cardiovascular effects (39, 40). Pirbuterol was 9-fold more selective for pulmonary tissue than albuterol and 1,520-fold more selective than isoproterenol.

The onset of pirbuterol activity occurs 5 minutes after aerosol administration and within 1 hour after oral administration. The peak activity is 30 minutes for aerosol use and 1 hour for oral use. The activity is equipotent to that of albuterol. The lowest doses that apparently produce maximum bronchodilation are 0.4 mg by aerosol and 15 mg of the oral preparation (40).

The usual MDI dose is two inhalations (200μg/puff) up to every 4 hours. The recommended oral dosage of pirbuterol is 10 to 15 mg given three to four times per day. The complication profile is similar to other β₂-agonists in which the neuromuscular side effects are more marked than the cardiovascular side effects.

Metaproterenol

Metaproterenol was the first synthetic noncatecholamine bronchodilator introduced into clinical practice in the United States. It has a duration of action of up to 4 hours. It was also the first oral agent to be introduced. It has fewer cardiovascular effects than isoproterenol but is a weak bronchodilator. Oral doses of 5 to 20 mg can be used every 4 to 6 hours. The major side effects are neuromuscular (eg, shakiness, tremor, and cramps) or cardiovascular (tachycardia). Peak effect usually occurs within 1 to 2 hours. It is delivered by MDI or as a solution for nebulization. The usual MDI dose is 1.3 mg (two puffs) given as needed up to every 3 or 4 hours for the onset of wheezing. The usual aerosolized dose is 10 to 15 mg (0.2–0.3 mL) diluted to 2 to 3 mL with sterile water or saline given every 3 to 4 hours.

Long-Acting Agents

The introduction of long-acting, inhaled β₂-agonists has been a major therapeutic development during the last number of years, and this has led to a fundamental reappraisal of β-agonist use in asthma management (36, 37). However, the long-acting agents are significantly slower than short-acting β₂-adrenergic receptor stimulators in reversing bronchoconstriction. Therefore, they should not be used as rescue medication during an acute asthmatic attack. Salmeterol and formoterol are highly selective β₂-agonists with a bronchodilating effect lasting for at least 12 hours after a single inhalation (37, 38).

Salmeterol is the result of a specific program to achieve prolonged duration of action by molecular modification of the short-acting β₂-agonist salbutamol (albuterol). Formoterol, a formanilide-substituted phenoethanolamine, was serendipitously found to be long-acting when given by inhalation (36, 38). Sufficient drug remains available in the aqueous biophase to allow immediate interaction with the active side of the receptor, thus accounting for the rapid onset of action. Formation of a depot within the plasmalemma seems to require high topical concentrations of formoterol in the bronchi. This finding may explain why inhaled formoterol has a longer duration of action than when given orally, because the inhaled route achieves higher topical concentrations in the pericillary fluid of the bronchi (41).

In addition to their different molecular structures, formoterol and salmeterol also have distinct pharmacologic features. Reflected in the routinely advocated dose for human use, formoterol has a higher potency than salmeterol (42). Comparative studies of healthy volunteers indicate that formoterol and salmeterol dose-dependently cause side effects with a potency ratio of approximately 5:1 (43). This is very similar to their difference in bronchodilator potency in patients with asthma. A few case reports have been published that show a significantly stronger bronchodilating effect with formoterol than with salmeterol in patients with severe asthma (44). However, in a larger comparative study involving patients with persistent severe asthma, no differences were observed in the bronchodilating effect of these agents (44). Also, chronic treatment with salmeterol does not hamper the bronchodilating effects of salbutamol during the acute phase in the emergency room.

Over the past 5 years, long-acting, inhaled β_2-agonists have gained acceptance as the preferred form of "add-on" treatment in persistent asthma. Combining these agents with inhaled glucocorticosteroids is the present standard formula of asthma care. In the majority of patients, these agents improve both lung function and symptoms.

Anticholinergics

The anticholinergic agents have been used in the treatment of asthma for several hundred years in the form of stramonium herbal preparations (46). Anticholinergic bronchodilators are competitive inhibitors of muscarinic receptors. Unlike β_2-agonists and theophylline, they are not functional antagonists; instead, they produce bronchodilation only in cholinergic-mediated bronchoconstriction. Normal bronchial tone is maintained through parasympathetic innervation of the airways via the vagus nerve. A number of well-known triggers of asthma and bronchospasm (eg, histamine, prostaglandins, sulfur dioxide, and allergens) produce bronchoconstriction (46, 47). Studies of patients with asthma consistently demonstrate that anticholinergics are effective bronchodilators, though not as potent as β_2-agonists.

The most commonly used agent is ipratropium bromide, which is a quaternary ammonium derivative. Ipratropium bromide consistently produces a 10% to 20% improvement in forced expiratory volume in 1 second (FEV_1) compared with use of β_2-agonists alone in acute, severe bronchospasm (47). Of note, however, is a significant interpatient variability, with some patients obtaining significantly greater (40–80%) improvement and others experiencing little or no improvement. This agent has also been shown not to improve outcome in chronic asthma compared with use of β_2-agonists alone (48).

The currently available anticholinergics are nonselective muscarinic-receptor blockers, and blockade of inhibitory muscarinic receptors could theoretically result in an increased release of acetylcholine and overcome the block on smooth muscle receptors. This important mechanism may explain why some patients have experienced paradoxical bronchoconstriction from nebulized anticholinergics. Only the quaternary ammonium-derivative ipratropium bromide should be used, because it has the advantage of poor absorption across the mucosae and the blood-brain barrier resulting from the charge associated with the five-valent tropane nitrogen atom. These agents result in only negligible systemic effects with a prolonged, desired local effect (ie, bronchodilation). They also do not have an effect on mucociliary clearance (46). These agents have a duration of action of 4 to 8 hours. Both the intensity and duration of action are dose-dependent. The optimal dose of ipratropium in adults is 500 ì g by nebulizer and 40 to 80 ì g by MDI in younger adults with asthma. The optimal MDI dose in older adults with severe airflow limitation is 2- to 4-fold higher. We should be cautious regarding use of high-dose ipratropium in older patients with prostate hypertrophy. Time to maximal bronchodilation is considerably slower than with aerosolized, short-acting â$_2$-agonists (2 hours vs 30 minutes). This, however, is of little clinical consequence, because some bronchodilation is seen within 30 seconds, 50% of maximum response occurs within 3 minutes, and 80% of maximum response is reached within 30 minutes (46).

In summary, the role of anticholinergics in the treatment of bronchospasm and asthma is limited. They are not currently recommended for long-term control of these disease processes (48). However, most studies show that anticholinergic agents provide at least as great and as prolonged an improvement in airflow of patients with COPD as do other agents, including long-acting β_2-agonists (49). Therefore, use of inhaled anticholinergics on a scheduled basis is recommended as first-line therapy in patients with COPD (50).

CROMOLYN SODIUM AND NEDOCROMIL SODIUM

Cromolyn sodium has been used in the prophylactic treatment of asthma for more than 20 years. A new, related agent, nedocromil sodium, which is a pyranoquinoline dicarboxylic acid, has only been released in the

United States in the last five years (48). The exact mechanism of action for these agents is still unknown. These agents have minor differences in activity; however, the principal differences appear to be in potency, with 4 mg of nedocromil by MDI being equivalent to 20 mg of cromolyn sodium by spinhaler (51). These drugs produce mast cell membrane stabilization. Both agents inhibit in vitro activation of human neutrophils, macrophages, and eosinophils (46, 51). These drugs also inhibit neurally mediated bronchoconstriction through C-fiber sensory nerve stimulation in the airways (51). These drugs, however, do not have any bronchodilatory effects.

Both are effective by inhalation only and are available as MDIs, whereas cromolyn also comes as a nebulizer solution. They are not bioavailable orally, but the portion of the drug that reaches the lung is completely absorbed (46). Absorption from the airway is slower than elimination (hours vs minutes). Both the intensity and the duration of protection against various challenges are dose-dependent (51).

These drugs have a highly nontoxic profile. The common side effects, cough and wheezing, have been reported following inhalation of each, as have bad taste and headache, especially for nedocrimal. The taste of nedocrimal is so bad that for some patients ($\approx$20%), it precludes them from taking the drug. Cromolyn has the best nontoxic profile of any compound to treat bronchospasm and asthma, with adverse effects occurring in less than 1 out of 10,000 patients (52).

Cromolyn and nedocromil are indicated for the prophylaxis of mild asthma, regardless of the cause, both in children and adults. They are particularly effective for patients with allergic asthma on a seasonal basis or just before an acute exposure (eg, entering a home with a pet). These drugs can be used in combination with β_2-agonists in patients with severe symptoms. The efficacy of these drugs is directly related to their degree of deposition in the lung. Therefore, these compounds do not work during active bronchospasm. Patients should initially receive cromolyn or nedocromil four times daily; and after stabilization, the frequency may be reduced to two times daily.

LEUKOTRIENE MODIFIERS

The newest treatment agents approved since 1996 address a new therapeutic pathway. They act by inhibiting the action of cysteinyl leukotrienes (LTC4, LTD4, and LTE4) (53). These medications—zafirlukast (Accolate), montelukast (Singulair), and zileuton (Zylfo)—all work by blocking the leukotriene receptor. Leukotrienes are proinflammatory modulators that increase microvascular permeability and airway edema, thus producing bronchoconstriction.

Zafirlukast has been shown to improve pulmonary function, increasing FEV_1 and reducing symptoms and bronchodilator medication requirements in patients (54). At doses of 20 mg twice daily, zafirlukast has been shown to reduce airway responses to inhaled allergen, platelet-activating factor, and exercise. Adverse effects are minimal, although experience with this medication is limited. Rare cases of hepatotoxicity and eosinophilic vasculitis have been reported. Food may impair absorption, and zafirlukast interacts with warfarin, resulting in prolonged prothrombin time.

Zileuton directly inhibits 5-lipoxygenase, whereas other drugs in development bind to and prevent translocation of 5-lipoxygenase-activating protein (53). Zileuton reduces bronchoconstriction caused by allergen, exercise, aspirin, and cold, dry air (53). Doses of 600 mg four times daily reduce symptoms and bronchodilator requirements and improve pulmonary function. Zileuton may produce elevated liver enzyme levels, and patients need to be monitored closely. This drug also affects hepatic isozymes and, therefore, also increases concentrations of warfarin and theophylline (48).

Neither zafirlukast nor zileuton completely attenuate induced bronchospasm in several challenge models (53). These new agents show great promise, but their place in the scheme of asthma management is still in evolution. National Heart, Lung and Blood Institute guidelines suggest that these compounds may be used as alternatives to low-dose inhaled steroids in patients with mild, persistent asthma. They also have the advantage of being oral medications, so compliance may be improved over that with inhaled medications.

MAGNESIUM SULFATE

Intravenous magnesium sulfate ($MgSO_4$), as a smooth muscle relaxant, had been advocated for patients with severe asthma who exhibit a suboptimal response. However, those initial trials did not use an adequate dose of inhaled β_2-agonists, and bronchodilation from $MgSO_4$ was only modest and did not exceed the β_2-agonist response (48).

GLUCORTICOIDS

Glucorticoid Therapy

The most important treatment for bronchospasm and asthma are the inhaled corticosteroids. Actions of this class of compounds include increasing the number of β_2-adrenergic receptors and improving the receptor responsiveness of β_2-adrenergic receptors to β_2-adrenergic stimulation, reducing mucous production and hypersecretion, and inhibiting the inflammatory response (55). The anti-inflammatory effects with possible benefit in asthma include decreasing the synthesis and release of several proinflammatory cytokines, such as interleukin-1, -3, -4, -5, -6, and -8 as well as granulocyte-macrophage colony-stimulating factor; reducing inflammatory cell activation, recruitment, and infiltration; and decreasing vascular permeability (55). Recently, regular use of a steroid inhaler in combination with long-acting, inhaled â$_2$-agonists was reported to improve lung function and to reduce the severity of dyspnea compared with individual drugs in patients with COPD (56).

Systemic Glucorticoid Therapy

In severe acute asthma, status asthmaticus, the standard of care is treatment with systemic glucocorticoids combined with frequent administration of inhaled â$_2$-agonists (48). Glucocorticoids can be administered by the parenteral route (methylprednisolone sodium succinate or hydrocortisone sodium succinate) or by the oral route (prednisone or methylprednisolone), either of which provides a rapid onset of action and a systemic effect (57).

The glucocorticoids used in asthma are compared in Table 14.1. Recommended dosages for acute asthma are listed in Table 14.2. No difference is observed in response between intravenous and oral administration of steroids (57, 58, 59). Evidence suggests that divided doses should be used initially. Following resolution of symptoms (decrease in obstruction achievement of >50% of predicted normal FEV_1, which generally occurs in the first 48 hours), the steroid dose is reduced as one or two doses orally (57, 58). The duration of treatment is dependent on the response of individual patients and on their response in the past. Tapering the dose after treatment is recommended, as with the use of all steroids, to prevent adrenal insufficiency.

Systemic glucocorticoids are also recommended for the treatment of impending episodes of severe bronchospasm unresponsive to bronchodilator therapy (48). Prednisone, 1 to 2 mg/kg/day (up to 40–60 mg/day) is administered orally in two divided doses for 3 to 10 days (48). If an adequate response is not achieved, administration of prednisone three times daily may be worthwhile.

The balance of control symptoms and toxicity is always in the forefront. Because short term (1–2 weeks), high-dose steroids (1–2 mg/kg/day of prednisone) do not produce serious toxicities, the ideal

TABLE 14.1 Comparison of Glucorticoids

Systemic	Relative anti-inflammatory potency	Relative sodium-retaining potency	Duration of biologic activity (hours)	Plasma elimination half-life (hours)
Hydrocortisone	1	1.0	8–12	1.5–2.0
Prednisone	4	0.8	12–36	2.5–3.5
Methylprednisolone	5	0.5	12–36	3.3
Dexamethasone	25	0	36–54	3.4–4–0

Aerosol	Topical potency	Receptor binding	Receptor complex	Oral bioavailability
Flunisolide	330	1.8	3.5	21
Triamcinolone acetonide	330	3.6	3.9	10.6
Beclomethasone dipropionate	600	13.5	7.5	20
Budesonide	980	9.4	5.1	11
Fluticasone propionate	1,200	18	10.5	<1

TABLE 14.2   Corticosteroids

Medications	Adult dosages	Comments
Prednisone Methylprednisolone Prednisolone	120–180 mg in three or four divided doses for 48 hours, then 60–80 mg/day until peak expiratory flow reaches 70% of personal best.	For outpatient "burst" use, 1–2 mg/kg/day to a maximum of 60 mg for 3 to 7 days. It is unnecessary to taper following the course.

use is to administer the glucocorticoids in a short "burst" and then to maintain the patient on appropriate long-term control therapy with extended periods between systemic glucocorticoid treatment (48).

Extended use may affect adrenal cortisol release. However, hypothalamic-pituitary-adrenal axis suppression is short-lived (1–3 days) and readily reversible following short bursts (=10 days) of pharmacologic doses (57, 58). Therefore, in patients who require chronic systemic glucocorticoids for control of disease, the lowest possible dose required to control symptoms should be used. An accepted method to decrease toxicity is to use alternate-day therapy or inhaled glucocorticoids.

Inhaled Glucocorticoids

The largest breakthrough in the treatment of bronchoconstriction is inhaled steroids, which are now considered to be first-line steroid therapy. As with all steroid use, a low to moderate dose carries a lower risk of systemic complications. The inhaled glucocorticoids demonstrate a favorable topical systemic potency ratio but are far from benign. If an "ideal" glucocorticoid were to be developed, it would have a high degree of topical potency, minimal systemic absorption of active drug, and minimal local or systemic side effects. No such agent is currently available.

The inhaled glucocorticoids have high topical anti-inflammatory effects and are either poorly absorbed or metabolized to less-active substances when they are absorbed (58). The systemic affects vary from agent to agent. Aerosol delivery of the preparations varies from 10% to 30%, which can make a difference in both topical potency and systemic activity (59, 60). Therefore, the delivery system can make a significant difference in the relative comparable dose (48).

Optimal dosing of inhaled steroids has not been thoroughly studied, but most patients may be controlled with twice-daily dosing. However, investigations have demonstrated an improved asthma response with decreased systemic effects by giving the same total daily dose four times daily as opposed to twice daily (48).

An apparent additive effect of long-acting β-agonists and inhaled glucocorticoids has been observed. A possible explanation is that steroids are anti-inflammatory, whereas the smooth muscle relaxing effect of long-acting β-agonists results in prolonged bronchodilation and bronchoprotection. It can be assumed that the combination of both pharmacologic activities is particularly beneficial clinically.

EXPERIMENTAL DRUGS

Potassium-Channel Openers

The plasma membrane of airway smooth muscle has a high density of potassium channels. The opening of potassium ion channels in the cell membrane would allow K^+ ions move out from cells, which is normally maintained by the ion-transporter K^+/Na^+-adenosine triphosphatase (ATPase). The opening potassium channels in cell membranes result in membrane hyperpolarization, which inhibits the cellular influx of calcium through voltage-dependent channels, thus leading to relaxation of airway smooth muscle cells (60). Few clinical trials have addressed the bronchodilatory effect of potassium-channel openers (KCOs). Cromakalim, a benzopyran prototype, when given orally significantly reduced the fall in early morning lung function of patients with asthma (61). However, levcromakalim, another KCO, did not produce a significant bronchodilation or changes in airway responsiveness in recent studies (62, 63). Therefore, whether KCOs will be useful bronchodilators remains to be determined.

Tachykinin- and Kinin-Receptor Antagonists

The tachykinins—substance P, neurokinin A, and neurokinin B—belong to a structural family of peptides. Bradykinin belongs to a family of short peptides. Tachykinin and bradykinin seem to be involved in the exaggerated neurogenic airway inflammation, such as bronchoconstriction and plasma extravasation (64, 65). Cold air-induced bronchoconstriction seems to be mediated by kinin and tachykinin (66). The biological actions of tachykinin and kinin are mediated by receptors: neurokinin $(NK)_1$, NK_2, and NK_3 receptors versus β_1 and β_2 receptors, respectively. Clinical studies regarding tachykinin- and kinin-receptor antagonists in human airways are scarce. In a double-blind, placebo-controlled, cross-over trial with nine patients having stable asthma, a selective NK_1-receptor antagonist, FK-888, did not attenuate the maximal fall by exercise in specific airway conductance (68). However, the recovery from exercise-induced airway narrowing was significantly faster after inhalation of FK-888 (67). Inhalation of a bradykinin-receptor antagonist, Hoe 140, had some protective effect in patients with moderate asthma during a 4-week study (68). Although tachykinin- and bradykinin-receptor antagonists are unlikely to play a major role in patients with asthma, they might be useful in the treatment of selected types of asthma, such as nocturnal asthma induced by gastroesophageal reflux (69) or hyperpnea-induced bronchoconstriction (70).

Antiallergic Drugs

Selective β_2-receptor agonists, glucocorticoids, disodium cromoglycate, and nedocromil are traditional antiallergic agents that block allergic response in several ways. As a new antiallergic drug, suplatast tosilate (IPD-1151T) modulates Th2-cytokine production (71). Oral administration of suplatast tosilate suppressed airway hyperresponsiveness in patients with asthma by reducing eosinophilic inflammation in the airways (72). A recombinant human monoclonal anti-IgE antibody (omalizumab), which forms complexes with free IgE, thereby blocking its interaction with mast cells and basophils and lowering free IgE levels in the circulation, provided clinical benefit in a dose-dependent fashion in patients with seasonal allergic rhinitis (73). Other antiallergic agents are under investigation.

Drugs Targeting Cell Signaling Pathways

Cellular inflammation is regulated by intracellular signaling pathways that control specific cell response. The overexpression of multiple gene-encoding inflammatory agents leads to diverse diseases. For example, the intracellular protein kinase C, which is a serine threonine protein kinase enzyme, has an important role in the genesis of pulmonary edema (74). Targeting key signaling component of intracellular transduction as a therapeutic measure would correct the underlying cause of disease, not simply modify the associated symptoms. Although many substances to block the signaling pathways are under investigation, no clinically proven multiple kinase inhibitors for lung disorders are available in the market at present.

NITRIC OXIDE

Nitric oxide (NO), in it role as an endothelial-derived relaxing factor, has been recognized as an important endogenous mediator for smooth muscle relaxation (75, 76). Therefore, exogenously administered, inhaled NO might be expected to cause vasodilation in well-aerated areas of the lung with no systemic hemodynamic effects. Inhaled NO-induced vasodilation of pulmonary vessels should increase blood flow to well-ventilated areas of the lung and preferentially shunt blood away from poorly ventilated areas.

Several years ago, interest arose in the use of NO for treatment of acute respiratory distress syndrome (ARDS). Early studies showed some promise (77), but in a large, multicenter study (75), no change in mortality rate was noted. The study did, however, show that NO was well-tolerated and improved oxygenation compared with placebo during the first 4 hours of treatment. The complex nature of ARDS and cytokine modulation may have lead to the failure to affect mortality. Nitric oxide is still used in several centers as a bridge therapy when traditional supportive therapy for ARDS is failing.

Nitric oxide does have a place in some neonatal centers. It lowers the need for extracorporeal membrane oxygenation in respiratory failure of the newborn (78). It also plays a role in the treatment of pulmonary hypertension of the newborn (78, 79). In this case, NO can increase oxygenation and decrease pulmonary arterial pressure. These studies, however, have typically involved few patients, examined only the acute physiologic changes associated with the administration of inhaled NO, and lacked concurrent placebo groups.

Further examination of using NO along with more advanced modes of mechanical ventilation that do not add to cytokine load may lead to better long-term survival. We must design more controlled trials in which we only study one aspect of the acute process and how specific tissues react to NO.

SURFACTANT

In 1959, when Avery and Mead (80) published direct evidence linking the absence of a surface active material in the lung to that of a substance that actively changes the surface tension of the alveoli of the lung. This material was later named pulmonary surfactant. Pulmonary surfactant is a complex of phospholipids (80–90%), neutral lipids (5–10%), and at least four specific surfactant-proteins (5–10%; SP-A, SP-B, SP-C, and SP-D), lying as a layer at the air-liquid interface in the alveoli (82, 83) and small airways, lowering surface tension. Surfactant is synthesized by the alveolar type II cells and is secreted into the alveolar spaces (82).

A further possible function of bronchial surfactant, which to date has not been studied, is its masking of receptors on smooth muscle with respect to substances that induce contraction and lead to airway obstruction. This means that surfactant also could possibly be involved in asthma (83). In addition, it has been demonstrated that surfactant plays a role in the lung's defense against infection (85). Surfactant (particularly SP-A) enhances the antibacterial and antiviral defense of alveolar macrophages.

Surfactant may also be important and involved in protecting the lung from lung-released mediators (eg, angiotensin II) and in protecting the cardiopulmonary system against mediators produced by the lung (85, 86).

Disturbances of the surfactant system can result from different factors. The most common is damage to the alveolar-capillary membrane, which leads to high-permeability edema with washout dilution of the surfactant and/or inactivation of the surfactant by plasma components, such as fibrinogen, albumin, globulin, and transferred hemoglobin as well as cell membrane lipids. Also, surfactant can be easily depleted by the cyclic opening and closing of alveoli during mechanical ventilation; this disturbed synthesis, storage, or release of surfactant is secondary to direct injury of Type II cells (85, 86). The diminished surfactant in mechanical ventilation may play an important role during respiratory failure in ARDS.

Diminished pulmonary surfactant has far-reaching consequences for lung function. Independent of the cause, decreased surfactant function will lead directly or indirectly to:

1. Decreased pulmonary compliance.
2. Decreased functional residual capacity.
3. Atelectasis and enlargement of the functional right-to-left shunt.
4. Decreased gas exchange and respiratory acidosis.
5. Hypoxemia with anaerobic metabolism and metabolic acidosis
6. Pulmonary edema with further inactivation of surfactant by plasma constituents.

Surfactant replacement therapy has been used in preterm infants for the last 20 years with great success (80). The rate of mortality has fallen as we have become better able to deliver surfactant to these preterm infants. After birth, these infants can have their respiratory distress prevented or its severity reduced by the intratracheal administration of synthetic or natural surfactants. Synthetic (eg, lecithin, tyloxapol, or hexadecanol) or natural (fortified extract of cow lungs) surfactant has also been administered repeatedly during the course of this disease process.

Ongoing research concerning surfactant replacement therapy in adults has not, as yet, lead to a decrease in the mortality rate. Several formulations are under investigation, along with systems to deliver the agent into the adult lung. Multiple technical problems in the delivery of surfactant into the adult lung in patients with ARDS have yet to be overcome. Also, the maturity of the immune system may play a role in the lack of positive outcomes during adult studies. New formulations are currently under development and may lead to more positive results in the adult population.

SUMMARY

Many agents are now available to maximize pulmonary function in multiple disease status (87). The physician who cares for these patients should be expert in the pharmacology of these drugs, from the older agents, such as theophylline and atropine, to the newer, long-acting β_2-agonists and leukotriene modulators. Most cases with severe airflow limitation require a combination therapy, such as glucocorticoids and β_2-agonists with or without theophylline and/or anticholinergics.

We should also be familiar with the new aerosol delivery systems. Aerosol delivery of drugs for asthma has the advantage of being site-specific. For example, inhalation of short-acting β_2-agonist provides more-rapid bronchodilation than is provided by oral agents. The various devices used to generate therapeutic aerosols include MDIs, jet nebulizers, ultrasonic nebulizers, and dry-powder inhalers. The single most important device factor determining the site of aerosol deposition is particle size. We as anesthesiologists should also review our ability to deliver these drugs down an endotracheal tube. Important determinants of aerosol deposition in ventilator-supported patients include the delivery system, particle size, amount of puffs or nebulization, characteristics of the ventilator circuit, ventilator mode, and patient-related factors. These factors require that we develop a treatment plan for each of our high-risk patients before bronchospasm.

References

1. Weibel ER, Taylor CR: Design and structure of the human lung. In: Fishman AP, ed: Pulmonary Diseases and Disorders. 2nd ed. New York: McGraw-Hill, York, 1988; 11–20.

2. Breeze RG, Wheelden EB: The cells of the pulmonary airways. Am Rev Respir Dis 1977; 116:705–77.
3. Cauldwell FW, Siebert RG, Lininger RE, et al.: Anatomic study of 150 human cadavers. Surg Gynecol Obstet 1948; 86:395–412.
4. Jerome EH: Pulmonary circulation. In: Hemmings IT, Hopkins P, eds: Foundations of Anesthesia: Basic and Clinical Sciences: London, Mosby, 2000; 465–81.
5. Barnes PJ: State of the art: neural control of the human airways in health and disease. Am Rev Respir Dis 1986; 134:1289–314.
6. Barnes PJ: New concepts in the pathogenesis of bronchial hyperresponsiveness and asthma. J Allergy Clin Immunol 1989; 83:1013–26.
7. Gross NJ, Skorodin MS: The place of anticholinergic agents in the treatment of airway obstruction. Immunol Allergy Pact 1986; 7:224–31.
8. Richardson JB, Farguson CC: Neuromuscular structure and function in the airways. Fed Proc 1979; 38:202–8.
9. Boushey HA, Holtzman MJ, Shellar JR, et al.: State of the art: bronchial hyperactivity. Am Rev Respir Dis 1980; 121:389–413.
10. Theodore AL, Beer DJ: Pharmacotherapy of chronic obstructive pulmonary disease. Clin Chest Med 1986; 7:657–71.
11. Lefkowitz RJ: Clinical physics of adrenoreceptor regulation. Am J Physiol 1982; 243:E43–7.
12. Seligman M, Chernow B: Use of adrenergic agents in the critically ill patient. Hosp Formul 1987; 223:348–60.
13. Richardson JO: Nonadrenergic inhibitory innervation of the lung. Lung 1982; 159:315–322.
14. Burgess C, Crane J, Pearce N, Beasley R: β_2-Agonists and New Zealand asthma mortality. Lancet 1991; 337:982–3.
15. Villar J, Petty TL, Slutsky AS: ARDS in its middle age: what have we learned. Applied Cardiopulmonary Pathophysiology 1998; 7:167–72.
16. So KL, Gommers D, Lachmann B: Bronchoalveolar surfactant system and intratracheal adrenaline. Lancet 1993; 341:120–1.
17. Kelly HW: Controversies in asthma therapy with theophylline and the β_2-adrenergic agents. Clin Pharm 1984; 3:386–95.
18. McFadden ER: Clinical use of β-adrenergic agonists. J Allergy Clin Immunol 1985; 76:352–6.
19. McFadden ER Jr: Methylxanthines in the treatment of asthma: the rise, the fall, and the possible rise again (editorial). Ann Intern Med 1991; 115:323–4.
20. Gora-Harper ML: The Injectable Drug Reference. Princeton, NJ: Society of Critical Care Medicine, Bioscientific Resources, 1998.

21. Weinberger M, Hendeles L: Slow-release theophylline: rationale and basis for product selection. N Engl J Med 1983; 308:64–76.
22. Persson CGA: Overview of effects of theophylline. J Allergy Clin Immunol 1986; 78:780–7.
23. Horrobin DF, Manku MS, Franks DJ, et al.: Methylxanthine phosphodiesterase inhibitors behave as prostaglandin antagonists in a perfuse rat mesenteric artery preparation. Prostaglandins 1977; 13:33–40.
24. Murphy CM, Coonce SL, Simon PA: Treatment of asthma in children. Clin Pharm 1992; 10:685–703.
25. Miech RP, Niedzwick JG, Smith TR: Effect of theophylline on the binding of cAMP to soluble protein from tracheal smooth muscle. Biochem Pharmacol 1979; 28:3687–8.
26. Hendeles L, Weinberger M: Theophylline: a state of the art review. Pharmacotherapy 1983; 32-44.
27. Ref. Kidney J, Dominguez M, Taylor PM, Rose M, Chung KF, Barnes PJ: Immunomodulation by theophylline in asthma. Demonstration by withdrawal of therapy. Am J Respir Crit Care Med 1995; 151:1907–14.
28. Ashutosh K, Sedat M, Fragale-Jackson J: Effects of theophylline on respiratory drive in patients with chronic obstructive pulmonary disease. J Clin Pharmacol 1997; 37:1100–7.
29. Parker JO, Kelkar K, West RS: Hemodynamic effects of aminophylline in cor pulmonale. Circulation 1966; 38:17–25.
30. McEvoy GK: Theophylline. In: McEvoy GK, ed: AHFS Drug Information 1993. Bethesda, MD: American Society of Hospital Pharmacists, 1993; 2278–85.
31. Bergstrand H: Phosphodiesterase inhibition and theophylline. Eur J Respir Dis 1980; 61(suppl 109):37–44.
32. Weinberger M, Hendeles L, Bighley L: Relationships of product formulation to absorption of oral theophylline. N Engl J Med 1978; 299:852–7.
33. Johnson M: The β-adrenoceptor. Am J Respir Crit Care Med 1998; 158 (Suppl 1):S146–53.
34. Nelson HS: β-Adrenergic bronchodilations. N Engl J Med 1995; 333:449–506.
35. Amory DW, Burnham SC, Cheney FW Jr: Comparison of the cardiopulmonary effects of subcutaneously administered epinephrine and terbutaline in patients with reversible airway obstruction. Chest 1975; 67:279–26.
36. Kips JC, Pauwels RA: Long-acting inhaled β_2-agonist therapy in asthma. Am J Respir Crit Care Med 2001; 164:923–32.
37. Ullman A, Suedmyr N: Salmeterol, a new long-acting inhaled β_2-

adrenoceptor agonist: comparison with solbutamol in adult asthmatic patients. Thorax 1988; 43:674–8.

38. Lofdahl CG, Suedmyr N: Formoterol fomarate, a new β_2-adrenoceptor agonist: acute studies of selectivity and duration of effect after inhaled and oral administration. Allergy 1989; 44:264–71.

39. Moore PF, Constantine JW, Barth WE: Pirbuterol selective β_2-adrenergic bronchodilator. J Pharmacol Exp Ther 1978; 207:410–8.

40. Littner MR, Tashkin DP, Culvarese B, Raotista M: Bronchial and cardiovascular effects of increasing doses of pirbuterol acetate aerosol in asthma. Ann Allergy 1982; 48:141–4.

41. Anderson GP, Linden A, Rabe KF: Why are long-acting β-adrenoceptor agonists long-acting? Eur Respir J 1994; 7:569–78.

42. Kallstrom BL, Sjoberg J, Waldeck B: The interaction between salmeterol and β_2-adrenoceptor agonists with higher efficacy on guinea pig trachea and human bronchus in vitro. Br J Pharmacol 1994; 113:687–92.

43. Guhan AR, Cooper S, Oborne J, et al.: Systemic effects of formoterol and salmeterol: a dose-response comparison in healthy subjects. Thorax 2000; 55:650–6.

44. Nightingale JA, Rogers DF, Barnes PJ: Comparison of the effects of salmeterol and formoterol in patients with severe asthma. Am J Respir Crit Car Med 2000; 161 (abstract):A190.

45. Noppen M, Vincken W: Bronchodilating effect of formoterol but not of salmeterol in two asthmatic patients (letter). Respiration 2000; 67:112–3.

46. Weiss EB, Stein M, eds: Bronchial Asthma: Mechanisms and Therapeutics. 3rd ed. Boston: Little, Brown, 1993.

47. Kelly HW, Murphy S: Should anticholinergics be used in acute severe asthma? Ann Pharmacother 1990, 24:409–16.

48. NHLBI, National Asthma Education and Prevention Program, Expert Panel Report 2. Guidelines for Diagnosis and management of Asthma. NIH Publication 97–4051, Bethesda, MD: U.S. Department of Health and Human Services, 1997.

49. Beeh K-M, Welte T, Buhl R: Anticholinergics in the treatment of chronic obstructive pulmonary disease. Respiration 2002; 69:372–9.

50. National Heart, Lung, and Blood Institute, World Health Organization: Global Strategy for the Diagnosis, Management, and Prevention of Chronic Obstructive Pulmonary Disease. NHLBI/WHO, Workshop Report, Publication 2701. Bethesda, MD: National Institutes of Health, National Heart, Lung, and Blood Institute, 2001.

51. Wasserman SI, ed: Nedocrimil sodium: a pyranoquinoline anti-inflammatory agent for the treatment of asthma. J Allergy Clin Immunol 1993; 92(suppl):143–216.

52. Murphy S, Kelly HW: Cromolyn sodium: a review of mechanisms and clinical use in asthma. Drug Intel Clin Pharm 1987; 21:22–35.

53. Hendeles L, Scheife RT, eds: New frontiers in asthma therapy: leukotriene-receptor antagonists and 5-lipoxygenase inhibitors. Pharmacotherapy 1997; 17(suppl):1S-54S.

54. Spector SL, Smith LJ, Glass M: Effects of six weeks of therapy with oral doses of ICI 204, 219, a leukotriene D_4-receptor antagonist. Crit Care Med 1994; 150:618–23.

55. Baraniuk JN, ed: Steroids in asthma: molecular mechanisms of glucocorticoid actions. J Allergy Clin Immunol 1996; 97(suppl):141–82.

56. Mahler DA, Wire P, Horstman D, Chang C-N, Yates J, Fisher T, Shah T: Effectiveness of fluticasone propionate and salmeterol combination delivered via diskus device in the treatment of chronic obstructive pulmonary disease. Am J Respir Crit Care Med 2002; 166:1084–91.

57. Kelly HW, Murphy S: Corticosteroids for acute severe asthma. Ann Pharmacother 1991; 25:72–9.

58. Barnes PJ: Inhaled glucocorticoids for asthma. N Engl J Med 1995; 332:868–75.

59. Kelly HW: Comparison of inhaled corticosteroids. Am Pharmacother 1998; 32:220–32.

60. Small RC, Berry JL, Burka JF, Cook SJ, Foster RW, Green KA, Murray MA: Potassium channel activators and bronchial asthma. Clin Exp Allergy 1992; 22:11–8.

61. Williams AJ, Lee TH, Cocnrane GM, Hopkirk A, Vyse T, Chiew F, Lavender E, Richards DH, Owen S, Stone P, et al.: Attenuation of nocturnal asthma by cromakalim. Lancet 1990; 336:334–6.

62. Kidney JC, Fuller RW, Worsdell YM, Lavender EA, Chung KF, Barnes PJ: Effect of an oral potassium channel activator, BRL 38227, on airway function and responsiveness in asthmatic patients: comparison with oral salbutamol. Thorax 1993; 48:130–3.

63. Faurschou P, Mikkelsen KL, Steffensen I, Franke B: The lack of bronchodilator effect and the short-term safety of cumulative single doses of an inhaled potassium-channel opener (bimakalim) in adult patients with mild to moderate bronchial asthma. Pulm Pharmacol Ther 1994; 7:293–7.

64. Joos G, Kips J, Pauwels R, Van der Straeten M: The respiratory effects of neuropeptides. Eur J Respir Dis 1986; 144:107–36.

65. Frossard N, Advenier C: Tachykinin receptors and the airways. Life Sci 1991; 49:1941–53.

66. Yoshihara S, Nadel JA, Figini M, Emanueli C, Pradelles P, Geppetti P: Endogenous nitric oxide inhibits bronchoconstriction induced by cold-air inhalation in guinea pigs: role of kinins. Am J Respir Crit Care Med 1998; 157:547–52.

67. Ichinose M, Miura M, Yamauchi H, Kageyama N, Tomaki M, Oyake T, Ohuchi Y, Hida W, Miki H, Tamura G, Shirato K: A neurokinin 1-receptor antagonist improves exercise-induced airway narrowing in asthmatic patients. Am J Respir Crit Care Med 1996; 153:936–41.

68. Akbary AM, Wirth KJ, Scholkens BA: Efficacy and tolerability of icatibant (Hoe 140) in patients with moderately severe chronic bronchial asthma. Immunopharmacology 1996; 33:238–42.

69. Ricciardolo FLM, Rado V, Fabbri LM, Sterk PJ, Di Maria GU, Geppetti P: Bronchoconstriction induced by citric acid inhalation in guinea pigs; role of tachykinin, bradykinin, and nitric oxide. Am J Respir Crit Care Med 1999; 159:557–62.

70. Solway J, Kao BM, Jordan JE, Gitter B, Rodger IW, Howbert JJ, Alger LE, Necheles J, Leff AR, Garland A: Tachykinin-receptor antagonists inhibit hyperpnea-induced bronchoconstriction in guinea pigs. J Clin Invest 1993; 92:315–23.

71. Furukido K, Takeno S, Ueda T, Hirakawa K, Yajin K: Suppression of the Th2 pathway by suplatast tosilate in patients with perennial nasal allergies. Am J Rhinol 2002; 16:329–36.

72. Yoshida M, Aizawa H, Inoue H, Matsumoto K, Koto H, Komori M, Fukuyama S, Okamoto M, Hara N: Effect of suplatast tosilate on airway hyperresponsiveness and inflammation in asthma patients. J Asthma 2002; 39:545–52.

73. Casale TB, Condemi J, LaForce C, Nayak A, Rowe M, Watrous M, McAlary M, Fowler-Taylor A, Racine A, Gupta N, Fick R, Della Cioppa G: Omalizumab Seasonal Allergic Rhinitis Trail Group: effect of omalizumab on symptoms of seasonal allergic rhinitis: a randomized controlled trial. JAMA 2001; 286:2956–67.

74. Siflinger-Birnboim A, Johnson A: Protein kinase C modulates pulmonary endothelial permeability: a paradigm for acute lung injury. Am J Physiol Lung Cell Mol Physiol 2003; 284:L435–51.

75. Dellinger RP, Zimmerman JL, Taylor RW, et al.: Inhaled nitric oxide in patients with acute respiratory distress syndrome: results of a randomized phase II trial. Crit Care Med 1998; 26:15–23.

76. Moncada S, Palmer RMJ, Higgs HA: Nitric oxide: physiology, pathophysiology and pharmacology. Pharmacol Rev 1991; 43:109–42.

77. Rossaint R, Falke KJ, López F, et al.: Inhaled nitric oxide for the adult respiratory distress syndrome. N Engl J Med 1993; 328:399–405.

78. The Neonatal Inhaled Nitric Oxide Study Group: Inhaled nitric oxide in full-term and nearly full-term infants with hypoxic respiratory failure. N Engl J Med 1997; 336:597–604.

79. Roberts JD, Polaner DM, Lang P, et al.: Inhaled nitric oxide in persistent pulmonary hypertension of the newborn. Lancet 1992; 340:819–826.

80. Avery MA, Mead J: Surface properties in relation to atelectasis and hyaline membrane disease. Am J Dis Child 1959; 97:517–23.
81. Lachmann B, Winsel K, Reutgen H: Der Anti-Atelektase-Faktor der Lunge. I Z Erkr Atm 1972; 137:267–87.
82. Van Golde LMG, Batenburg JJ, Robertson B: The pulmonary surfactant system: Biochemical aspects and functional significance. Physiol Rev 1988; 68:374–455.
83. Lachmann B, Becher G: Protective effect of lung surfactant on allergic bronchial constriction in guinea pigs. Am Rev Respir Dis 1986; 133 (abstract):A118.
84. Van Iwaarden F: Surfactant and pulmonary defense system. In: Robertson B, Van Golde LMG, Battenburg JJ, eds: Pulmonary Surfactant. Amsterdam, Elsevier 1992; 215–53.
85. Verbrugge SJC, Lachmann B: Mechanisms of ventilation-induced lung injury and its prevention: role of surfactant. Applied Cardiopulmonary Pathophysiology 1998; 7:173–98.
86. Papadakos PJ: Artificial ventilation. In: Hemmings H, Hopkins P, eds: Foundations of Anesthesia: Basic Clinical Sciences. London, Mosby, 2000; 507–14.
87. Tobin N: Asthma, airway biology and nasal disorders. Am J Respir Crit Care Med 2002; 165:598–618.

Index

Note: Italic numbers indicate figures; numbers followed by t indicate tables.